Language: normal and pathological development

Fondazione Pierfranco e Luisa Mariani ONLUS
viale Bianca Maria 28
20129 Milan, Italy

Telephone: +39 02 795458
Fax: +39 02 76009582
Publications Coordinator: Valeria Basilico
e-mail: publications@fondazione-mariani.org
www.fondazione-mariani.org

Language: normal and pathological development
Remembering Elisabeth Bates

Edited by

D. Riva, I. Rapin and G. Zardini

Mariani Foundation Paediatric Neurology Series: 16
Series Editor: Maria Majno

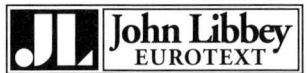

ISSN: 0969-0301
ISBN: 2-7420-0638-9

Cover illustration: design by Costanza Magnocavallo.
Technical and language editor: Oliver Brooke.

(Second book of the series dedicated
to *Developmental cognitive neurosciences* – the first was vol. 13)

Published by

Éditions John Libbey Eurotext
127, avenue de la République, 92120 Montrouge, France.
Tél.: 33 (0)1 46 73 06 60; Fax: 33 (0)1 40 84 09 99
e-mail: contact@jle.com
http//www.jle.com

© 2006 John Libbey Eurotext. All rights reserved.

Unauthorized duplication contravenes applicable laws.

Il est interdit de reproduire intégralement ou partiellement le présent ouvrage sans autorisation de l'éditeur ou du Centre Français d'Exploitation du Droit de Copie, 20, rue des Grands-Augustins, 75006 Paris.

Contents

Normal language development

Chapter 1   Language and the brain: the contributions of Elisabeth Bates
Frederic Dick   3

Chapter 2   Early language acquisition: typical and atypical processes
Maria Cristina Caselli, Silvia Stefanini   15

Chapter 3   The development of grammar
Antonella Devescovi, Daniela Marchione   27

Chapter 4   Pragmatic development
Loredana Hvastja-Stefani   39

Language and neurofunctional correlates

Chapter 5   Auditory comprehension of language in young children
Madison M. Berl, Erin N. Moore, Chandan Vaidya, Gerard A. Gioia, Bernstein Ratner, William Davis Gaillard   51

Chapter 6   The language production-comprehension network in functional imaging
Stefan Heim   61

Chapter 7   Developmental changes in human cerebral functional organization for word generation
Timothy T. Brown, Heather M. Lugar, Rebecca S. Coalson, Fran M. Miezin, Steven E. Petersen, Bradley L. Schlaggar   77

Chapter 8   Functional magnetic resonance imaging in normal and pathological language development
William D. Gaillard, Erin N. Moore, Deborah A. Weber, Eva K. Ritzl, Madison M. Berl   105

Language in congenital and acquired brain lesions/maldevelopment

Chapter 9   Language and its development in the autism spectrum disorders
Isabelle Rapin   121

Chapter 10	Language regression in autism: pathogenesis and differential diagnosis *Barıs Korkmaz*	139
Chapter 11	Language disorders in cerebellar pathology *Daria Riva, Chiara Vago, Federica Aggio, Chiara Pantaleoni,* *Stefano D'Arrigo, Arianna Usilla, Sara Bulgheroni*	157
Chapter 12	Cortical specialization for language in childhood: evidence from negative cases *Isabel Pavão Martins*	169
Chapter 13	Language in Italian children with Williams syndrome *Virginia Volterra, Olga Capirci, Arianna Bello*	183
Chapter 14	Verbal and non-verbal communication disorders in children with bilateral perisylvian polymicrogyria *Veronica Saletti, Sara Bulgheroni, Daria Riva*	195

Developmental language disorders (DLD)

Chapter 15	Specific language impairment: definition and diagnostic criteria *Giovanna Zardini*	207
Chapter 16	Developmental language delay in early childhood: differential diagnosis between specific language delay and language delay secondary to other communication disorders *Bruno Molteni, Gloria Airaghi, Giulia Mantegazza, Daniela Sarti*	217
Chapter 17	The natural history of early language delay: from late talking to specific language impairment *Anna Maria Chilosi, Paola Cipriani, Lucia Pfanner, Chiara Pecini,* *Tiziana Fapore*	229
Chapter 18	A follow-up study of reading and writing in Italian children with specific language impairment *Daniela Brizzolara, Claudia Casalini, Filippo Gasperini, Silvia Roncoli,* *Sara Mazzotti, Paola Cipriani, Anna Maria Chilosi*	239
Chapter 19	The relationship between developmental language disorders and behavioural disorders *Charles Njiokiktjien*	253

Normal language development

Chapter 1

Language and the brain: the contributions of Elizabeth Bates

Frederic Dick

School of Psychology, Birkbeck College, University of London, Malet Street, London WC1E HQX, UK and Center for Research in Language, University of California – San Diego, California, USA
fdick@crl.ucsd.edu

Preface

On 13 December 2003, Elizabeth Bates died, after a courageous year-long struggle with pancreatic cancer. In passing away, Liz leaves an enormous hole, both in the field and in the lives of her many friends. But she leaves an enormous legacy as well. Over the course of more than 30 years, Liz established herself as a world leader in a range of fields – child development, language acquisition, aphasia research, cross-linguistic research, and adult psycholinguistics. She was passionate about science and about ideas. Her contributions to the field of cognitive science were rich and varied, and defy any simple categorization. A summary of just the research initiatives and empirical instruments she produced would fill many pages of this volume. The following list may give a sense of the breadth of her achievement in multiple areas:

- MacArthur Communicative Development Inventory. *This instrument has become one of the most widely used tools in the field for assessing communicative development. There are now versions of the CDI in 35 languages, based on a total population of tens of thousands of children.*
- The International Picture Naming Project. *Liz initiated and headed the International Picture Naming Project, which has provided the field with a wealth of developmental and adult behavioural data on action and object naming in seven languages.*
- Voxel-based lesion-symptom mapping. *Liz led the team that developed this important tool for correlating the site of a lesion with the degree of behavioural deficit.*
- The UCSD Project in Cognitive and Neural Development. *For nearly two decades, Liz directed this multimillion dollar NIH-funded project to study the longitudinal development of language, learning, and behaviour in children with neurological disorders. It remains a unique and productive international centre for the study of these important and challenging questions about development.*

- International Cross-Linguistic Consortium. *Liz established an international network of researchers that made possible large scale collaborative research into cross-linguistic comparisons of aphasia and normal language processing.*
- Founding member of the UCSD Cognitive Science Department. *Liz was one of the pioneering faculty who established the first cognitive science department in the world.*
- Founding co-director of the Joint Doctoral Program in Language and Communicative Disorders (SDSU/UCSD). *Liz played a key role in the creation of one of the most innovative PhD programmes in the USA in the area of language and communicative disorders.*
- Scholarly record. *In a prolific career over three decades, Liz conducted studies in over 20 languages on four continents. She was author, or co-author, of 10 books and more than 200 articles.*

As important as each of these has been, and as great the impact each has had on the everyday scientific lives of students and researchers around the world, they cannot be properly understood in isolation. Rather, they need to be placed in the context of the larger legacy that constituted the full breadth of Liz's career achievements – achievements that will continue to influence the course of scientific discourse and practice for many years to come. In an important sense, underlying all of Liz's work is a unified view of language, cognition, and the brain that motivates the work in different areas. But although one can separate Liz's work into areas – development, aphasia, cross-linguistic studies, and so on – this obscures the deep theoretical insights that cut across the various domains.

Liz was a true developmentalist. She understood that what is interesting about development is change – the forces that drive change, the shape of change, and the mechanisms that underlie it. She viewed life as dynamic, and development as emergent, deriving from the interaction of the organism with its environment.

Liz was an ardent theorist. Beginning with her early work with Brian MacWhinney on the Competition Model and continuing – literally – to the end of her life, she developed well articulated positions on some of the most central issues in cognitive science, from modularity to embodied cognition, to brain plasticity, to questions about innateness and the origins of knowledge. She saw behaviours such as language as reflecting important, interesting, and novel traits that are unique to humans; but she also understood that even the most complex behaviours are rooted in a shared biological history. She believed that big changes – like the emergence of language – developed out of many small changes. As she often said, 'Language is a new machine built out of old parts.' Liz did not believe in a language module in the human brain. Instead she saw functional modularity as an outcome rather than a starting condition.

Liz was the consummate empirical scientist (her students often referred to her as a data junkie). The many tools and instruments she created – for quantifying dissociations, studying small samples, and interpreting multivariate analyses – bear witness to her passion for data. In many ways, Liz viewed her experimental results as an explorer might see a newly discovered continent – a vast terrain ready to be poked, prodded, and encouraged to reveal its underlying structure.

Finally, Liz was a generous and energetic collaborator. She was a one-woman force for scientific globalization, forging lasting and productive partnerships with linguists and psychologists working in many countries, including Bulgaria, the United Kingdom, Germany, Hungary, India, Italy, Mexico, Russia, Taiwan, and Tanzania. She also built bridges across an extraordinary array of disciplines, with long-time collaborators hailing from fields as disparate as biology, computer science, medicine, physics, primatology, and statistics. Liz has left a particularly rich legacy of collaborations and friendships in Italy – above all in Rome, the city she and her family considered their true home.

The following few pages (adapted from a larger chapter (Dick et al., 2005) trace out some of the background issues and current studies informing our understanding of the relation between language and the developing – and damaged – brain, with particular reference to studies by Elizabeth Bates and her colleagues.

Introduction

For centuries, opinions about the fundamental character of neural organization have swung between two often caricatured poles: a phrenological view (Gall, 1810; Fodor, 1983), where each sensorimotor and cognitive function is subserved by a single region of neural tissue, and an equipotential view (Goldstein, 1948; Lashley, 1950), where the functions of particular brain regions are not sharply defined, and contribute to multiple mental processes. Over the last 40 years, the field of language research has been particularly polarized by an analogous debate regarding mental organization, with both generative linguistics and psycholinguistics often taking an explicitly modular and phrenological position (Mauner et al., 1993; Grodzinsky, 2000), in which mental processes are subserved in specific 'loci' of information processing systems or specific brain regions. By contrast, some psycholinguistic and neuropsychological research has moved away from this extreme position, but without resorting to a theory of equipotentiality. This alternative is consistent both with neurobiological notions of regional specialization and with the observed overlap in the regional responsibilities toward high-level computations. This major revision, known as 'embodied cognition', reflects a change in the functional primitives used to characterize the mental processes produced by the brain.

Embodied cognition is an approach originally charted by early researchers in affect (James, 1994), perception (Gibson, 1951), and cognitive development (Piaget, 1928). Here, the primate brain is acknowledged to have significant functional and anatomical divisions of labour; however, the brain's parcellation is driven not by abstract psychological constructs (such as those proposed by Gall and Fodor), but by the body that inhabits it. In this view, language (as well as other abstract or higher-order skills) emerges from, and is intimately linked to, the more evolutionarily entrenched sensorimotor substrates that allow us to comprehend and produce it.

Indeed, results from a half century of research strongly suggest that the ability to comprehend and produce language is based upon an interwoven constellation of skills that emerges from everyday human behaviour: social, physical, and linguistic interactions with the environment (exogenous) combined with the consequent interactions among neural systems (endogenous). Studies of language development and breakdown suggest that sensorimotor and language processes develop with similar trajectories (that is, the ability to manipulate an object in a certain way emerges at the same time in development as does production of a certain language structure); conversely, lesions causing language deficits often cause problems with other sensorimotor skills (that is, patients with aphasia are very likely to have problems producing gestures or interacting with objects – for a review and discussion see Bates & Dick, 2002).

Such an 'emergentist' view (MacWhinney, 1999) of language evolution, development, and processing is often paired with a commitment to a distributive or connectionist account of language processing and its neural instantiation (Elman et al., 1996). In connectionist accounts, complex skills like language (or even simple ones) are subserved by a 'vast neuronal conspiracy' of locally and distally connected computational units that also contribute to processing of other domains with similar underlying perceptuo-motor demands. A key tenet of this approach is that the pattern of connections underlying knowledge or skill representations is *dynamic* or *plastic*, continually adjusting to new contingencies in the internal and external milieu.

Below are summarized findings from a variety of studies that support this new perspective. First we review recent findings from studies of adult aphasia, suggesting that the relation between the character of language breakdown and the locus of brain damage is much less straightforward than had previously been believed; indeed, the divisions that are revealed seem to have more to do with language's conceptual or sensorimotor processing demands than with abstract linguistic distinctions such as syntax *vs.* semantics. We contrast these with results from studies of children with early-occurring focal lesions that shed new light on issues of plasticity, neural reorganization, and developmental processes more generally.

Brain and language: evidence from aphasia

Systematic studies of the language breakdown that can occur after neurological injury are the bedrock supporting our understanding of the relation between brain and language. By investigating the linguistic changes that result from injuries such as stroke, head trauma, tumour, or dementia, we are better equipped both to treat people with aphasia and to understand better the language system itself. The wide variation in the manifestations of aphasia can inform us about the individual components of the language system that may be differentially affected. Further, the relation between the observed deficits and the areas of the brain that are affected can inform us about how the brain supports language functions. Investigations of aphasia have grown exponentially over the past several decades. These studies have begun to change the 19th century view that language consisted of two simple parts, production and comprehension, localized in Broca's and Wernicke's areas of the brain, respectively. After a period of abandonment, this localizationist perspective returned years later with the idea that it was functional modules defined by linguistic theory, such as syntax and semantics, that were supported by these brain regions. Broca's area was believed to subserve syntactic processing because patients with perceived deficits in processing grammatical information had damage to this part of the brain. Similarly, Wernicke's area was believed to be a centre for semantic processing, as patients with Wernicke's aphasia had lexical processing deficits and many had damage to Wernicke's area. It was assumed that these patterns would be observed worldwide, in all aphasic patients, regardless of the languages they spoke, and that these functions were therefore hard wired into the brains of humans.

There is now a significant body of evidence suggesting that the relation between function – be it clinically or linguistically defined – and a specific brain region is considerably more complicated, and more variable, than was previously believed. For instance, lesions confined entirely to Broca's area do not lead to a persisting Broca's aphasia, nor do lesions affecting only Wernicke's area lead to a persisting Wernicke's aphasia (Mohr, 1976; Dronkers *et al.*, 2001). Furthermore, the classical theory that production and comprehension are subserved by Broca's and Wernicke's areas, respectively, cannot be supported. For example, Bates *et al.* (2003) used a new system of lesion-symptom mapping to demonstrate the effects of lesions to the brain on general performance in fluency and auditory comprehension in 101 chronic aphasic patients (see below for further details). The investigators showed that when involvement in other brain regions was co-varied out (the anterior insula and middle temporal gyrus, respectively), damage to Broca's area was not strongly associated with reduced fluency, and damage to Wernicke's area likewise did not correlate robustly with impairments in auditory comprehension.

Indeed, the original speech articulation deficit described by Broca – *aphemia*, roughly, a severe disruption in the patient's voluntary speech production ability, associated with 'recurring utterances' such as 'tan tan tan' – is associated not with injury to a specific cortical area, but with damage to the left superior arcuate fasciculus, a major fibre tract passing from the temporal lobe over the lateral ventricle to the anterior cortical regions (Dronkers *et al.*, 1993). A related deficit typically seen in patients with Broca's aphasia – namely a loss of articulatory agility, or apraxia of speech – also appears not to be associated with the third frontal convolution as previously thought, but rather with damage to the superior portion of the left precentral gyrus of the insula. In a study of 44 aphasic patients with left hemisphere damage, Dronkers (1996) showed that all 25 patients with speech apraxia suffered from a lesion extending into this portion of the anterior insula, while the remaining 19 aphasic patients without speech apraxia had approximately equivalently sized lesions, but ones that spared exactly this region of cortex.

We should emphasize that mapping symptoms to lesions does *not* presume that the associated brain area is solely responsible for the function in question. Metter, Kempler, and colleagues have elegantly demonstrated this fact in a series of positron emission tomography (PET) studies, showing that the locus and extent of structural lesions (as detected by computed tomography) often vastly underestimate the functional impact of seemingly focal damage, and that functional changes (as demonstrated by the presence of brain hypometabolism) are often more tightly yoked to the resulting behavioural deficits than are the lesions themselves. As an example, Kempler *et al.* (1991) showed that structural damage to the classical 'language areas' – the left inferior frontal gyrus ('Broca's area') and left superior and middle temporal gyri ('Wernicke's area') – correlated only weakly with the degree of syntactic deficit observed in the 43 aphasic patients they studied. However, examination of the same patients' PET data showed that comprehension deficits in morphology and syntax were highly correlated with hypometabolism in the left occipital and temporal regions; syntactic deficits were further correlated with hypometabolism in the parietal lobe. Such findings suggest not only that the effect of 'focal' brain lesions is considerably less circumscribed than is generally believed, but also that language may rely upon a much broader confederacy of cortical and subcortical regions than those classically associated with language function.

Not surprisingly, claims regarding the specificity of mapping between discrete linguistically defined abilities and particular (if loosely defined) brain regions or aphasia syndromes have been difficult to uphold. For instance, Grodzinsky (1995; 2000) has claimed that Broca's area '... is neural home to mechanisms involved in the computation of transformational relations between moved phrasal constituents and their extraction sites' (Grodzinsky, 2000, p. 2), a computation posited by some linguists to be crucial for comprehension of sentence types such as passives and object relatives, but not for comprehension of 'canonical' sentence types such as simple transitives. However, the results of several large studies of aphasic patients' syntactic comprehension have in fact found no systematic relation between damage to *any* single brain region and the presence of syntactic comprehension deficits (Caplan *et al.*, 1985; Caplan *et al.*, 1996; Dick *et al.*, 2001a; Dronkers *et al.*, 2004). What is more, the signature profile of syntactic deficits cited by Grodzinsky (2000) as evidence for the modularity and localizability of syntactic operations can be reproduced both qualitatively and quantitatively in neurologically intact college students operating under 'stressful' or degraded conditions – a finding that holds for speakers of both English (Dick *et al.*, 2001a) and German (Dick *et al.*, 2003). Similarly, Wilson & Saygin (2004) re-examined Grodzinsky & Finkel's (1998) claim that individuals with agrammatic aphasia are selectively impaired in their ability to process syntactic structures involving 'traces of maximal projections' in grammaticality judgment tasks. Wilson & Saygin found no evidence that agrammatic aphasic subjects (or any other aphasic subgroup) are selectively impaired on structures involving traces. In fact, groups of patients had remarkably similar profiles of performance across sentence types, regardless of whether the grouping was made by aphasia type, screening for agrammatic comprehension, or lesion site. Furthermore, Wilson *et al.* (2003) examined grammaticality judgment on sentences with and without traces of maximal projections when healthy young controls performed the task under 'stressful' conditions, and found that the breakdown of performance under non-optimal processing conditions closely resembles the breakdown observed in aphasic patients.

In summary, the lesion correlates of 'specific' linguistic deficits in adult aphasic patients are much more variable and complicated than was previously thought, supporting the view that higher level language skills are dynamic, and distributed throughout the brain. On the other hand, there are obviously quite dramatic global differences in the character of linguistic deficits depending on lesion site – for example, left hemisphere injury in adults is much more apt to cause severe and lasting language problems, damage to frontal regions tends to be correlated with production and articulation difficulties, while posterior damage correlates with comprehension difficulties. Moreover, these coarse mappings tend to be quite consistent over individuals (indeed, around 95 per cent of neurologically intact right-handed adults appear to be 'left-dominant' for language, based on the results of WADA tests – Rasmussen & Milner, 1977). Does this quasi-inevitability of left-hemisphere-dominated processing of language imply not only that the left hemisphere is 'purpose-built' for processing language, but in addition, that a special mechanism or mechanisms are needed for successful language acquisition and processing? Or is the typical adult profile of language organization a result of softer constraints or regional biological predispositions to undertake certain types of computations? Perhaps the emerging processing biases of the constituent regions of the left hemisphere are more suited to the demands of language (for example, rapid coordination of effectors, analyses of fast formant transitions), but given enough time and learning, alternate organizations for language production and comprehension could arise. Such plasticity might be anticipated *a priori*, given the significant individual variability in language organization found in typically developing children and adults (Dick *et al.*, 2001b). These issues are addressed in the following section.

Learning language after early brain injury

Results from 30 years of studies of children with early-onset brain injury (for example, caused by congenital arteriovenous malformation, prenatal or perinatal stroke, chronic seizures, or later hemispherectomy) suggest a remarkable potential for alternative modes of language organization in the brain. As reviewed by Bates & Roe (2001), the overall picture from the published reports on children with early focal lesions and hemispherectomy tends *not* to show consistent differences between early left and right hemisphere injury in terms of language abilities. If differences are observed, they are much smaller than those observed in adults with commensurate injuries, and generally are noted for only a few language subscales. As Bates and Roe point out, these are particularly thorny studies to conduct and to evaluate – the variability over patients and over studies in lesion onset time, seizure history, type and extent of injury, sample sizes, and statistical methods complicates the interpretation of putative differences tremendously. Indeed, when sample sizes are large, and direct statistical comparisons between lesion groups are made [for example, right hemisphere damage (RHD) *vs.* left hemisphere damage (LHD), controlling for seizure history and lesion onset time], lesion side and site appear not to predict language proficiency (Bates & Roe, 2001).

For instance, in a study of 43 English-speaking and 33 Italian-speaking children aged 5 years and upwards with focal lesions of prenatal and perinatal onset, Bates *et al.* (1999) found that there was an overall delay in language acquisition associated with *any* lesion, with IQ scores in the low to normal range. In contrast to the expected adult profile (where LHD patients show more pronounced language deficits, and RHD patients show more pronounced spatial deficits), Bates *et al.* observed no difference between children with RHD and LHD on standard IQ measures (both verbal and non-verbal), or on all language comprehension/production measures (available for the Italian sample only). With regard to the latter result, the overall differences between Italian-speaking patients and control children in language comprehension and production disappeared after controlling for mental age.

Bates and her colleagues have also directly compared school-age children and adults with comparable focal lesions on various different measures. For instance, Kempler *et al.* (1999) tested comprehension of familiar *versus* novel phrases in adults and children (aged 6 to 12). Results with adult patients revealed a classic double dissociation, with RHD patients showing impaired comprehension of familiar phrases and idioms, and relatively preserved comprehension of novel phrases, while LHD patients showed the opposite pattern of deficits. In stark contrast, in the child patients not only was there no difference in either measure between LHD and RHD, but both groups performed within the low normal range for their age-matched controls, whereas their adult aphasic counterparts were massively impaired relative to healthy age-matched controls.

Dick *et al.* (1999; 2003) tested the online syntactic comprehension of 20 children aged 7 to 18 years with RHD or LHD, comparing them with a large sample of typically developing children. Children with lesions to either hemisphere showed developmental delays in both accuracy and reaction time, though their comprehension was similar to that of the youngest typically developing children. Again there was little evidence for an RHD/LHD difference in accuracy or response times. Similar results were found by Feldman *et al.* (2002), where children with focal lesions were delayed, and not deviant, in a standard competition model task. Direct comparisons between adults and children revealed a substantial quantitative but marginally significant interaction between lesion and age, where RH-damaged adults and RH- or LH-damaged children performed roughly equivalently, while LH-damaged adult aphasic patients fared considerably worse, with massive intersubject variability.

The dramatic differences between language comprehension skills after early- and late-onset focal lesions are echoed in a recent study of language production (Bates *et al.*, 2001). Here, children and adults with right or left hemisphere focal brain damage were asked to narrate brief biographical sketches; these narratives were transcribed and further analysed in terms of patterns of error (omission *versus* commission), propositional content, sentence length, and so forth. As would be expected, adults with LHD were significantly more impaired than their RHD counterparts, with each group showing a very different pattern of relative strengths and weaknesses. But comparisons between children with RHD and LHD showed absolutely no differences on any production measures; moreover, this sample of children with early-onset lesions differed very little from age-matched controls, where children with lesions used fewer words and made more omission errors than their age-matched controls.

In short, the results of these studies of school-age children with early-onset focal lesions provide compelling evidence for the plasticity of the developing brain. Although these children do tend to have language processing delays relative to their age-matched peers, they show remarkably spared comprehension and production relative to adults with comparable focal lesions. What is more, these results suggest that the usual pattern of brain organization for language – for example, left hemisphere dominance – is neither inevitable nor even necessary for successful language processing. In tandem with a bevy of behavioural results with neurologically intact subjects, these results further suggest that there is considerable change in children's neural underpinnings for language, even well into the school-age years.

In this regard, the few functional magnetic resonance imaging (fMRI) studies that have been directed at typical language development have shown interesting differences between activation patterns for adults and school-age children, even when very simple tasks are employed. Using a variety of word-generation tasks (verb/rhyme/opposites), Schlaggar *et al.* (2002) found that young adults showed activation in a left dorsal prefrontal region that was completely absent in children; conversely, children showed increased activation in a left fusiform region that was significantly greater than that evoked in adults. Saccuman *et al.* (2002) showed similar findings, where young adults in a covert picture-naming task showed significantly more activation in left lateral prefrontal and superior temporal regions than children aged 10 to 12. These differences in activation could not easily be attributed to group differences in behaviour, suggesting that as learning and development progress there are qualitative changes in the way in which our brains structure themselves to process language, even after much of the 'heavy lifting' in language acquisition has taken place.

It might be anticipated that significant neural circuit modifications take place early on and concomitantly with the development of language skills. Unfortunately there are as of now no functional imaging studies of typically developing children under the age of 5 that bear on this issue [but see a recent study of young infants by Dehaene-Lambertz *et al.* (2003)]. However, Bates and colleagues have conducted prospective cross-sectional studies of children with perinatal focal lesions at the dawn of language comprehension and production, allowing a direct contrast between various 'stages' of brain organization for language. In three similar studies of English- and Italian-speaking children with either LHD or RHD (Thal *et al.*, 1991; Bates *et al.*, 1997; Vicari *et al.*, 2000) data from several communicative inventories (MacArthur Communicative Development Inventories (CDI); Fenson *et al.*, 1993) and free-speech samples were collected from children from 10 to 40 months, a period beginning with early language comprehension and word production (10 to 17 months) and continuing to multiword utterances and grammatical development (18 to 40 months). The results of these studies serve as *prima facie* evidence against the theoretical notion that the developing brain is a conglomeration of inexorably maturing modules devoted to different processing needs. In the next section, we summarize these data, and suggest that the developing brain is best understood as a dynamic and self-organizing system that cannot be parcelled up according to abstract psychological or linguistic principles. For example, Thal *et al.* (1991), Bates *et al.* (1997), and Vicari *et al.* (2000) showed that early in the development of language skills (10 to 18 months), some children with perinatal focal lesions show delays in language comprehension as well as gestural communication. However, this delay was observed only in children with *right* hemisphere injury; those with LHD (even with left temporal damage) were within the normal range on word comprehension. Not only is this the opposite of what one would expect from an adult model of language comprehension – where left temporal damage tends to correlate with comprehension disorders – but it is also opposite to the usual lesion correlate of deficits in gesture production and comprehension, which in adults are strongly associated with left hemisphere damage (see Bates & Dick, 2002 for extended discussion, as well as Wang & Goodglass, 1992).

For early single-word production in the same cohort of children (again aged 10 to 18 months), lesions to either hemisphere provoke delays in development, but are particularly severe in children with left *temporal* damage; this is again in contrast to the adult model, where language production deficits tend to correlate with left frontal damage.

Results from all three studies showed that left temporal damage continues to be a predictor of delayed language production somewhat later in development (for example, 19 to 31 months). Here, toddlers with left temporal damage show impaired lexical production, with commensurate delays in grammatical development (as measured in free speech and the toddler version of the MacArthur CDI). With regard to this unexpected finding, Bates *et al.* (1997) suggested that whereas successful naturalistic auditory language comprehension relies on a wide range of partially redundant cues (such as temporal and spectral structure, prosody, gesture, and environmental cues) that allow for good comprehension in the face of incomplete or imperfect perception, language production requires a more fine-tuned and detailed set of acoustic representations – ones that would take longer to develop in the face of disrupted acoustic processing. In contrast to the left temporal findings, frontal damage to *either* hemisphere was also implicated in production delays – again unlike the adult model of left frontal damage leading to production difficulties.

Interestingly, these lesion-specific (left temporal) deficits are observed in somewhat older or more advanced children [at the stage of multiword production in Vicari *et al.* (2000), and at age 5 in Reilly *et al.* (1998)]. At this point in development, children with focal lesions are on average slightly delayed relative to their age-matched peers, but still function in the low-to-normal range overall.

Clearly these children's brains are organizing themselves differently than they would in typical development. Does this indicate that the brain is equipotential for language, or – as might be expected from an embodied account – that there are early-forming connections and architectures that make some developing brain regions more hospitable to language than others? More concretely, if left frontal and temporal regions are damaged early in development, will the brain regions enabling language function emerge throughout the brain (as one might predict, given strict equipotentiality) or will contralateral regions homologous to those characteristically associated with language be recruited for language tasks?

Axel Müller and colleagues (Müller *et al.*, 1998a; 1998b; 1999) have investigated this question using PET imaging in patients with early-onset lesions that resulted in intractable epilepsy. Using sentence listening and repetition tasks (Müller *et al.*, 1998a), they compared activation profiles for children with perinatal left and right focal lesions (with the functional deficit confirmed by resting hypometabolism in the affected hemisphere). Here, children and adolescents with early LH lesions showed extensive right lateralization of activation in both traditional perisylvian 'language' areas, as well as much of the right temporal lobe (particularly the anterior temporal lobe), the angular gyrus, the precuneus, and the anterior cingulate. Roughly the opposite pattern was seen for the group with RH lesions – see Müller *et al.* (1998a) for details. A more recent fMRI study (Staudt *et al.*, 2002) of five children with left periventricular lesions (causing hemiplegia but not epilepsy) showed a similar mirroring of typical left-lateralized activation in a covert verb generation task.

In an imaging analogue to the behavioural studies of Bates and colleagues discussed above, Müller *et al.* (1999) directly compared typical adult language-related activation to children and adults with, respectively, early- and late-onset left hemisphere focal lesions – with the expectation that earlier injuries would allow greater potential for reorganization of function. Here, neurologically intact adults showed the usual left-lateralized perisylvian activation profile for sentence comprehension, while patients with early-onset focal lesions showed a mirrored, right-lateralized profile, and late-onset patients showed highly symmetrical perisylvian activation. The dramatic lateralization difference between the early and the late lesion groups suggests that at least some of the remarkable capacity of the early lesion group to acquire normal language may reflect the development of these functions (or closely related ones) in the right hemisphere. These findings argue against the view that language functions are inexorably hard wired within specific left hemisphere regions, but rather, that the brain has some flexibility to reorganize such cognitive functions if necessary.

Interestingly, this early-lesion-induced shift in interhemispheric activation is not seen in all domains, even in the face of early cerebral insult. In this regard, Müller *et al.* (1998b) directly compared left-right fluorodeoxyglucose PET activation asymmetries for sentence listening and repetition *versus* a basic motor task (finger tapping) in a sample of nine patients with relatively early-onset left hemisphere lesions. The difference in activation asymmetry was striking: for the language tasks, patients showed strong rightward activation asymmetries in the regions typically associated with these tasks (for example, the superior and middle temporal gyri, inferior frontal gyri) – again, a pattern opposite that of healthy control subjects. However, the same patients showed strong leftward activation asymmetries in the motor task, asymmetries very similar to controls. As with the behavioural studies discussed above, these results suggest that the development and commitment of neural resources for language is a protracted process, and one that might be more flexible than that of more developmentally and evolutionarily entrenched capacities such as the motor system. However, it is worth emphasizing that lesion-induced reorganization of language function appears to recruit roughly homologous regions in the right hemisphere rather than, for instance, co-opting left hemisphere visual and somatosensory regions to accomplish language tasks. This suggests that regions with certain patterns of cortical and subcortical connections may be more amenable than others to cooption or 'shared use' by language – an area of research that Elizabeth Bates was particularly interested in exploring at the beginning and at the end of her career.

Conclusions

The field of brain and language has veered back and forth between the Scylla of phrenological determinism and the Charybdis of *tabula rasa* empiricism, with neither account providing a sufficient explanatory framework for more than a century of data from behavioural, neuropsychological, and neuroimaging experiments. Elizabeth Bates has done the field a great service by showing us a 'third way' of thinking about language in the brain – one that takes into consideration basic phylogenetic, developmental, and anatomical constraints on the brain while also acknowledging both the extraordinary plasticity of the mammalian nervous system (during development and throughout the life span) and the information-processing capacities afforded by a distributive processing system.

Acknowledgments: The preface to this chapter is a revised version of "Elisabeth Bates: a scientific obituary" in: *Developmental Science* **7** (2), iii-iv, Frederic Dick, Jeffrey Elman and Joan Stiles (authors).

References

Bates, E. & Roe, K. (2001): Language development in children with unilateral brain injury. In: *Handbook of developmental cognitive neuroscience*, eds. C.A. Nelson & M. Luciana, pp. 281–307). Cambridge, MA: MIT Press.

Bates, E. & Dick, F. (2002): Language, gesture, and the developing brain. *Dev. Psychobiol.* **40**, 293–310.

Bates, E., Thal, D., Trauner, D., Fenson, J., Aram, D., Eisele, J. & Nass, R. (1997): From first words to grammar in children with focal brain injury. *Dev. Neuropsychol.* **13**, 275–343.

Bates, E., Vicari, S. & Trauner, D. (1999): Neural mediation of language development: perspectives from lesion studies of infants and children. In: *Neurodevelopmental disorders*, ed. H. Tager-Flusberg, pp. 533–581. Cambridge, MA: MIT Press.

Bates, E., Reilly, J., Wulfeck, B., Dronkers, N., Opie, M., Fenson, J., Kriz, S., Jeffries, R., Miller, L. & Herbst, K. (2001): Differential effects of unilateral lesions on language production in children and adults. *Brain Lang.* **79**, 223–265.

Bates, E., Wilson, S.M., Saygin, A.P., Dick, F., Sereno, M.I., Knight, R.T. & Dronkers, N.F. (2003): Voxel-based lesion-symptom mapping. *Nat. Neurosci.* **6**, 448–450.

Caplan, D., Baker, C. & Dehaut, F. (1985): Syntactic determinants of sentence comprehension in aphasia. *Cognition* **21**, 117–175.

Caplan, D., Hildebrandt, N. & Makris, N. (1996): Location of lesions in stroke patients with deficits in syntactic processing in sentence comprehension. *Brain* **119**, 933–949.

Dehaene-Lambertz, G., Dehaene, S. & Hertz-Pannier, L. (2003): Functional neuroimaging of speech perception in infants. *Science* **298**, 2013–2015.

Dick, F., Wulfeck, B., Bates, E., Saltzman, D., Naucler, N. & Dronkers, N. (1999): Interpretation of complex syntax in aphasic adults and children with focal lesions or specific language impairment. *Brain Lang.* **69**, 335–336.

Dick, F., Bates, E., Wulfeck, B., Utman, J., Dronkers, N. & Gernsbacher, M.A. (2001a): Language deficits, localization and grammar: evidence for a distributive model of language breakdown in aphasics and normals. *Psychol. Rev.* **108**, 759–788.

Dick, F., Saccuman, C., Sereno, M., Müller, R.A., Bates, E. & Wulfeck, B. (2001b): Language production and comprehension in fMRI: consistency and variability over individuals and group averages. Poster presented at the Meeting of the Society for Cognitive Neuroscience, New York.

Dick, F., Bates, E. & Ferstl, E.C. (2003): Spectral and temporal degradation of speech as a simulation of morphosyntactic deficits in English and German. *Brain Lang.* **85**, 535–542.

Dick, F., Dronkers, N., Pizzamiglio, L., Saygin, A.P., Small, S.L. & Wilson, S. (2005): Language and the brain. In: *Festschrift for Elizabeth Bates*, ed. M. Tomasello & D. Slobin. Mahwah, NJ: Lawrence Erlbaum.

Dronkers, N. (1996): A new brain region for coordinating speech articulation. *Nature* **384**, 159–161.

Dronkers, N., Redfern, B. & Shapiro, J. (1993): Neuroanatomic correlates of production deficits in severe Broca's aphasia. *Exp. Neuropsychol.* **15**, 59–60.

Dronkers, N.F., Wilkins, D.P., Van Valin, R.D., Redfern, B.B. & Jaeger, J.J. (2004): Lesion analysis of the brain areas involved in language comprehension. *Cognition* **92**, 145–177.

Elman, J.L., Bates, E.A., Johnson, M.H., Karmiloff-Smith, A., Parisi, D. & Plunkett, K. (1996): *Rethinking innateness: a connectionist perspective on development*. Cambridge, MA: MIT Press.

Feldman, H., MacWhinney, B. & Sacco, K. (2002): Sentence processing in children with early unilateral brain injury. *Brain Lang.* **83**, 335–352.

Fenson, L., Dale, P.S., Reznick, J., Thal, D., Bates, E., Hartung, J.P., Pethick, S. & Reilly, J.S. (1993): *The MacArthur Communicative Development Inventories: user's guide and technical manual*. San Diego, CA: Singular Publishing Group.

Fodor, J.A. (1983): *The modularity of mind: an essay on faculty psychology*. Cambridge, MA: MIT Press.

Gall, F.J. (1810): *Anatomie et physiologie du système nerveux* (vol. 1). Paris: Librairie grecque-latine-allemande.

Gibson, J.J. (1951): What is form? *Psychol. Rev.* **58**, 403–412.

Goldstein, K. (1948): Language and language disturbances: aphasic symptom complexes and their significance for medicine and theory of language. New York: Grune & Stratton.

Grodzinsky, Y. (1995): A restrictive theory of agrammatic comprehension. *Brain Lang.* **50**, 27–51.

Grodzinsky, Y. (2000): The neurology of syntax: language use without Broca's area. *Behav. Brain Sci.* **23**, 1–71.

Grodzinsky, Y. & Finkel, L. (1998): The neurology of empty categories: aphasics' failure to detect ungrammaticality. *J. Cogn. Neurosci.* **10**, 281–292.

James, W. (1994): The physical basis of emotion (1894). *Psychol. Rev.* **101**, 205–210.

Kempler, D., Metter, E.J., Curtiss, S., Jackson, C.A. & Hanson, W.R. (1991): Grammatical comprehension, aphasic syndromes, and neuroimaging. *J. Neurolinguistics* **6**, 301–318.

Kempler, D., Van Lancker, D., Marchman, V. & Bates, E. (1999): Idiom comprehension in children and adults with unilateral brain damage. *Dev. Psychol.* **15**, 327–349.

Lashley, K.S. (1950): *In search of the engram*, vol. 4. New York: Academic Press.

MacWhinney, B. (1999): *The emergence of language*. Mahwah, NJ: Lawrence Erlbaum.

Mauner, G., Fromkin, V.A. & Cornell, T.L. (1993): Comprehension and acceptability judgments in agrammatism: disruptions in the syntax of referential dependency. *Brain Lang.* **45**, 340–370.

Mohr, J.P. (1976): Broca's area and Broca's aphasia. In: *Studies in neuro-linguistics*, vol. 1, eds. H. Whitaker & H. Whitaker, pp. 201–233. New York: Academic Press.

Müller, R.-A., Rothermel, R., Behen, M., Muzik, O., Chakraborty, P. & Chugani, H. (1999): Language organization in patients with early and late left-hemisphere lesion: a PET study. *Neuropsychologia* **37**, 545–557.

Müller, R.-A., Rothermel, R., Behen, M., Muzik, O., Mangner, T., Chakraborty, P. & Chugani, H. (1998a): Brain organization of language after early unilateral lesion: a PET study. *Brain Lang.* **62**, 422–451.

Müller, R.-A., Rothermel, R., Behen, M., Otto Muzik, O., Mangner, T. & Chugani, H. (1998b): Differential patterns of language and motor reorganization following early left hemisphere injury. *Arch. Neurol.* **55**, 1113–1119.

Piaget, J. (1928): *Le jugement et le raisonnement chez l'enfant*. (Judgement and reasoning in the child). London: Kegan Paul Trench Trubner.

Rasmussen, T. & Milner, B. (1977): The role of early left-brain injury in determining lateralization of cerebral speech functions. *Ann. N.Y. Acad. Sci.* **299**, 355–369.

Reilly, J., Bates, E. & Marchman, V. (1998): Narrative discourse in children with early focal brain injury. *Brain Lang.* **61**, 335–375.

Saccuman, C., Dick, F., Bates, E., Müller, R.A., Bussiere, J., Krupa-Kwiatkowski, M. & Wulfeck, B. (2002): Lexical access and sentence processing: a developmental fMRI study of language processing. Poster presented at the Meeting of the Cognitive Neuroscience Society, April, 2002.

Schlaggar, B., Brown, T.T., Lugar, H., Visscher, K., Miezin, F. & Petersen, S. (2002): Functional neuroanatomical differences between adults and school-age children in the processing of single words. *Science* **296**, 1476–1479.

Staudt, M., Lidzba, K., Grodd, W., Wildgruber, D., Erb, M. & Kraegeloh-Mann, I. (2002): Right-hemispheric organization of language following early left-sided brain lesions: Functional MRI topography. *Neuroimage* **16**, 954–967.

Thal, D., Marchman, V., Stiles, J., Aram, D., Trauner, D., Nass, R. & Bates, E. (1991): Early lexical development in children with focal brain injury. *Brain Lang.* **40**, 491–527.

Vicari, S., Albertoni, A., Chilosi, A., Cipriani, P., Cioni, G. & Bates, E. (2000): Plasticity and reorganization during early language learning in children with congenital brain injury. *Cortex* **36**, 31–46.

Wang, L. & Goodglass, H. (1992): Pantomime, praxis, and aphasia. *Brain Lang.* **42**, 402–418.

Wilson, S.M. & Saygin, A.P. (2004): Grammaticality judgment in aphasia: deficits are not specific to syntactic structures, aphasic syndromes or lesion sites. *J. Cogn. Neurosci.* **16**, 238–252.

Wilson, S.M., Saygin, A.P., Schleicher, E., Dick, F. & Bates, E. (2003): Grammaticality judgment under non-optimal processing conditions: deficits induced in normal participants resemble those observed in aphasic patients. *Brain Lang.* **87**, 67–68.

Chapter 2

Early language acquisition: typical and atypical processes

Maria Cristina Caselli[*] and Silvia Stefanini[*#o]

[*] *Institute of Cognitive Sciences and Technologies – CNR, Via Nomentana 56, 00161 Rome, Italy*
[#] *Centro per la ricerca sui disturbi neurocognitivi del bambino, Parma, Italy*
[o] *Department of Neurosciences, University of Parma, Parma, Italy*
cristina.caselli@istc.cnr.it

Summary

In this chapter we will summarize some recent research on early language acquisition. We will focus on the continuity both across modalities (from gestures to gesture and words), and intramodally (from lexicon to grammar). The chapter mainly focuses on the work conducted by our Italian team at the Institute of Cognitive Sciences and Technologies of the CNR and comprises four sections. In the first we discuss the role of gesture, its interplay with first words and combinations in typically developing children. These studies were carried out both in Italian and in cross-linguistic comparisons. In the second section we briefly analyse the results of some research on the link between gestures and speech in children with cognitive impairment (Down syndrome). In the third section we focus on the relation between vocabulary and grammar in typical populations, also referring to results obtained by research in different languages. In the final section, we summarise some recent work on the development of lexicon and grammar in children with Down syndrome. The entire chapter is a tribute to Elizabeth Bates's scientific work, which has strongly influenced our research on language acquisition.

Introduction

Our aim in this chapter is to present a survey of the current body of knowledge on early language acquisition. We will discuss this topic by focusing on the continuity from prelinguistic to linguistic development, and from lexicon to grammar. The main feature of these processes is universality – that is, the language learning process remains very similar across different languages and is characterized by precise and common changes. However, all children follow their own approach to achieving mature linguistic and communicative abilities, and language experts are familiar with the wide variability resulting from individual differences and dissimilarities between typical and atypical development.

In the following pages we report some recent studies on the role of gesture and its relation to first words and combinations, and on the interdependence of vocabulary and grammar in children acquiring different languages (for example, Italian and English). We will consider data from these studies as they refer to normally developing children and children with Down syndrome.

With regard to the first topic – the continuity from prelinguistic to linguistic development – our aim is to provide evidence on the continuity between prelinguistic and linguistic development, and on the interplay between the gestural and vocal modalities in both typical and atypical development. As we will suggest, our results appear to highlight a strong interrelation between language and other cognitive domains: in our view language is solidly linked to more general cognitive and neuro-sensory-motor structures that language shares with other domains (for example, memory and sensorimotor coordination), and that are put in the service of language in a unique way, as proposed by Bates (Bates & Goodman, 1997; Bates & Dick, 2002) and other leading researchers (Elman *et al.*, 1996; Deacon, 1997; Tomasello, 1999).

The second topic – the continuity from lexicon to grammar – aims to highlight the interplay between universal and language-specific factors in lexical development in the second year of life, a crucial period in which children make the passage from first words to grammar. As we shall see, cross-linguistic studies and comparisons between different populations (typical *vs.* atypical) provide strong evidence for universal constraints on the development and composition of vocabulary, although subtle variations are observed between different languages and populations.

Gestures and speech in typical development

According to McNeill (McNeill, 1992; 2000) gesture and speech co-occur during production because they are linked to one another and are also connected to the same underlying system of thought (though each modality may express a different aspect of that thought). Hence there are links between gesture and speech throughout the process of speech production.

Nevertheless, the general public and many scientific observers find it hard to distinguish between language and speech, and thus it has been difficult to build up a perspective on language acquisition and development that includes gestures. A consideration of the deep link between vocal and gestural components in communication systems could be an interesting starting point to answer a recurring question in language development research – are linguistic and cognitive abilities independent? In Bates's opinion, language and cognitive development are strictly interconnected: "Language emerges from a nexus of skills in attention, perception, imitation, and symbolic processing that transcend the boundaries of 'language proper'" (Bates & Dick, 2002). The fact that all typically developing infants communicate gesturally before using a language shows this developmental continuity between these two modalities in the early appearance and construction of symbols.

The onset of intentional communication between the ages of 9 and 13 months is partially marked by the emergence of a series of gestures – ritualized request, showing, pointing – which precedes the appearance of the first words. These gestures, formerly called *performatives* and recently renamed *deictic gestures*, are used to refer to external objects or events and express communicative intents on the part of the child. The specific referents of these gestures can only be interpreted by referring to the extralinguistic context in which communication occurs. These deictic gestures are often accompanied by vocalizations or words, or both. In approximately the same age range, children show other gestures – called *referential* gestures – in order to communicate a more meaningful content. By using this kind of gesture, children not only refer to a present object but also try to express a comment about the whole situation, by naming, asking, or telling something. In this category we also put representational gestures, which mainly derive from actions or referent functions (for example, *sleeping, aeroplane, dancing*), and conventional gestures. Most of the meanings expressed by referential gestures (for example, *eat*) are equivalent to those conveyed by first words (for example, *'pappa'* <lunch>) (Volterra, 1981; Volterra *et al.*, 1993).

Some studies have recently examined the role that both deictic and representational gestures play in the transition to two-word speech (Morford & Goldin-Meadow, 1992; Capirci et al., 1996; Butcher & Goldin-Meadow, 2000). This issue is fundamental for an understanding of whether there is any continuity between an earlier 'preverbal' and a later functionally 'equivalent' linguistic form, or even more between the structuring of gestures and cross-modal combinations and later word combinations.

To analyse this topic, two related studies were conducted on the spontaneous communication of 12 Italian children, observed at the age of 16 months, when the children's vocal communication consisted largely of one-word utterances, and at 20 months, when two-word utterances were produced in an appreciable number (Iverson et al., 1994; Capirci et al., 1996). Extensive communication in both gestural and vocal modalities, including deictic and referential elements, was observed in all the children. A substantial amount of variability among individual children was also evident, especially at 16 months, but more in their repertoire of words (range 1 to 73) than in their gestures (range 5 to 14).

A substantial difference between 16 and 20 months was also found. All the 16-month-old children produced gestures more frequently than words. At 20 months all the children produced words more often than gestures.

All the children's combinations were first categorized into three major classes according to their modality of production. At both 16 and 20 months, *cross-modal* combinations (combinations of a gesture and a word) were produced more often than *unimodal* ones (gesture-gesture or word-word combinations), and the most frequently produced subtype was the combination of pointing with a referential word. Unimodal combinations, which were almost absent at 16 months, increased markedly in the 20-month group and were expressed in particular by two-word combinations.

According to the informational content conveyed it was also possible to classify the combinations into *unireferential* and *bireferential*. In the unireferential combinations the two elements express the same meaning (for example, moving the hand to the mouth while producing the word for 'eating'); in the bireferential combination the two elements express two different meanings and one adds information to one another (for example, pointing and saying 'other', referring to a biscuit; producing two words like: 'pappa più' – meal all gone). At 20 months the bireferential gesture-word combination increased and the bireferential word-word combination appeared frequently.

These findings underscore the fact that the two types of gestural elements (deictic and representational) appear to make different contributions to the informational content of combinations. Deictic gestures were often combined with representational words in bireferential utterances, even at 16 months. Representational gestures, on the other hand, were primarily employed in unireferential combinations, in which two signals were superimposed to 'reinforce' the same meaning that one of the two could also convey alone. When children produced biferential combinations of two representational elements, they did so by combining two representational words.

In conclusion, it is important to underline how vocabulary size at 20 months was predicted by the gestural (deictic and referential) repertoire measured at 16 months – a result that confirms the clear link between words and gestures (Capirci et al., 1996).

Apart from direct observations, as presented above, some studies have explored gestural and spoken repertoire sizes, as well as the relation between vocal comprehension and gesture-word production, using indirect measures (Casadio & Caselli, 1989; Fenson et al., 1994; Caselli & Casadio, 1995). The results collected on a sample of about 300 Italian children aged 8 to

17 months by the parental questionnaire *Primo Vocabolario del Bambino*, the Italian version of the American MacArthur Communicative Development Inventory (CDI) hereafter referred to as the PVB (see also Caselli & Casadio, 1995), have highlighted the fact that receptive vocabulary in the age range considered is significantly larger than expressive vocabulary. Furthermore, children are reported to produce more action and gestures than words, and, in the same period, there is an interesting correlation and correspondence of meaning between words comprehended and gestures produced. Finally, in the months that follow, action or gestures and words appear to develop in parallel up to the age of 17 months: at around 16 to 17 months children are reported to use a mean of about 40 action or gestures and 32 words. The range of meanings conveyed and the size of the gestural and vocal repertoire are comparable (Caselli & Volterra, 1999).

These findings are coherent with the data collected using the same instrument (the parental questionnaire CDI) in other languages [for example, English (Fenson *et al.*, 1994) and Swedish (Eriksson & Berglund, 1999)], confirming that many languages are characterized by similar developmental processes.

However, less research has been conducted with observational techniques allowing direct comparisons among different languages. Some years ago a cross-linguistic study was carried out to clarify whether gestures had a special developmental role in particularly 'gestural' cultures (such as Italian), or if their relevance was common to many cultures (Bates *et al.*, 1979). The findings showed strong similarities between Italian and English: gestural and vocal symbols emerged in children around the same time (1 year of age), they were correlated across the sample in the frequency of use and rate of acquisition, and both kinds of symbols (gestural and vocal) followed a similar process of progressive decontextualization.

At this time other studies are under way, comparing the emergence and the role of gestures in different cultures. For example, two recent studies compared Swedish and Italian children using observation data or parental reports, and found strong similarities between the two cultures, even though they are traditionally described as using gestures with different frequencies and intensities (Volterra & Berglund, 2004).

Gestures and words in children with Down syndrome

Although there are now numerous descriptions of the relation between gesture and the developing language system in typically developing children, relatively little is known about the nature and early development of the gesture-language system in children with developmental disorders involving delayed or deviant language. Studies of such populations would contribute to our understanding of the link between gesture and language by providing information on the development of gesture in the context of specific profiles of language delay or impairment. Questions to be answered involve the role of gesture in relation to language when language is developing atypically, and how patterns of gesture use may vary in relation to specific profiles of language impairment. An interesting possibility for responding to these points could come from research on language development in children with Down syndrome. Many investigators have highlighted the retarded development of language production in this population, as well as describing asynchrony between the different linguistic subdomains. In particular, morphology and phonology have been found more seriously impaired than lexicon and syntax.

However, very few studies have considered the role of gesture in language acquisition in these children. Caselli and colleagues (Caselli *et al.*, 1998) administered the PVB, Words and Gestures scale (Caselli & Casadio, 1995) to the parents of 40 Italian children with Down syndrome with an average chronological age of 28 months. Comparing the children's scores on the 'actions and gestures' section of the PVB with those of a group of typically developing children from the normative sample matched on the basis of comprehension vocabulary size, the investigators reported that the children with Down syndrome had a significantly larger gestural repertoire than the control group.

Nevertheless, inventories such as the PVB and CDI only provide information about whether or not a particular behaviour is in a child's repertoire. The data cannot give information about the frequency with which children produce gestures while communicating. This issue was addressed in a qualitative study of word and gesture production on five children with Down syndrome with an average mental age of 22.4 months and an average language age of 18 months (Iverson *et al.*, 2003). Each child with Down syndrome was matched to a typically developing child on the basis of sex, language age, and observed expressive vocabulary size. Each child was videotaped for 30 minutes in interaction with their mothers. The findings provide evidence for a tight link between gesture and language in children with Down syndrome, a link that holds despite specific difficulties with some aspects of expressive language that are characteristic of this population. Relative to their language-matched typically developing peers, children with Down syndrome had a significantly smaller repertoire of representational gestures, fewer bireferential combinations (gesture and word), and did not combine two words. Nevertheless, children with Down syndrome produced representational gestures with a frequency similar to their controls. It is possible that Down syndrome children may have a specific delay in making the transition from one-word to two-word speech. It may be important to conduct more research on this topic in order to explore the organization of the developing gesture-language system and to assess gesture in young children with communicative delays and disorders. At the end of their research, the investigators found that during the early stages of communicative development, the relation between gesture and language in children with Down syndrome is very similar to that observed in typically developing children with similar language production abilities.

To summarize so far, several studies have shown that language is characterized by continuity across modalities (for example, from gesture to vocal language) in different cultures and populations (that is, in typically developing children as well as in children with Down syndrome). We will now report data showing that there is also continuity within the traditional language domains of lexicon and grammar.

Lexicon and grammar

The correct use of grammar in the first years of life has traditionally been thought to depend on innate and domain-specific systems of rules – that is, Universal Grammar (Chomsky, 1975; Pinker, 1999). The alternative hypothesis, recently called *emergentist* (for a review see Marchman & Thal, 2005), proposes that 'children can create their own grammatical systems harnessing an impressive array of domain-general skills and mechanisms, e.g. linguistic, communicative, perceptual and cognitive.' The consequence is that language acquisition is a long and complicated process and children have an essential duty to learn from social interactions with adults and to construct efficient grammar structures for communication. In the Chomskyian perspective the study of individual differences in acquisition was rarely investigated, but in the emergentist view it gets a special role, thus allowing exploration of many possible routes in order to achieve the same final target. The emergentist perspective suggests that we could find the same mechanisms underlying the emergence of language across different periods of development and special tasks that children constantly have to solve, such as the learning of words and the understanding of grammar rules. The findings on the interdependence of vocabulary and grammar reported in children acquiring English (Bates *et al.*, 1994; Fenson *et al.*, 1994; Marchman & Bates, 1994; Bates & Goodman, 1997) are very relevant with regard to the continuity of development mechanisms. These include the proportional increase in the number of function words described for children with vocabularies over 400 words, but also a tight non-linear correlation between vocabulary size and sentence complexity. Other studies support these findings from the CDI – for example, Bates *et al.* (1988) reported that the best predictor of mean length of utterance was the size of vocabulary observed 10 months earlier. Marchman & Bates (1994) found that the size of verb vocabulary strongly predicted the number of verb overregularization errors. These 'mistakes' are typically viewed as a major milestone in the development of grammatical rule-based knowledge.

Bates and Goodman propose that the non-linear relation between vocabulary size and grammar may be a universal property of language development. Nevertheless, some possible universal stages in the composition of early vocabulary have been proposed, which are hypothesized to reflect universal cognitive and social constraints that override language-specific variations in content. Perhaps the best known proposal of this kind comes from Gentner (1982), who argued that verbs must develop later than nouns in all human languages, because nouns are easy to grasp while verbs reflect relational meanings that are harder to perceive and (more importantly) are defined by a network of meanings that are subject to language-specific and situation-specific variations.

Two studies (Caselli *et al.*, 1995; Caselli *et al.*, 1999) sought to provide a cross-linguistic test of the transition from nouns to verbs (Gentner & Boroditsky, 2001). Both cross-linguistic studies used the MacArthur CDI to compare language development in large samples of Italian and American children from 8 to 30 months of age. The principal questions posed in these studies related to the passage from first words to grammar. First, are there cross-linguistic differences in the composition of vocabulary within and across this age range, with special reference to hypothesized differences in the onset and growth of nouns and verbs? Second, are there cross-linguistic differences in the pace and shape of grammatical development and its relation to vocabulary size?

With regard to the first question, Caselli *et al.* (2001) presented an expanded version of Gentner's noun-verb proposal in a four stage model of lexical development that includes hypotheses about lexical content before and after the noun-verb transition. It is as follows (Caselli *et al.*, 2001, pp. 77–78):

(1) *Routines and word games*: In the very first phase of lexical development, when expressive vocabularies range from 0 to 10 words, children tend to produce words that are difficult, if not impossible, to classify in adult part-of-speech categories ('noun' and 'verb'), including sound effects for animals ('woof-woof') and vehicles ('brumm'), and social routines ('bye') (Ninio, 1993; Tomasello, 1992).

(2) *Reference*: When expressive vocabulary grows to a range of about 50 to 200 words, the overwhelming majority of words are nominals (broadly defined). Even when we restrict the definition of nominals to common nouns (that is, names for classes of concrete objects), it is still evident that nouns predominate and grow sharply, both in absolute numbers and as a proportion of all word types. For most children this period of development revolves primarily around words that establish reference.

(3) *Predication*: Verbs and adjectives are very rare in the first two periods of lexical development, comprising 0 to 5 per cent of all words for most English-speaking children. These categories undergo a notable increase after the first 100 words, both in absolute numbers and as a proportion of all word types. It has been argued that this change in vocabulary composition

reflects the emergence of predication – that is, the ability to encode relational meanings. Such an ability is strictly related to the emergence of word combinations, appearing when children's vocabulary achieves between 100 and 200 words (Fenson *et al.*, 1994).

(4) *Grammar*: Grammatical function words are also extremely rare in the first stages of lexical development. These terms constitute fewer than 5 per cent of all words in the first and second year of life, and do not display proportional growth until children achieve a total expressive vocabulary of between 300 and 500 words (Bates *et al.*, 1994). This point coincides and correlates with various indices of grammatical productivity, including mean length of utterance in morphemes and alternative measures of inflectional productivity.

However, this proposed 'universal noun advantage' has recently been challenged in cross-linguistic studies of the Korean (Choi & Gopnik, 1995) and Chinese languages (Tardif, 1996), with numerous implications for the whole chain of events leading up to grammar. These analyses argue that the proposed universal transition from nouns to verbs may be an epiphenomenon of the fact that most studies of early lexical development have been based on English. The investigators suggest that differences among languages could reflect differences in linguistic structure (for example, word order variation, morphosyntactic complexity). In Korean verbs are often in a salient position or are the only content words in sentences spoken to young children. Italian has some analogous characteristics: in Italian verbs are often easier to perceive than nouns for children (because of their positions in the sentence and subject omission), but, unlike Korean and Chinese, Italian has an extremely rich system of verb morphology. Caselli & colleagues (2001) also suggest that differences between findings for Italian and for Chinese and Korean could reflect the methods used to assess language production (parental report *vs.* free speech). Parental report seems to highlight strong universal constraints on the development of *lexical knowledge*, but these universals coexist with language-specific profiles of *lexical use*, which emerge better from free speech samples. This claim was proposed by Bates and colleagues (1988) who compared the percentage of verbs over all word types in parent report *vs.* free speech and found remarkably low correlations between these two measures. These investigators proposed that the two measures were tapping into different abilities – to account for the differences between methodologies, they suggested that free speech tells us about what the child likes to do, while parent report tells us more about what the child knows. Based on these and other findings, Caselli *et al.* (2001) suggested a related hypothesis for cross-linguistic research: *cross-linguistic differences in lexical and grammatical development will be greater in studies using methods that are sensitive to the statistical probabilities and contextual preferences that characterize everyday language use.*

Let us now consider the second question posed above: Are there cross-linguistic differences in the pace and shape of grammatical development and in its relation to vocabulary size? The answer to this question depends on which aspect of the data we choose to focus on. In the study by Caselli *et al.* (1999), closed-class words in both English and Italian were reported to appear consistently when vocabularies were under 200 words. The subsequent growth in the function word category is tightly correlated with overall vocabulary size. However, the shape of the relation between closed-class development and vocabulary size is somewhat different in English and Italian. The data collected for American children are best characterized by a non-linear function, with little or no effect of vocabulary size under 400 words and a visible acceleration after that point, while the data on Italian children are more gradual and linear across this period of development so that there appears to be a slight closed-class advantage for Italian in the early stages. Switching from function word counts to a more comprehensive measure of grammatical complexity (for example, telegraphic *vs.* complete sentences; nuclear *vs.* expanded sentences), it is possible to see a striking similarity between English and Italian in the non-linear function that ties grammatical complexity to overall vocabulary size.

Despite the host of similarities in grammatical and lexical development revealed in their study, Caselli *et al.* (1999) suggest that it is well known that Italian children have to acquire a much richer array of morphological contrasts. A measure that is more sensitive to these differences would undoubtedly pick up measurable differences in grammatical development between English and Italian. By analysing the longest sentences of a small group of children as reported by parents on the CDI or PVB, it is evident that when children were matched for both age and vocabulary size, sharp differences were evident in the sheer amount of grammatical morphology that Italian children produced, reflecting the greater morphological load that they have to acquire.

We conclude by emphasizing that the cross-linguistic results discussed here are largely compatible with findings obtained using free speech methods in the past two decades of cross-linguistic research by other investigators. Some new perspectives on this issue are provided, but the overall picture remains the same.

In view of this claim it seems important to investigate the correlations among different language domains in atypical populations, and how these correlations change as a function of age and cognitive developmental stage. The literature on children with language disorders gives us reason to expect some peculiarities in the relation between vocabulary and morphosyntactic abilities.

Lexicon and grammar in children with Down syndrome

Some of the most interesting evidence comes from studies conducted on children with Down syndrome. Studies on populations with genetic syndromes such as Down syndrome allow us to explore interesting relations between defined cognitive characteristics and language development. As previously reported, numerous studies have shown that many children with Down syndrome have inferior linguistic ability in certain areas compared with what would be expected for their mental age. In a recent study, Vicari *et al.* (2000) investigated linguistic development in children with Down syndrome during the very first acquisition stages to identify asynchronies between linguistic and cognitive development, and among various aspects of language (lexical, morphological, and syntactic), and the possible dissociations among them.

Fifteen children with Down syndrome (aged from 4 to 7 years) and 15 normally developing children matched on mental age (average of 30 months) participated in the study. Linguistic measures included a parental questionnaire to assess vocabulary (PVB), a verbal comprehension test, a sentence repetition test, and mean length of utterance calculated on spontaneous production.

Results indicate that children with Down syndrome had much poorer overall linguistic performance than normally developing children. This points to a discrepancy between cognitive and linguistic abilities to the detriment of the latter. However, the differences between the two groups were significant only for grammar; in fact, results on the PVB showed a comparable level of lexical production in the two groups. This shows that, at least at the developmental stage considered, children with Down syndrome and normal children of equivalent mental age produce a comparable number of words. That is, children with Down syndrome show no specific dissociation between cognitive level and lexical development. In comparison with typically developing children of the same mental age and lexical repertoire, children with Down syndrome have specific problems in controlling morphological elements in all the tasks used (PVB, phrase repetition test, and mean length of utterance analysis): the Down syndrome children produced significantly shorter and more telegraphic utterances, and made far more mistakes in all the verbal morphological categories investigated.

According to Fowler (1990), these results confirm the emergence of an apparent dissociation between mental age and morphosyntactic abilities and, within the area of linguistic skills, a dissociation between morphosyntactic development and lexical ability at the expense of the former. But is this really a dissociation, or a selective disadvantage? In typically developing children, morphological and syntactic abilities are strongly correlated with vocabulary size. If grammar and the lexicon were truly dissociated in the Down syndrome population, then we should not expect to find a correlation of this kind. However, a robust correlation between grammatical and lexical performance was found within the Down syndrome sample. In other words, children with Down syndrome have a selective disadvantage in grammar, but grammar is not dissociated from other aspects of language. One possible explanation for the selective disadvantage in grammar noted in children with Down syndrome involves more general perceptual and motor skills – specific deficits in the morphological area are believed to reflect perceptual/articulatory problems (in the processing of acoustic information), leading to atypical results in the construction of suitable morpho-phonological models.

This hypothesis suggests that language problems and the relations among linguistic subdomains do not remain constant over time, but vary as a function of the subjects' developmental level, the characteristics of the language they are learning, and individual differences in the rate and nature of this learning process. For example, in children with Down syndrome, the dissociation between lexical and morphosyntactic abilities that is so evident in the early stages of development gradually decreases with age, leading to a pattern of residual deficits in both domains (Miller, 1992). Such findings invalidate the notion of static and specific deficits in language in favour of a dynamic approach to disorders and their progress over time – a dynamic profile that involves complex relations among cognitive, linguistic, and (perhaps) perceptual-motor domains (Karmiloff-Smith, 1997).

Concluding remarks

In this chapter we have reviewed several studies on early language acquisition (including some conducted within our own laboratory). We have focused on continuities across modalities (from gestures to the 'gesture *and* words' period), as well as between modality (from lexicon to grammar).

As regards the gesture-word relation, we can summarize the principal results as follows. Before one year of age, children begin to communicate intentionally, mainly through gestures, and these gestures are often accompanied by vocalizations. Vocalizations become progressively more sophisticated and similar to the words used in the adult language to which the children are exposed. Around 14 months there is a basic 'equipotentiality' between the gestural and vocal channels (Abrahamsen, 2000). Words and gestures appear to encode similar meanings, and go through a similar decontextualization process. In the following months, the repertoire of spoken words increases dramatically, but gestures are not simply replaced by speech. Rather, both the vocal and the gestural modalities are used together, and cross-modal combinations mark the transition to the two-word stage.

The main hypotheses underlying much current work on the interplay between gesture and speech is that there is a continuity between an earlier 'preverbal' and a subsequent, somehow functionally 'equivalent' linguistic form, and that the use of gesture is a robust developmental phenomenon, with similar features across different children and cultures. The output systems of speech and gesture may draw on underlying brain mechanisms common to both language and motor functions (Iverson & Thelen, 1999). Within this broad framework, evidence on children with atypical patterns of language and cognitive development may be particularly relevant for assessing the resilience of gesture as a developmental phenomenon.

In the studies conducted on children with Down syndrome, we found that the gesture-speech developmental patterns during the early stages of language learning are on the whole similar to those observed in typically developing children with similar language production abilities. Relevant differences are also observable: in children with Down syndrome a greater use of redundant unireferential combinations of gestures and words was noted. The studies on the gesture-word relation reviewed in this chapter strongly support the view that there is remarkable continuity between prelinguistic and linguistic development. Furthermore, the symbolic skills that are most evident in vocal linguistic production are inextricably linked to, and co-evolve with, more general cognitive and representational abilities, as is most apparent in the tight relation between gestures and words that continues through adulthood (McNeill, 1992; McNeill, 2000). This view appears to be particularly plausible in the light of the neurophysiological studies on 'mirror neurons' (Gallese *et al.*, 1996; Rizzolatti & Arbib, 1998). These have shown powerful links between motor and representational abilities in both monkey and human brains, with implications for a clearer understanding of the relation between structured action, gestures, and vocal language in humans.

The second topic addressed in this chapter aimed to highlight the interplay between universal and language-specific factors in lexical development in the second year of life, a crucial period in which children make the passage from first words to grammar. As we have shown, cross-linguistic studies and comparisons between different populations (typical *vs.* atypical) provide strong evidence for universal constraints on the development and composition of vocabulary, as well as a strong relation between lexicon and grammar, despite differences due to cultural factors (in typical development) or biological factors (in children with Down syndrome).

Recently a 'lexicalist' approach has been proposed which claims that grammar is an inherent part of the lexicon. The same mechanisms for learning and processing are supposed to underlie both aspects (Bates & Goodman, 2001). The data that we have reviewed so far may be relevant only to the early stage of language development. It is possible that a modular distinction between grammar and lexicon will emerge later in development, in accordance with the 'modularization' processes described by Bates *et al.* (1988) and Karmiloff-Smith (1992). However, many recent studies have demonstrated a strong relation between lexicon and grammar not only in infancy but also in later stages of development and in adults with typical or atypical linguistic profiles.

In conclusion, we would like to emphasize the enormous contribution that Elizabeth Bates's studies have made in improving our understanding of the complex relation between language and cognition. Many years ago she convinced us that 'the emergence of symbols in human children may reflect the resulting interaction of old parts in the creation of a new system' (Bates *et al.*, 1979). This theory is still modern and has recently been re-proposed in many scientific contexts. We agree with her point of view that "language emerges from a nexus of skills in attention, perception, imitation, and symbolic processing that transcends the boundaries of 'language proper'" (Bates & Dick, 2002).

Acknowledgments: We wish to thank Aaron Shield and Cristina Massaccesi for their helpful comments on the manuscript. This work, as part of the European Science Foundation EUROCORES Programme OMLL, was supported by funds from the Italian National Research Council and the EC Sixth Framework Programme under Contract No. ERAS-CT-2003-980409

References

Abrahamsen, A. (2000): Explorations of enhanced gestural input to children in the bimodal period. In: *The signs of language revisited: an anthology to honor Ursula Bellugi and Edward Klima*, eds. K. Emmorey & H. Lane, pp. 357–399. Mahwak: Erlbaum.

Bates, E. & Goodman, J.C. (1997): On the inseparability of grammar and the lexicon: evidence from acquisition, aphasia and real-time processing. *Lang. Cognitive Proc.* **12**, 507–584.

Bates, E. & Goodman, J.C. (2001): On the inseparability of grammar and the lexicon: evidence from acquisition. In: *Language development*, eds. M. Tomasello & E. Bates, pp. 124–161. Oxford: Blackwell.

Bates, E. & Dick, F. (2002): Language, gesture, and the developing brain. *Dev. Psychobiol.* **40**, 293–310.

Bates, E., Benigni, L., Bretherton, I., Camaioni, L. & Volterra, V. (1979): *The emergence of symbols: cognition and communication in infancy*. New York: Academic Press.

Bates, E., Bretherton, I. & Snyder, L. (1988): *From first words to grammar: individual differences and dissociable mechanisms*. New York: Cambridge University Press.

Bates, E., Marchman, V., Thal, D., Fenson, L., Dale, P., Reznick, S., Reilly, J. & Hartung, J. (1994): Developmental and stylistic variation in the composition of early vocabulary. *J. Child. Lang.* **21**, 85–124.

Butcher, C. & Goldin-Meadow, S. (2000): Gesture and the transition from one- to two-word speech: when hand and mouth come together. In: *Language and gesture*, ed. D. McNeill, pp. 235–257. Cambridge: Cambridge University Press.

Capirci, O., Iverson, J.M., Pizzuto, E. & Volterra, V. (1996): Gestures and words during the transition to two-word speech. *J. Child. Lang.* **23**, 645–673.

Casadio, P. & Caselli, M.C. (1989): Il primo vocabolario del bambino. Gesti e parole a 14 mesi. *Età Evolutiva* **33**, 32–42.

Caselli, M.C. & Casadio, P. (1995): *Il primo vocabolario del bambino. Guida all'uso del questionario MacArthur per la valutazione della comunicazione e del linguaggio nei primi anni di vita*. Milano: FrancoAngeli.

Caselli, M.C. & Volterra, V. (1999): Acquisire il linguaggio: competenze di base e differenze individuali. In: *Manuale di psicologia dell'educazione*, ed. C. Pontecorvo, pp. 91–114. Bologna: Il Mulino.

Caselli, M.C., Bates, E., Casadio, P., Fenson, J., Fenson, L., Sanderl, L. & Weir, J. (1995): A cross-linguistic study of early lexical development. *Cogn. Dev.* **10**, 159–201.

Caselli, M.C., Vicari, S., Longobardi, E., Lami, L., Pizzoli, C. & Stella, G. (1998): Gestures and words in early development of children with Down syndrome. *J. Speech. Lang. Hear. Res.* **41**, 1125–1135.

Caselli, M.C., Casadio, P. & Bates, E. (1999): A comparison of the transition from first words to grammar in English and Italian. *J. Child. Lang.* **26**, 69–111.

Caselli, M.C., Casadio, P. & Bates, E. (2001): Lexical development in English and Italian. In: *Language development: essential readings*, eds. M. Tomasello & E. Bates, pp. 76–110. Oxford: Blackwell.

Choi, S. & Gopnik, A. (1995): Early acquisition of verbs in Korean: a cross-linguistic study. *J. Child. Lang.* **22**, 497–529.

Chomsky, N. (1975): *Reflections on language* New York: Pantheon Books.

Deacon, T. (1997): *The symbolic species. The co-evolution of language and the human brain*. New York: Norton & Co.

Elman, J.L., Bates, E., Johnson, M.H., Karmiloff-Smith, A., Parisi, D. & Plunkett, K. (1996): *Rethinking innateness*. Cambridge, MA: MIT press.

Eriksson, M. & Berglund, E. (1999): Swedish early communicative development. *First Lang.* **19**, 55–90.

Fenson, L., Dale, P., Reznick, J., Bates, E., Thal, D. & Pethick, S. (1994): Variability in early communicative development. *Monogr. Soc. Res. Child.* **59**, Serial No. 242.

Fowler, A. (1990): Language abilities in children with Down syndrome: evidence for a syntactic delay. In: *Children with Down syndrome*, eds. D. Cicchetti & M. Beeghly, pp. 302–328. Cambridge: Cambridge University Press.

Gallese, V., Fadiga, L, Fogassi L. & Rizzolatti, G. (1996): Action recognition in the premotor cortex. *Brain* **119**, 593–609.

Gentner, D. (1982): Why are nouns learned before verbs: linguistic relativity versus natural partitioning. In: *Language development, Vol. 2. Language, thought and culture*, ed. S. Kuczaj, pp. 301–334. Hillsdale, NJ: Lawrence Erlbaum.

Gentner, D. & Boroditsky, L. (2001): Individuation, relativity and early word learning. In: *Language acquisition and conceptual development*, eds. M. Bowerman & S. Levinson, pp. 215–256. Cambridge: Cambridge University Press.

Iverson, J.M. & Thelen, E. (1999): Hand, mouth, and brain: the dynamic emergence of speech and gesture. *J. Consciousness Stud.* **6**, 19–40.

Iverson, J.M., Capirci, O. & Caselli, M.C. (1994): From communication to language in two modalities. *Cogn. Dev.* **9**, 23–43.

Iverson, J., Longobardi, E. & Caselli, M.C. (2003): The relationship between gestures and words in children with Down syndrome and typically developing children in the early stages of communicative development. *Int. J. Lang. Comm. Dis.* **38**, 179–197.

Karmiloff-Smith, A. (1992): *Beyond modularity: a developmental perspective on cognitive science*. Cambridge, MA: MIT Press.

Karmiloff-Smith, A. (1997): Crucial differences between developmental cognitive neuroscience and adult neuropsychology. *Dev. Neuropsychol.* **13**, 513–524.

Marchman, V. & Bates, E. (1994): Continuity in lexical and morphological development: a test of the critical mass hypothesis. *J. Child. Lang.* **21**, 339–366.

Marchman, V. & Thal, D. (2005): Word and grammar. In: *Beyond nature-nurture: essays in honor of Elizabeth Bates*, eds. M. Tomasello & D.I. Slobin, pp. 139-164. Mahwah, New Jersey: Erlbaum Lawrence.

McNeill, D. (1992): *Hand and mind – what gestures reveal about thought*. Chicago: University of Chicago Press.

McNeill, D. (2000): *Language and gesture*. Cambridge: Cambridge University Press.

Miller, J. (1992): Lexical acquisition in children with Down syndrome. In: *Child talk: advances in language acquisition*, ed. R.S. Chapman, pp. 202–216. St. Louis: Mosby Year Book Inc.

Morford, M. & Goldin-Meadow, S. (1992): Comprehension and production of gesture in combination with speech in one-word speakers. *J. Child. Lang.* **19**, 559–580.

Ninio, A. (1993): On the fringes of the system: children's acquisition of syntactically isolated forms at the onset of speech. *First Language* **13**, 291–313.

Pinker S. (1999): *Words and rules: the ingredients of language*. New York: Basic Book Co.

Rizzolatti, G. & Arbib, M.A. (1998): Language within our grasp. *Trends Neurol. Sci.* **21**, 188–194.

Tardif, T. (1996): Nouns are not always learned before verbs: evidence from Mandarin speakers' early vocabularies. *Dev. Psychol.* **32**, 492–504.

Tomasello, M. (1992): *First verbs: a case study in early grammatical development*. Cambridge: Cambridge University Press.

Tomasello, M. (1999): *The cultural origins of human cognition*. Cambridge, MA: Harvard University Press.

Vicari, S., Caselli, M.C. & Tonucci, F. (2000): Asynchrony of lexical and morphosyntactic development in children with Down Syndrome. *Neuropsychologia* **38**, 634–644.

Volterra, V. (1981): Gestures signs and words at two years: when does communication become language? *Sign Lang. Stud.* **33**, 351–362.

Volterra, V. & Berglund, E. (2004): *Gestures and words in early language development: cultural and linguistic variations*. First OMLL conference, Max Planck Institute for Evolutionary Anthropology, Leipzig, April 3–6, 2004.

Volterra, V., Caselli, M.C., Longobardi, E. & Camaioni, L. (1993): Sviluppo gestuale e vocale nei primi due anni di vita. *Psicologia Italiana* **IV**, 62–67.

Chapter 3

The development of grammar

Antonella Devescovi and Daniela Marchione

*Department of Psychology of Developmental and Socialization Processes,
University 'La Sapienza', via dei Marsi 78, 00185 Rome, Italy*
antonella.devescovi@uniroma1.it
daniela.marchione@uniroma1.it

Summary

Children begin to speak around the end of their first year of life, and between 3 to 4 years of age most of them master the basic grammatical structures of language, using them correctly and productively in novel contexts. Given the speed of this achievement a broad theoretical debate has raged for centuries about the nature of the language development processes in human children. In this chapter, we discuss the theoretical positions on the origin of grammar and define the analysis unit that we use in describing language development processes. We also discuss grammar development at various stages of life, with special reference to the Italian language development research data, and reflect on the methodological aspects of assessing children's language.

Introduction

When children begin to speak, they generally produce one-word utterances. Around the end of their second year of life, most children start producing utterances containing more than one word. The emergence of two-word combinations is preceded by a long preparation stage during which the child produces utterances where different elements are combined: words, gestures, sound sequences that are not true words yet, and types of word combinations that will disappear over time. With time, children's utterances become longer and more complex; it is at this stage that the gradual 'grammatization' of their verbal expressions can be observed. This means the appearance of those aspects of human verbal language that set it apart from other communication systems: *morphology*, the set of rules to modify word form and meaning, and *syntax*, the set of principles governing the way words and other morphemes are ordered to make up a possible sentence in a given language. These features of language have led to a heated theoretical debate on the origin of grammar – whether it is innate or results from the organism/environment interaction – and on the mechanisms responsible for its development – whether they are domain-specific or domain-general (Karmiloff-Smith, 1995). Chomsky is currently considered the most distinguished representative of the first theoretical position, which dates back to Plato and Kant – that is, 'nativism', according to which knowledge stems from human nature. Chomsky clearly supported this view from the time of his first book in 1957 and continues to support it now. Chomsky's version of innatism is based on two logically and empirically distinct claims: the first is that human language does not look like any other type of behaviour – it cannot be derived from experience, and our brains contain a dedicated, specialized device that has developed exclusively for language; the second is incorporated in the doctrine that has been called 'domain specificity', 'autonomy', or 'modularity'.

The human language capacity is attributed to Universal Grammar which describes the structural aspects shared by all natural languages (Chomsky, 1969). Such a description includes the elements (for example, noun and verb, phrases) and the operations (for example, rules to move the phrases in the sentence) that are shared by all languages. According to Chomsky, symbols and language operations cannot even be derived from a more general cognitive capacity, because they are completely different from what pertains to other cognitive domains. It is in this light that Chomsky adopted and further developed Fodor's 'modularity theory'. Chomsky believes that the mind is made up of a set of distinct computational mechanisms, specifically devoted to the various cognitive domains. Each domain, in turn, works in a modular manner so that the various language components – phonetics and phonology, lexicon, grammar, and pragmatics – are encapsulated; that is, they make up a closed system and operate autonomously.

The second position, currently called 'interactionism', 'constructivism', 'emergentism' or 'epigenetic approach', has been associated with the psychologist Jean Piaget. More recently, this concept has emerged in a new approach to learning, called 'connectionism', 'distributed parallel processing', or 'neural networks' (Rumelhart & McCelland, 1986). According to the epigenetic approach, the result of a problem-solving process is obtained from any processing system input, for reasons that are not necessarily obvious or predictable. For example, beehives are hexagonal in shape because this represents the ultimate solution to the problem of pressing circles together (Bates & MacWhinney, 1982). Jean Piaget said that logic and knowledge emerge exactly in the same way, from subsequent interactions between sensory-motor activity and a structured world.

A similar argument was presented to explain the birth of grammars that represent the possible solutions to the problem of mapping a rich set of meanings onto a speech channel heavily constrained by the limits of memory, perception, and motor planning. Grammar abstract principles are not given in the word but neither are they given in the genes. They were discovered by humans because they represented the best possible solution to specific problems that other species do not care about and which, in any case, they could not solve even if they did. Proponents of the epigenetic approach recognize that in the human brain there is something innate that makes language emergence possible. Language can be something that we can realize thanks to a big and sophisticated brain that has developed to handle the numerous and complex objectives of human society and culture (Tomasello, 1998). In other words, following Elizabeth Bates, language is a new machine built out of old parts and reconstructed from those parts by every human child (Bates, 2003). In this scenario, the acquisition of individual words and grammar configurations is guided by the same learning principles and representational mechanisms (MacWhinney, 1987).

Unit of analysis: utterance *vs.* sentence

Traditionally, the unit of analysis used to describe the grammatical aspects of language is an abstract theoretical category called the *sentence*. The problem is to identify the minimum conditions that allow a linguistic sign to function as a sentence. The notions we more often refer to for its definition are *presence of predicate, autonomy*, and *intonation* (Bloomfield, 1933). According to the nativist theory, the sentence is considered an autonomous unit, the completeness of which is determined by the presence of formal units (certain grammar categories such as noun and verb) connected to certain syntactic functions (such as subject and verb). In other words, the production context is not considered relevant for recognition of the sentence, and no reference is made to the semantic or communicative aspects of the utterance. Sentences are either well formed or ill formed in relation to mere grammatical principles.

Instead, the reality that emerges when we observe spoken language in daily life is very complex and cannot be fully explained by traditional grammar categories (Renzi, 1991; Serianni, 1997). Indeed, while in a written communication the text is preplanned and information is governed by an explicit and articulated syntactic structure (Chafe & Tannen, 1987), the production of spoken texts proceeds in a 'jolting' manner through the production of short information units (Benveniste, 1996; Cresti, 1987). Spoken language thus prefers semantic consistency, with a quantitative reduction in phraseal structures that require explicit syntactical markers (Halliday, 1987). Syntax in the spoken language is also affected by the pragmatic aspects of discourse, such as conversational turn organization, the number of speakers, and their proximity. In particular, the proximity of the speakers affects the number of interruptions and the number of topics and planning changes (Goodwin, 1981; Bazzanella, 1994; Baumgartner & Devescovi, 2001; Veneziano, 2001). These phenomena are reflected in the distribution of the various proposition types – that is, in the ratio between propositions containing verbs and nominal propositions – and in the matching of syntactic units and intonational units. Indeed, as the turn-taking frequency increases, the noun-proposition frequency increases as well, and the syntactic-intonational unit matching decreases (Voghera, 1992).

Another feature implied in the definition of utterance is intonation (Ferguson *et al.*, 1993; Cresti *et al.*, 1998). In the Italian language, it is possible to identify significant changes in the fundamental frequency or tone associated with certain syntactic constructs and, in particular, with some significant functional units. The hypothesis is that each significant unit, expressed by a different modulation of the tone of voice, represents a significant segment of discourse and the way a speaker organizes it on-line (Halliday, 1992). On the basis of intonation (fundamental frequency) and semantics (information units), the utterance was defined as equivalent to a speech act (Austin, 1962) that is implemented in two ways: first, a linear complex utterance; second, a patterned complex utterance. In the first, words are linked together by a predicate holistically expressing the utterance's pragmatic power (illocutive act). However, one word pronounced with pragmatic emphasis can also represent an illocutive act and consequently an utterance (Cresti & Firenzuoli, 1999; Cresti & Firenzuoli, 2002). Intonation, in this case, expresses a modality that can be declarative, interrogative, jussive, and so on, and the instrumental analysis of the wave shows a continuous ascending-descending line (Cresti, 1993, 2000; Moneglia & Cresti, 1997). The second way of implementation requires that words have a different relevance on the basis of the pragmatic information we intend to convey. Speakers manage tone modulation so as to obtain as many tone units as the pieces of information conveyed by the message. This means that an information unit, called *comment*, is present that implements illocution, as well as a second information unit, called *topic*, that is the referent for the illocution expressed by the comment. Also in this case, intonation expresses a modality that can be declarative, interrogative, jussive, and so on. However, the sound wave shown by the instrumental analysis appears fragmented, indicating that within the same intonation profile two different tone units are prodused (Moneglia, 1994). A patterned complex utterance is made up by at least two words, each carrying one tone unit. This approach therefore takes the utterance into the sphere pertaining to syntax, taking into account verbal elements, formal properties, and their communication value (Givon, 1983; Serianni, 1997; Searle, 1975; Simone, 1995).

From this point of view, intonation can be considered as one of the parameters used to decide word grouping objectively, irrespective of and before the existence of syntactic relations.

As a result of this renewed interest in spoken language intonation, over the past 30 years the study of the prosodic component has played an important role in research on language comprehension and production processes. The utterance prosodic contour can convey syntactical information, thus favouring adult speakers' formulation of grammaticality or non-grammaticality judgements about utterances (Bates et al., 1982; Bates et al., 1984; Tomlin, 1995). The prosodic component is also relevant in the language addressed to children. Numerous researches on different languages have shown that when adults speak to children they more often put the verb in a relevant position from the perception point of view (Camaioni & Longobardi, 2001) and generally use a language in which the prosodic component is extremely marked (Cruttenden, 1994; Chouinard & Clark, 2003). A child seems to perceive the characteristics related to the fundamental frequency form as crucial elements for the acquisition of the structural properties of language (Albin & Echols, 1996; Jacob & D'Odorico, 2002). Furthermore, discrimination of the relevant part of an utterance might play a role in the word comprehension processes in an early phase (Caselli & Devescovi, 1982) as well as in the sentence structure identification processes during the subsequent language development stage (Hirsh-Pasek et al., 1987).

From early words to complex utterance

The study of intonation has also turned out to be very useful in so far as the assessment analysis of early childhood verbal production is concerned. The functional differentiation expressed by linear and patterned complex utterances could indeed be related to the formation of syntax. So far research has demonstrated that the intonation profiles produced by children in the early language development stage are only partially comparable to those produced by adults (D'Odorico & Carrubbi, 2001; D'Odorico & Carrubbi, 2003; D'Odorico, 2005) and might represent transitional forms. This means that the utterance formation strategies could have a developmental nature. More specifically, patterned complex utterances, a partial form of which appears around 19 months of age, could represent an early linguistic functional distinction as well as the first grammar structure. However, a vocabulary of at least 100 words is necessary to produce protolinear complex utterances. The increase in the number of words mastered by the child would seem to be correlated with the children's achievement of the adult's melodic forms. Children who reach a 200-word vocabulary are indeed capable of producing patterned complex utterances and more sophisticated linear complex utterances (D'Odorico et al., 2004; Marchione et al., 2004). The 200-word threshold is also correlated with the appearance of the early grammar skills which generally begin to emerge between 18 and 24 months of age (Caselli et al., 1999). At this stage, the language repertoire mainly comprises nouns and undifferentiated phonetic elements or prototypical forms that can be expressed individually, making up one-word utterances, or in combination, making up longer utterances (Braine, 1976; Caselli & Casadio, 1995; Caselli et al., 1995; D'Odorico et al., 2001; Slobin, 1985). Syntactic, grammar, and prosodic characteristics of productions differ from more advanced language productions (Barret, 1982; Clark, 1995; D'Odorico & Carrubi, 1997; Blake, 2000). Their existence and importance in the subsequent language development was reported by Bloom (1970), who observed the elements present in utterances produced by children in a short time succession and identified two different combination modes. In some cases each expression has a precise referent and is separated by a short pause. In other cases utterances may contain a significant expression, with a clear referent, preceded or followed by a non-significant element. In other transitional forms, the child repeats the same word, referred to the same context element in the same conversation turn (horizontal repetition), or he can produce the word in subsequent turns, giving rise to vertical utterance sequences (Scollon, 1976). The analyses carried out so far indicate that the child gets ready in this way for the production of complex utterances where two or more words are present (Veneziano et al., 1990; Cresti & Moneglia, 1996; Marchione & Devescovi, 2005). Furthermore, during the second year of life, language production is often rich in stereotyped expressions called 'frozen phrases', 'formulas' or 'amalgams' (Hickey, 1993; D'Odorico & Carrubi, 1997; Dore et al., 1976), which are apparently more linguistically advanced compared with the current skills and which are used by the child as if they were individual words. In this phase we frequently find combinations of words and sound elements that are not true words yet. They precede lexical elements of various types and are made up of vowel segments – for example, /a/, /e/, /i/, and sometimes of single or multisyllable segments /en/, /pa/, /ella/, to which it is impossible to assign a referential meaning. However, in other cases, although their position makes their functional interpretation possible, there is no phonetic similarity with adult morphemes (Bottari et al., 1993). During the third year of life, all transitional forms will be replaced by true word combinations thanks to the gradual increase in the number of words present in the child's lexical repertoire. From a structural point of view, utterances do not generally have a verb or free morphemes (articles, pronouns, prepositions), and can express a range of semantic relations that may be identified in different languages in the early phases of language acquisition. Table 1 shows some English and Italian examples of children's utterances.

Some investigators call this stage 'presyntactic' to distinguish it from the ensuing stage where a verb predicate systematically appears (Parisi & Antinucci, 1973; Taeschner & Volterra, 1986; Cipriani et al., 1993). These are simple sentences, made up of a predicate with at least one nominal element, subject, or complement and initially incomplete, where some complements and most free morphology – that is articles, pronouns and prepositions – may be missing (Taeschner & Volterra, 1986; Cipriani et al., 1993) (for example, Pette cache, 'I put the keys'; Francesco, 24 months). Later, adjectives and adverbs and some free morphemes, namely articles, appear (for example, Ecco si mette qua la minestrina al fuoco, 'Here you are, you put here the soup on the fire'; Diana, 25 months).

On the whole, published reports suggest that children's language production could be better analysed if the number of utterances rather than of sentences is assessed (Bloom, 1970, 1973; Beninca et al., 1991; Clark, 2003; Tomasello, 1998; Devescovi & Bates, 2000; Tomasello,

Table 1. Semantic relations underlying first word combinations in English and Italian (adapted from Braine, 1976)

Relation	English examples	Italian examples
Attention to x	See doggie	Gadda bau
Properties of x	Big doggie	Grande bau
Ownership	My truck	Mia Brum-brum
Plurality	Two shoes	Due pappe
Recurrence	Other cookie	Attto bototto
Disappearance	Daddy bye bye	Papà via
Denial	No bath	Bagno no
Actor-action	Mommy do it	Mamma fa
Location	Baby home	Bimbo casa
Request	Have dat	Dà chetto

2003). Furthermore, the literature stresses the role played by the prosodic component in the study of early language acquisition stages and in investigating the creation of complex utterances, because it groups words together regardless of the existence of traditionally defined syntactic relations, and includes – among analysable expressions – all those additional expressions that are not generally considered sentences and which instead represent the greater part of young children's language.

From a methodological point of view, it is crucial for those who analyse and assess children's language to use measures that allow one to verify the level of development achieved by a specific child. It is well known that the rate at which children extend their utterances quantitatively, learning at the same time the lexical and morphological elements that allow them to produce an increasingly complex and articulated language, may vary remarkably, and it is very difficult to foresee or assess the degree of grammar development in a child on the sole basis of their chronological age. From a purely quantitative point of view, a relatively reliable grammar development index is the increase in the mean length of utterance (MLU) (Brown, 1973; Crystal, 1985). This measure is based on the assumption that the production of an increasing number of elements in an utterance reflects a greater grammar and syntactic complexity. This claim has numerous theoretical and application-related components. One important aspect is the choice of the type of element on which the MLU calculation should be based: morphemes or words. The modality originally introduced by Brown based such calculations on morphemes: the English expression 'the dogs' contains two words but three distinct morphemes: the definite article, the noun dog, and the morpheme '-s' indicating plurality. The Italian corresponding expression 'I cani' is always made up of two words, but the number of morphemes is greater: the article '-i', indicates not only the plural, but also conveys information that is not present in the English noun morphemes – that is, gender information, masculine in this case; the noun root 'can-' and the morpheme '-i' in this case convey two meanings: the masculine gender and the plural noun (five morphemes in all).

It is clear that whenever we use a morphological criterion, the cross-language comparison between an English child and an Italian child in relation to the production of a simple two-word combination (noun + article) implies a disparity between the two children, ascribable to the nature of the two languages rather than to a different competence level. In a recent cross-linguistic study comparing English and Italian children, the MLU was calculated using different computing units: content words alone (nouns, verbs, adjectives), content words plus function words (articles, prepositions, pronouns, copula, auxiliary verbs), and morphemes (roots, bound morphemes, function words). The aim was to identify a modality that made the English measure more comparable to the Italian one, to see whether variations in MLU can be explained by the language (English *vs.* Italian), by the age of the child, or by the quantity of words known by the child (Caselli *et al.*, 2005). The results showed that the most conservative measure to verify interindividual MLU variability is 'total words' (content words plus function words), which is a measure that is already fairly widely used in Italian (Bottari *et al.*, 1993; Cipriani *et al.*, 1993; Caselli *et al.*, 1995; Devescovi & Pizzuto, 1995). They also confirm the numerous studies that show how MLU variations are explained by the children's vocabulary level rather than by their age. Moreover, the study shows that language differences are evident in the early stages, until children know around 300 words, and then they disappear.

Qualitative development of utterances

Cipriani and collaborators (1993), in their analysis of spontaneous language in 12- to 36-month-old children, correlated the increase in mean length of utterance with the development of various utterance types and found significant results. The MLU, taken as independent variable, turned out to be correlated with complex sentences. An increase in the MLU was reflected in an ascending curve in all children in the sample, although the pattern was discontinuous.

It should be noted, however, that after 3 years of age, although the presence of increasingly complex utterances is documented (Bates *et al.*, 1992; Karmiloff-Smith, 1995; D'Amico & Devescovi, 2003; Tomasello & Slobin, 2005), the MLU does not show equivalent changes (MacWhinney, 1987; Bates & Devescovi, 1989; Marchione, 2000) (Fig. 1).

In other words, although this measure is particularly suited to the evaluation of language development during the first 3 years of life and to the identification of quantitative regularities, it appears unsuited to such assessments at subsequent ages, because it does not take into account that two utterances of the same length may contain language structures of different syntactical complexity.

Some investigators, following Halliday (1992), suggested using the presence of the verb in the utterance as an indicator of syntactical complexity; the verb in fact represents the core of the aggregation of lexical elements and function words in a broader grammar unit, the *clause* (Berman & Slobin, 1994). Halliday introduced the 'lexical density' concept, referring to the complexity that is found when words are put together. From his point of view, what determines complexity in a spoken passage is the percentage of combinations of lexical and grammar items in larger language forms. Thus a spoken text would be made up of structurally connected sets or proposition sequences, 'clauses'.

Baumgartner & Devescovi (2001) believe that, within a spoken text, an utterance can contain one or more propositions bound together by coordination, juxtaposition, or subordination relations. The suggested complexity measure is represented by the clause/utterance ratio as an indicator of the average number of information units a speaker is able to contain in an utterance.

A recent study by Marchione *et al.* (2003) compared different syntactic complexity measures in a sample of 50 children aged 2 to 4 years, including the MLU and the number of verb-containing clauses, in order to assess which measure was most suited to describing the linguistic skills of children in this age group. The results confirmed that between 3 and 4 years of age MLU does not undergo any significant change, while the number of clauses increases between 2 and 4 years of age (Table 2). This measure seems particularly useful for assessing qualitative changes in the utterances produced by children after 3 years of age. Moreover, the investigators found a considerable number of propositions containing a verb linked by implicit or explicit syntactic relations but produced in different utterances.

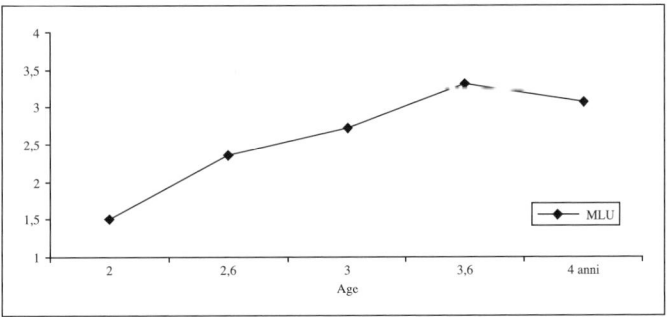

Fig. 1. Mean length of utterance in 2- to 4-year-old children (Marchione et al., 2003).

Table 2. Examples of language structures observed in Italian children's spontaneous speech (adapted from Marchione *et al.*, 2003)

Observed language structures	Examples
Two subsequent utterances joined by the verb that is found either in the first or in the second utterance	1) Adult: guarda! (Look!) Child: la bimba fa. (the little girl does). Child: il bagno. (the bath). 2) Adult: e qui? (and here?) Child: qui c'è. (here is). Child: la mamma. (mummy).
Two subsequent utterances both containing a verb, joined by a grammatical connective connector in the second utterance	1) Adult: che succede? (what happens?) Child: c'è la bimba. (there is the little girl). Child: che dorme.(who sleeps). 2) Adult: mi racconti? (can you tell me?) Child: qua piange. (here she cries). Child: perché ha la bua. (because she hurt herself).

This phenomenon appears to be similar to that identified in the transition from one-word to two-word utterances: in some cases semantically linked words are produced in subsequent different utterances (vertical construction) and are later combined into a single utterance.

Towards the end of preschool age, syntactic units such as semantically or syntactically connected clauses are produced in subsequent utterances. These structures do not contribute to extending the MLU because they are found in subsequent utterances; however, they favour the development of discourse syntax and, although they are numerous throughout all the childhood sample, they significantly differentiate the 4-year-old group (Fig. 2).

Complex utterances containing several clauses connected by syntactic coordination and subordination relations appear in children's language from the end of the second year of life. D'Amico *et al.* (2002) compared the use of simple utterances and complex utterances (coordinates and subordinates) and revealed that the productivity of these language structures increased significantly after 5 years of age (Fig. 3). These data show that access to and frequency of use of this type of utterance become significant only when children reach school age.

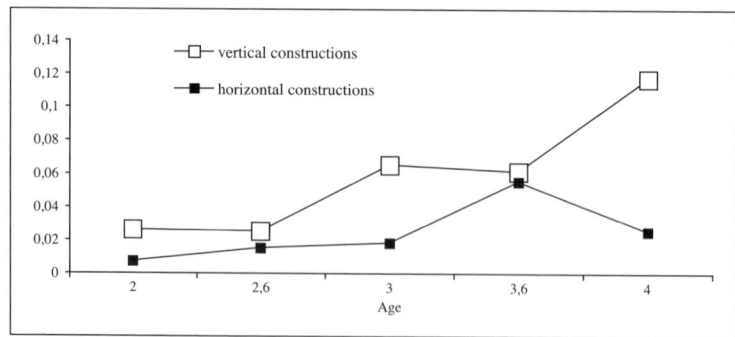

Fig. 2. Syntactic links within the same utterance (horizontal constructions) compared with syntactic links between different utterances (vertical constructions) observed in 2- to 4-year-old children (Marchione et al., 2003).

Conclusions

Anyone who is involved in the study of language, without necessarily sharing the assumptions or the theoretical models developed by Chomsky in his long and productive career, has to

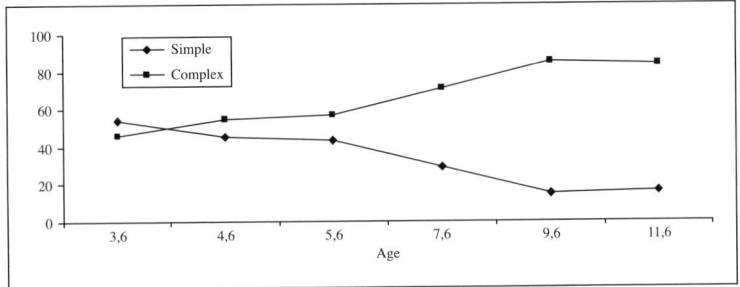

Fig. 3. Simple and complex sentences in children's story telling (D'Amico et al., 2002).

recognize the fundamental influence of his work on subsequent theoretical and empirical research on the development of grammar. Many of the studies that were later carried out resulted from comparisons with his model and with his powerful and provocative claims. However, the research we have presented in this chapter shows that the development of syntactic aspects is better explained by a non-modular language model where the definition of different syntactic complexity levels also contributes to lexical, grammar, and pragmatic aspects.

Our overview allows us to identify the criteria that characterize different language complexity levels which can be assessed by these various measures:

• At 2–3 years: increasingly systematic and productive use of various grammar morphemes; a significant increase in the use of the verb reflected in an increase in the MLU.
• At 3–4 years: the presence of complex syntactic structures marks the beginning of syntactic planning that takes into account the discourse dimension.
• After 5 years, grammar is structured at the service of discourse and improves access to complex grammar structures, as shown by a significant increase in the use of coordinate and subordinate clauses.

References

Albin, D.D. & Echols, C.H. (1996): Stressed and word final-syllables in infant directed speech. *Infant Behav. Dev.* **19**, 401–418.

Austin, L.J. (1962): *How to do things with words*, p. 166. Oxford: Oxford University Press.

Barret, M. (1982): The holophrastic hypothesis: conceptual and empirical issues. *Cognition* **11**, 47–76.

Bates, E. (2003). Natura e cultura nel linguaggio [On the nature and nurture of language]. In: *Frontiere della biologia. Il cervello di Homo sapiens* [Frontiers of biology. The brain of homo sapiens], eds. E. Bizzi, P. Calissano & V. Volterra, pp. 241–265. Rome: Istituto della Enciclopedia Italiana fondata da Giovanni Treccani.

Bates, E. & MacWhinney, B. (1982): Functionalist approach to grammar. In: *Language acquisition: state of the art*, eds. E. Wanner & L. Gleitman, pp. 89–121. New York: Cambridge University Press.

Bates, E. & Devescovi, A. (1989): Crosslinguistic studies of sentence production. In: *The crosslinguistic study of sentence processing*, eds. B. MacWhinney & B. Bates, pp. 225–253. New York: Cambridge University Press.

Bates, E., McNew, S., MacWhinney, B., Devescovi, A. & Smith, S. (1982): Functional constraints on sentence processing: a cross-linguistic study. *Cognition* **11**, 245–299.

Bates, E., MacWhinney, B., Caselli, C., Devescovi, A., Natale, F. & Venza, V. (1984): A cross-linguistic study of the development of sentence interpretation strategies. *Child Dev.* **55**, 341–354.

Bates, E., Bretherton, I. & Snider, L.S. (1992). *From first words to grammar*. Cambridge: Cambridge University Press.

Baumgartner, E. & Devescovi, A (2001): *I bambini raccontano. Lettura, interazione sociale e competenza narrativa.* Trento: Erickson.

Bazzanella, C. (1994): *Le facce del parlare.* Firenze: La Nuova Italia.

Beninca, P., Salvi, G. & Frison, L., (1991): L'ordine dei costituenti della frase e le costruzioni marcate. In: *Grande grammatica italina di consultazione*, vol. 1, *La frase. I sintagmi nominale e preposizionale*, a cura di L. Renzi, pp. 115–225. Bologna: Il Mulino.

Benveniste, E. (1996): *Problemi di linguistica generale*. Milan: Il Saggiatore.

Berman, R. & Slobin, D. (1994): *Relating events in narrative: a crosslinguistic developmental study*. Hillsdale, NJ: Lawrence Erlbaum.

Blake, J. (2000): *Routes to child language. Evolutionary and developmental precursors*. New York: Cambridge University Press.

Bloom, L. (1970): *Language development: form and function in emerging grammars*. Cambridge, MA: MIT Press.

Bloom, L. (1973): *One word at a time. The use of single word utterances before syntax*. Mouton: The Hague.

Bloomfield, L. (1933): *Language*. London: Allen & Unwin.

Bottari, P., Cipriani, P., Pfanner, L., Chilosi, A. (1993): Inferenze strutturali nell'acquisizione della morfologia libera italiana. In: *Ricerche sull'acquisizione dell'italiano. Giornata di studio sull'acquisizione del linguaggio in bambini normali e patologici*, eds. M. Moneglia & E. Cresti, pp. 189–215. Rome: Bulzoni.

Braine, M.D.S. (1976): Children's first word combinations. *Monographs of the Society for Research in Child Development*, **41**, 164.

Brown, R. (1973): *A first language: the early stages*. Cambridge, MA: Harvard University Press.

Camaioni, L. & Longobardi, E. (2001): Noun versus verb emphasis in Italian mother to child speech. *J. Child Lang.* **28**, 773–785.

Caselli, C. & Devescovi, A. (1982): Sentence comprehension in Italian children from 2 to 5 years of age. *J. Ital. Linguistics* **2**, 1–17.

Caselli, M. C. & Casadio, P. (1995): *Il primo vocabolario del bambino. Guida all'uso del questionario MacArthur per la valutazione della comunicazione e del linguaggio nei primi anni di vita*. Milan: FrancoAngeli.

Caselli, M. C., Bates, E., Casadio, P., Fenson, L., Fenson, J., Sanderl, L. & Weir J. (1995): A cross-linguistic study of early lexical development. *Cogn. Dev.* **10**, 59–199.

Caselli, M. C., Casadio, P. & Bates, E. (1999): A comparison of the transition from first words to grammar in English and Italian. *J. Child Lang.* **26**, 69–111.

Caselli, C.M., Devescovi, A., Marchione, D., Reilly, J. & Bates, E. (2005): A cross-linguistic study of the relationship between grammar & lexical development. *J. Child Lang.* **32**, 759–786.

Chafe, W. & Tannen, D. (1987): The relation between written and spoken language. *Annu. Rev. Anthropol.* **16**, 383–407.

Chomsky, N. (1969): *Filosofia del linguaggio. Saggi linguistici*, vol. 3. Torino: Boringhieri.

Chouinard, M. M. & Clark, E. V. (2003): Adult reformulations of child errors as negative evidence. *J. Child Lang.* **30**, 637–669.

Cipriani, P., Chilosi, P., Bottari, P. & Pfanner, L. (1993): *L'acquisizione della morfosintassi in italiano*. Fasi e processi. Padova: Unipress.

Clark, E.V. (1995): Later lexical development and word formation. In: *The handbook of child language*, eds. P. Fletcher & B. MacWhinney, pp. 393–412. Oxford: Blackwell.

Clark, E.V. (2003): *First language acquisition*. Cambridge: Cambridge University Press.

Cresti, E. (1987): L'articolazione dell'informazione nell'italiano parlato. In: *Gli italiani parlati*, AA.VV., pp. 27–90. Firenze: Accademia delle Crusca.

Cresti, E. (1993): Dalla linearizzazione alla formazione del predicato. In: *Ricerche sull'acquisizione dell'italiano, Giornata di studio sull'acquisizine del linguaggio in bambini normali e patologici*, eds. M. Moneglia & E. Cresti, pp. 115–164. Rome: Bulzoni.

Cresti, E. (2000): *Corpus di italiano parlato*. Firenze: Accademia della Crusca.

Cresti, E. & Moneglia, M. (1996): Monological repetitions in very early acquisition. In: *Repetition in dialogue*, ed. C. Bazzanella, pp. 50–65. Tübingen: Max Niemeyer Verlag.

Cresti, E. & Firenzuoli, V. (1999): Illocution et profils intonatifs de l'italien. *Rev. Franc. Ling. Appl.* **IV**, 77–98.

Cresti, E. & Firenzuoli, V. (2002): L'articolazione informativa topic-comment e comment-appendice: correlati intonativi. In: *Atti delle XII giornate del GFS*, ed. A. Regnicoli, pp. 153–160. Rome: Il Calamo.

Cresti, E., Martin, P. & Moneglia, M. (1998): L'intonazione delle illocuzioni naturali rappresentative: analisi e validazione percettiva. In: *Atti delle IX giornate GFS*, ed. R. Del Monte, pp. 51–63. Padova: Unipress.

Cruttenden, A. (1994): Phonetic and prosodic aspects of Baby Talk. In: *Input and interaction in language acquisition*, eds. C. Gallaway & B.J. Richards, pp. 135–152. Cambridge: Cambridge University Press.

Crystal, D. (1985): *A dictionary of linguistics and phonetics*. Oxford: Oxford University Press.

D'Amico, S., Devescovi, A. & Tonucci, F. (2002): La capacità narrativa di bambini con sviluppo tipico e con sindrome di Williams. In: *I disturbi dello sviluppo. Neuropsicologia clinica e ipotesi riabilitative*, eds. S. Vicari & M.C. Caselli, pp. 70–103. Bologna: Il Mulino.

D'Amico, S. & Devescovi, A (2003): *Comunicazione e linguaggio nei bambini*. Rome: Carocci.

Devescovi, A. & Pizzuto, E. (1995): Lo sviluppo grammaticale. In: *Manuale di neuropsicologia dell'età evolutiva*, ed. G. Sabbadini, pp. 260–285. Bologna: Zanichelli.

Devescovi, A. & Bates, E., (2000): Psicolinguistica. In: *Psicologia. Introduzione per le scienze umane*, eds. N. Dazzi & G. Veltrone, pp. 239–276. Rome: Carocci.

D'Odorico, L. (2005): *Lo sviluppo del linguaggio*. Bari: Laterza.

D'Odorico, L. & Carrubbi, S. (1997): Dalle espressioni di una sola parola alle prime combinazioni di parole. *Età Evolutiva* 57, 26–39.

D'Odorico L. & Carrubbi, S. (2001): Early multi-word utterances in Italian-speaking children. In: *Research on child language acquisition*, eds. M. Almgrem, A. Barrena, M.J. Ezeizabarrena, I. Idiazabal & B. MacWhinney, pp. 1124–1142. Sommerville, MA: Cascadilla Press.

D'Odorico, L., Carrubbi, S. (2003): Prosodic characteristics of early-multiword utterances in Italian children. *First Lang.* 23, 97–116.

D'Odorico, L., Carrubbi, S., Salerni, N. & Calvo, V. (2001): Vocabulary development in Italian children: a longitudinal evaluation of quantitative and qualitative aspects. *J. Child Lang.* 28, 351–372.

D'Odorico, L., Fasolo, M. & Marchione, D. (2004): Caratteristiche prosodiche delle prime strutture sintattiche. Poster presented at the XVIII Congresso AIP Sviluppo Comunicativo e Linguistico. Sciacca, 20–23 September.

Dore, J., Franklin, M., Miller, R. & Ramer, A.L. (1976): Transitional phenomena in early language acquisition. *J. Child Lang.* 3, 13–29.

Ferguson, B.G., Gezundhajt, H. & Martin, P. (1993): *Accent, intonation et modelès phonologique*. Toronto: Editions Mélodie.

Givon, T. (1983): Topic continuity in discourse: an introduction. In: *Topic continuity in discourse: a quantitative cross-language study*, ed. T. Givòn, pp. 1–41. Amsterdam: Benjiamins.

Goodwin, C. (1981): *Conversational organization: interaction between speakers and hearers*. New York: Academic Press.

Halliday, M.A.K. (1987): *Sistema e funzione del linguaggio*. Bologna: Il Mulino.

Halliday, M.A.K. (1992): *Lingua parlata e lingua scritta*. Bologna: Il Mulino.

Hickey, T. (1993): Identifying formulas in first language acquisition. *J. Child Lang.* 20, 27–41.

Hirsh-Pasek, K., Kemler Nelson, D., Jusczyk, P. W., Cassidy, K.W., Druss, B. & Kennedy, L. (1987): Clauses are perceptual units for young infants. *Cognition* 26, 269–286.

Jacob, V. & D'Odorico, L. (2002): Prosody in maternal input addressed to early expressive language delayed children. The other side of infant perception. Poster presentation at Euresco Conference 'Brain development and cognition in human infants', Acquafredda di Maratea, 7–12 June.

Karmiloff-Smith, A. (1997): *Oltre la mente modulare. Una prospettiva evolutiva sulla scienza cognitiva*. Bologna: Il Mulino.

MacWhinney, B., editor (1987): *Mechanism of language acquisition*. Hillsdale, NJ: Lawrence Erlbaum.

Marchione, D., (2000): Sviluppo della complessità sintattica tra i 3 e i 4 anni. Poster presented at the XIV Congresso AIP, L'attività cognitiva nei primi anni di vita e i processi di sviluppo. Alghero, 26–28 September.

Marchione, D. & Devescovi A. (2005): Aspetti della ripetizione monologica in bambini di età prescolare. *Riv. Psicoloinguistica Appl.* 1–2, 9–18.

Marchione, D., Devescovi, A., D'Amico, S. & Bentrovato S. (2003): Strategie di costruzione dell'enunciato complesso: valutazione di corpora di linguaggio parlato tra i 2 e i 4 anni. Poster presented at the XVII Congresso AIP Acquisizione del linguaggio in età prescolare e scolare. Bari, 22–25 September.

Marchione, D., Fasolo, M. & D'Odorico, L. (2004): Studio comparato di tre software e l'orecchio per la rilevazione degli aspetti prosodici del parlato adulto. Poster presented at the XVIII Congresso AIP Sezione di Psicologia Sperimentale. Sciacca, 18–20 September.

Moneglia, M. (1994): *Intonation, the property of distantiation, the mastering of complex utterance in Italian spoken language. Quaderni del dipartimento di linguistica*. Firenze: Unipress.

Moneglia, M. & Cresti, E. (1997): L'intonazione e i criteri di trascrizione del parlato adulto e infantile. In: *Il progetto CHILDES: strumenti per l'analisi del linguaggio parlato*, eds. U. Bortolini & E. Pizzuto, vol. 2, pp. 57–90. Pisa: Edizioni del Cerro.

Parisi, D. & Antinucci F. (1973): *Elementi di grammatica*. Torino: Boringhieri.

Renzi, L. (1991): *Grande grammatica italiana di consultazione*, vol. 1. Bologna: Il Mulino.

Rumelhart D.E. & McCelland, J.L. (1986): *PDP Microstruttura dei processi cognitivi*. Bologna: Il Mulino.

Scollon, R. (1976): Conversation with a one year old, the origins of construction. University of Hawaii. Working Paper of Linguistics **6** (5), 118–184.

Searle, J. (1975): A taxonomy of illocutionary acts. In: *Minnesota studies in the philosophy of language*, ed. K. Gunderson, pp. 344–369. Minneapolis: University of Minnesota Press.

Serianni, L. (1997): *Italiano. Grammatica, sintassi, dubbi*. Milan: Garzanti Editore.

Simone, R. (1995): *Fondamenti di linguistica*. Bari: Laterza.

Slobin, D. (1985): *The cross-linguistic study of language acquisition*. Hillsdale, NJ: Lawrence Erlbaum.

Taeschner, T. & Volterra, V. (1986): *Strumenti di analisi per una prima valutazione del linguaggio infantile*. Rome: Bulzoni.

Tomasello, M., (1998): *The new psychology of language. Cognitive and functional approaches to language structure*. London: Lawrence Erlbaum.

Tomasello, M. (2003): *Constructing a language. A usage-based theory of acquisition*. Cambridge, MA: Harvard University Press.

Tomasello, M & Slobin, D.J. (2005): *Beyond nature-nurture. Essays in honour of Elizabeth Bates*. Mahwah, NJ: Lawrence Erlbaum.

Tomlin, R.S. (1995): Focal attention, voice, and word order. In: *Word order in discourse*, eds. P. Downing & M. Noonan, pp. 517–554. Amsterdam: Benjiamins.

Veneziano, E. (2001): Interactional processes in the origins of the explaining capacity. In: *Children's language, 10: developing narrative and discourse competence*, eds. K. Nelson, A. Aksu-koc & C. Johnson, pp. 113–141. Mahwah, NJ: Erlbaum.

Veneziano, E., Sinclair, H. & Berthoud, J. (1990): From one word to two words: repetition patterns on the way to structured speech. *J. Child Lang.* **17**, 633–650.

Voghera, M. (1992): Sintassi e intonazione nell'italiano parlato, pp. 335. Bologna: Il Mulino.

Chapter 4

Pragmatic development

Loredana Hvastja-Stefani

Department of Psychology, University of Trieste, via S. Anastasio 12, 34134 Trieste, Italy
hvastja@univ.trieste.it

Summary

Pragmatics in language concern a wide range of phenomena, such as text analysis, speech acts, interactions and conversations, as well as processing of oral and written texts. Research on pragmatic development refers to the child's fundamental knowledge and skills needed for the social uses of language. Children learn to use language within and by means of highly structured social contexts.

The main stages of pragmatic development in the preschool years are described in this chapter: the acquisition of communicative intentions and their prelinguistic and linguistic expressions, the development of communicative acts, and the acquisition of conversational and narrative skills. Complexity of morphology and syntax evolves quickly in the preschool years, when communicative functions become more stable. Conversational skills require the capacity to request attention, take turns, and understand referencing. These skills progress, in familiar contexts and about familiar topics, from the age of 2 to 4–5 years and onwards. Narrative capacity means the description of at least two events in such a way that their relationship can be followed. This skill begins to emerge at about 3 years of age.

Some results of two studies concerned with pragmatic development in preschool Italian children are presented in this chapter and are compared with the development of communicative acts in American and Israeli children.

Introduction: what is pragmatics?

Pragmatics is concerned with the core of communication, 'the study of language in context' (Bates, 2003). The term refers to very complex systems of competencies and rules, which allow the creative and adequate use of verbal and non-verbal language, according to situations, interlocutors, and personal style. These last factors require evaluation of the 'effects' of what the speaker says, which are connected with the partner's interpretation. Creativity is very important for ensuring communicative variation and flexibility, while adequacy is also important for achieving communicative comprehension and sharing situation meanings.

The answer to the question 'what is pragmatics?' is complex, because the study of language is concerned with a large range of phenomena – for instance *structural analysis* of texts, *functional aspects* of language usage, and the description of *linguistic events*. Pragmatics is concerned also with *analysis of speech acts* – that is, how utterances are used to accomplish social actions; with social *interactions* and everyday *conversation rules*; and with *processing* of verbal and written texts. Green (1989) defined pragmatics as 'the study of understanding intentional human action' – that is, the study of human intentions, desires, beliefs, and projects, which are typical psychological fields.

If we speak to someone with the intention of 'persuading' them to do something, we are carrying out a social action. This kind of social action has been referred to as a *speech act*. Speech act theory was elaborated by Austin in 1962; for Austin, *to say* something is always *to do* something. Speakers may express their intentions *indirectly*; in this case the speech act form does not correspond to speech act function (or *force* according to Austin's terminology). For instance, one can utter an indirect request for action by expressing it as a statement: 'It is hot here', rather than 'Open the window'. Indirect speech acts are more complex and refer to shared knowledge and information between social actors. They generally require reference to the social actor's culture, reasoning, and social skills, where inferential processes assume crucial importance. Making inferences implies, for instance, that we use our information and competence to create a connection between words in text or discourse, so that we can comprehend the meaning of the words in the given context, and make explicit what is implicit. Interactional and cultural aspects of language use are thus in the foreground. According to Bates (2003), pragmatic mastery requires a great deal of sociocultural information. This relates to feelings and internal states, and to knowledge of how the listener can interpret the speaker's discourse in accordance with that person's point of view. The asymmetrical or intimate relationships between dialogue partners determine the formal or explicit character of conversational moves.

Cultural psychology (see Bruner, 1990) refers to the study of pragmatics and to pragmatic development as fundamental psychological questions. In this perspective, pragmatics is a cultural tool with which people in a group, community, or society combine to develop a system of shared meaning systems to explain the world.

Pragmatic development

Research on pragmatic development refers to the fundamental knowledge and skills needed by the child for the social uses of language. Children learn to use language within and by means of highly structured social contexts, thereby becoming quickly (from 2 to 3 years) adequate and efficient 'communicators', despite the need for further progress. Pragmatic development explains 'how children acquire the knowledge necessary to appropriate, effective, rule-governed employment of speech in interpersonal situations' (Ninio & Snow, 1996, p. 4). This domain is very complex, and its study involves many other developmental domains and the whole cultural context. Assigning the correct meaning to a word, utterance, or discourse requires mastering, remembering, and monitoring an encyclopaedic system of facts in both linguistic production and linguistic comprehension. We can interpret language 'only with considerable knowledge of the world, society, and human psychology' (Ninio & Snow, 1996, p. 9).

Some of the main topics of pragmatic development research in pre-school years are as follows (see Hvastja Stefani, 1998; Ninio & Snow, 1999; Hvastja Stefani, 2004).

• The study of the *acquisition of communicative intents* and their prelinguistic and linguistic *expressions*, including vocalisations and gestures (Camaioni *et al.*, 1986; Ninio & Snow, 1996). The continuity from the prelinguistic to the linguistic phase – that is, from vocalisations and gestures to first words – would permit, for instance, very early assessment and intervention in cases of delay or difficulty in communication, as might be present in autism (Bonifacio & Hvastja Stefani, 2004).

- The study of the development of *conversational skills* and the acquisition of rules that permit adequate conversation. Conversation requires referring to (and the acquisition of capacities for) conversational postulates – principles that govern conversation as a social activity, studied by Grice (1989).
- The study of the developmental skills that control communicative/linguistic devices for organisation of discourse in *cohesive* (that is, to the point) and *genre-specific* ways (Ninio & Snow, 1996). The study of discourse implies the study of discourse types, text cohesion, co-reference relations (Bates, 2003), *narrative skills*, and *decontextualized discourse* skills (Hvastja Stefani, 2004).
- The study of other pragmatic acquisition factors which are fundamental for linguistic and communicative development and which determine it. These are the interactive context within and by which language use is permitted (Hvastja-Stefani, 1998, 2004); the role of maternal/parental input; and the role of *scaffolding* as determinants of language development (Ninio *et al.*, 1994; Bonifacio & Hvastja-Stefani, 1998; Tomasello, 1999; Bonifacio & Hvastja-Stefani, 2004). We can use these factors very early on as risk indicators, clinical assessment indices, and clinical intervention fields in all types of developmental problems, difficulties, or disorders that involve interaction, communication, and language disturbances (Bonifacio & Hvastja-Stefani, 1998, 2004).

To summarize, according to the socio-constructionist and the socio-pragmatic points of view of cultural psychology (for example, Bruner, 1990), children must develop competencies and skills that allow them to create and to interpret shared social meanings. They must learn the 'art' of conversation and develop capacities that allow them to appreciate, in interactions and communications, the points of view of the people they are interacting with. They must also develop narrative competence and skills and interconnected 'narrative thought'. On some of these topics there is scanty information in Italian children in their first 3 years of life.

The development of communicative acts

The main task for anyone who intends to use language is to understand the interlocutor's intent and to develop the ability to communicate one's own intent. This task is very demanding because communicative intents do not have a direct one-to-one relation with forms of utterance. Furthermore, some rules of social interaction or courtesy require certain ambiguities or lack of transparency relative to the interlocutor's intent (Ninio *et al.*, 1994). Finally, interlocutors can lie or dissimulate so that their true intent is obscured.

The expression of verbal communicative acts is determined by an overall capability involving many different individual types of competence. First there is the communicative *intent*, which is the will to influence an interlocutor by purposeful behaviour, and the *control* (that is, mastering) of intentionality. Then there is the *mastery* of a large range of different communicative acts, and the communicative and linguistic *capability* to express one's intentions in a conventional, effective, and polite way (Ninio & Snow, 1996).

The number of communicative acts in children increases rapidly between the age of 8 and 32 months. Within these two years the child has been able to master most of the crucial communicative moves, particularly *discussions* about many topics and *action negotiations*. Twelve-month-old toddlers can call one's attention and direct it to an object or a person, express distress or surprise, show effort, and agree or refuse to do something, in both verbal and non-verbal ways.

Some crucial communicative functions or intentions emerge before the child is able to express them verbally – for instance, communicative pointing, showing, and ritualized requests. These communicative gestures are highly correlated with linguistic development, so they can be used as predictors of lexical development (Camaioni *et al.*, 1986). The communicative pointing gesture is especially predictive.

Later during their third year, children acquire more complex linguistic skills that are less frequent and increasingly specialized. Morphology and syntax grow rapidly in complexity, while the system of pragmatic communicative acts seems to show few changes. We can therefore emphasize the *continuity* in communicative functions (Ninio & Snow, 1996) during a developmental phase that involves great changes in linguistic expression and linguistic forms, and in the complexity of utterances. An important factor that determines the order of acquisition among the different types of communicative acts seems to be their strict or poor connection with concrete and current settings. Acts that refer to abstract or non-present situations and are context independent (for example, the act of 'promising') are acquired later.

Wells (1985) noticed a relatively slight increase in new communicative acts between 30 and 60 months of age, but during this time children increase their lexical and grammatical means of verbal expression markedly.

According to Ninio & Snow (1996), the verbal communicative system extends in an orderly way according to different 'stages and substages characterized by distinct levels of organization'. In a first phase, the child is able to master the verbal means of *directing attention* and learns to participate verbally in *game interaction*. Successive phases are built on the preceding ones. The *discussion* system results from moves of *object denomination* games; the *action negotiation* system is based on the system of *attention direction*. The order of emergence of communicative acts is determined by many factors, such as the importance of the act itself for achieving the child's communicative and interactive goals, and its relative complexity as regards its formal and conceptual characteristics. Other determinants of acquisition order are as follows:

- The adequacy of the child's role as such: child-role acts (for instance, requests or verbal moves during games) are acquired before adult-role acts (for instance, comforting or scolding).
- The complexity of general cognitive prerequisites implied by verbal acts.
- The direct and concrete connection of what one says with the interactive context.

Thus game verbalizations that 'build' a given context are developed before action directives, which 'govern' it. The latter in turn precede clarification requests related to 'definition' or 'interpretation' in the situation of social actors (meta-communicative modalities). Another important factor is the complexity of the particular social concept implicated in a verbal act. Further factors are the phonological skills required for the act, and the syntactic or formal complexity of utterance used in expressing it.

Conversational skills

Becoming a competent partner in conversations – that is, an 'adequate conversationalist' – requires diverse and complex capacities. Conversation requires the coordination of what we say with what the conversational partner says, and with the whole conversation, with respect to contents, dialogue, and general context.

Some conversational components are purely linguistic, others are social and interactive. Children are able to show very early the simpler ones and those components more directly connected to a concrete situation, but they are unable to deal with more complex competencies and with ones requiring multilevel or abstract references.

As a first step, conversation requires calling the attention of the conversational partner – that is, initiating the conversation with the first move of turn-taking. The child is able to do this verbally from the second year of life, and makes progress at ages 2 to 3. Four-year-old children are able to adapt their conversational style according to an adult or child partner. With a younger child they indeed use simpler speech, as they are sensitive to lower linguistic skills. A 3-year-old child can converse only by referring to present actions; at about 5 years dialogues emerge which contain references to past or future plans.

An important requisite of conversation is turn-taking, which in the case of adult conversation is fluent, avoiding overlaps and pauses. Here too, cultural differences will matter. Children can show turn-taking in conversations with their peers beginning from the age of 3 years. In children, inability to turn-take may depend on factors that are independent of the process itself, such as the lack of comprehension of what the speaker is saying, or being unable to say anything about that conversational topic.

In conversation, it is very important that the listener identify the *topic*. Two-year-old children are able to facilitate the identification of referents by non-verbal devices, and they repeat what was just said if the listener seems to not to understanding. From about $2^1/_2$ years, children are able to signal that they have not understood what the speaker said, and by the age of 3 they can request repetition and clarification.

Information interchanges by dialogue begin during the second year of life, but only at 3 to 4 years can children develop a topic through conversation, especially if the topic is a familiar one. Four-year-old children can exchange information or discuss complex topics with support from an adult. At 5 years, conversational skills seem very articulate, but at this age children cannot always consider the possibility of discrepancies between their viewpoints, information, and opinions and the conversational partner's (Orsolini, 1995; Ninio & Snow, 1996). The capacity to consider possible differences between one's own knowledge and opinions and the ones of others involves social and cognitive processes that are very complex, involving a progressive 'decentralisation' which increases at school age, as noted by Piaget.

Narrative skills

Units of conversations may be analysed as 'turns' or as longer 'sequences of turns', but connected discourse implies a different and more complex level of organisation of communicative interchange. Therefore we need a new and more complex level of analysis; its units are *narratives*, *arguments*, *explanations*, and *definitions* which are socially and culturally defined units.

Among several topics concerning connected discourse, I will refer here only to narratives. However, all kinds of connected discourse require the child to take into consideration information, expectations, and the characteristics of the partner and of the situation, showing the related capacities of decontextualized language production without adult support.

In order to achieve this level of appropriateness, the child must master the pragmatic skills required to evaluate the conversational partner's expectations about the relevant information, and to produce a structure of discourse based on these expectations. The child must evaluate what the partner knows and cannot know. They must understand that many people are not inclined to agree with their perspectives and for that reason they must learn to support these perspectives by effective arguments.

Some of these competencies are developed long after the preschool age, and also depend on other factors such as education and cultural level. For instance, the experience of reading and writing may be helpful to develop competencies connected with meta-communication and meta-language (Camaioni, 2001).

Narratives represent a basic type of connected discourse. They are defined in general as forms of connected discourse in which the speaker describes at least *two events* so that their relation appears evident. This relation may be a temporal one (before-after), a causal one ('I did it for this reason'), a contrasting one, and so on. Narrative capacities are fundamental for the production of discourses or texts of all sorts. At first they are only 'vocal', but afterwards, during school age, they may become written texts.

According to cultural psychologists, narration represents a fundamental and universal model of human thinking and of 'thinking about how the world works' (Ninio & Snow, 1996). The fundamental components of narration are the *control* of the action by the agent, the *sequential nature* of events and psychological states, the *sense* of what is canonical and what is exceptional (as we mostly narrate exceptionality), and the *narrator's perspective* – that is, the feelings and evaluations of the storyteller about what is being narrated. The last element is the main purpose of the speaker in narrative production.

Narrative abilities involve mastering various cognitive, social, and communicative skills at a higher level of complexity (Paul *et al.*, 1996). These include the ability to produce a cohesive text through the use of explicit linguistic markers or forms, and to use a precise, specific lexicon; the ability to achieve communication of ideas unrelated to extra-linguistic means (that is, ideas not tied to a concrete situation), and to understand cause–effect relations. Finally, there is the ability to organize the structure of narration along the specific directives of 'story schemata' prescribed by an individual culture, enabling the listener to understand the story.

At about 3 years of age, and sometimes before, children can describe or label events or actions, but a main theme is absent. Children aged 18 months can converse with parents about events which 'just happened': for instance they can tell that a bus has just passed. This is the first step towards talking about 'non-present' things, leading to decontextualized language.

Narrative skills, measured by a story-retelling task, are one of the best predictors of school success in 4-year-old children with language disabilities. Thus the achievement level in this ability can be considered an important risk index for subsequent cognitive, linguistic, and academic difficulties in children with either a specific language impairment or delayed language development – for instance in the case of 'late talkers'. Through an intervention directed to improve communicative skills, significant improvements may follow in the areas of language, social communication, and self-esteem (Law & Sivyer, 2003).

Canonical schemes of stories and fundamental rules for elaborating an adequate story are defined by a 'grammar of stories'. The main components of a story are a *setting* or *scenery* (which includes some characters and time and place of action) plus a *plot* or *succession of incidents*, with a few or many *episodes*.

Next to these components we can add a beginning ('once upon a time there was...') and a conventional end ('and they lived happily ever after'). We have obvious differences according to story genres (tale, spy story, comedy, thriller, and so on).

We can distinguish many kinds of narrative forms. The following forms have been studied more widely in developmental psychology relating to pragmatic development, and in developmental psycholinguistics:

- A *script* is a narrative about usual, routine events.
- A *personal events narrative* can consist of a simple answer to a question about school, or in complex reports about specific exciting life events or anecdotes. Autobiography may be included in this kind of narrative.

- *Fantasy narratives* inspire the structure of many fantasy games played by children, although the early fantasy play (playing house or doctor) shows a script form rather than a plot form (Ninio & Snow, 1996). Adult fantasy narratives are the ones we find in books or movies, the ones we play in role games, and the ones we write (or read) in chat-lines.

From about 3 years of age (or perhaps a little before), the narrative capacity of children can be assessed with the 'narrative stage scoring system' proposed by Paul *et al.* (1996, p. 1299), which has five levels.

(1) *Heap*: stories where the child labels or describes events and actions. A central theme is missing.
(2) *Sequence*: the child labels or describes events concerning a central theme.
(3) *Primitive narrative*: this contains the three main components of story grammar: the initiating event, the attempt or action (of leading character), and the consequence, relating to a central theme.
(4) *Chain*: there are four components of story grammar, three of which are the preceding ones. The child may produce an ending, but it is disjointed.
(5) *True narrative*: this comprehends at least five components of story grammar, three of which are the main components (initiating event, attempt or action, consequence). The ending constitutes a resolution of story problem.

The more complex levels of narration, for instance presenting the point of view of many characters, are developed at about 9 to 10 years of age.

Some research data about pragmatic development in Italian children

The following data refer to two of my own still unpublished researches on early pragmatic development, specifically about the acquisition of communicative acts in Italian children aged 1 to 3 years.

Study 1 – An initial longitudinal study of lexical and pragmatic development in the second year of life involved two samples of 24 children (sample 1 and sample 2). They were assessed at ages 12–14, 16–18, and 24 months with the 'PVB' test ('Primo vocabolario del bambino'; Caselli & Casadio, 1995), the Italian version of McArthur Communicative Development Inventories, and with a preliminary Italian version of Parental Interview on Communicative Acts (PICA). This interview on the first 100, functionally different, communicative acts was first elaborated by Ninio & Goren (1993) and then translated and adapted by Hvastja-Stefani in a preliminary format. Table 1 presents the mean values of the different communicative acts (verbal and non-verbal) and their standard deviations for different age levels. Italian 2-year-olds achieve almost 70 per cent of PICA communicative acts. The variability shown by the standard deviations in Table 1 is less than that measured in the development of vocabulary.

Pragmatic development is highly correlated with lexical development. In sample 1, the total number of diverse kinds of communicative acts at 12 months correlated with lexical production at 16–18 months and at 24 months (Pearson's test, $p = 0.000$ and $p = 0.004$). The total number of different communicative acts at 16–18 months correlated with lexical production at 24 months ($p = 0.002$). In sample 2, vocabulary at 14 months was correlated with the level of different communicative acts at 14 ($p = 0.01$), 18 ($p = 0.001$), and 24 months ($p = 0.03$). Therefore we can suggest that the pragmatic development level could be used as an early risk index of communicative–linguistic development as well as of vocabulary development – for instance, in cases of speech delay.

Table 1. Means and standard deviations at four different age levels

Age (months)	n	Mean	SD
12	24	36.10	4.10
14–15	24	37.87	7.75
17–19	48	50.37	10.69
24	48	68.92	11.25

Study 2 – Data from a second, semilongitudinal study show more specific aspects of pragmatic development, concerning the first 100, functionally different, communicative acts in Italian children during their first 3 years of life. This study was also concerned with lexical development as well as with the assessment of the quality of stimulation and support available to the child in the home environment, tested with HOME Inventory (Home Observation for the Measurement of the Environment, Caldwell and Bradley, 1984).

Four small samples of children of different ages participated in the study (n = 16). The age range was 3 to 36 months, and the children were grouped by age as follows: four were aged 3 months (sample 1), four were aged 6 months (sample 2), four were aged 18 months (sample 3), and four were aged 24 months (sample 4) at the beginning of the study. Sex ratios were similar in different samples (eight girls and eight boys).

Education levels of families were as follows: 5 mothers and 3 fathers had a lower level of education, 6 mothers and 11 fathers had a middle level, and 5 mothers and 2 fathers had a higher level (university degree).

Methods

The PICA Parental Interview (Ninio & Goren, 1993) was administered to the parents in their homes, beginning when their children were about 6 months old. The PICA was then applied monthly from 6 to 18 months in sample 1 and sample 2; at 18, 24, and 30 months in sample 3; and at 24, 30, and 36 months in sample 4. The total number of different communicative acts reported by parents was 87/100 (the PICA item 'other' was never brought up by these parents).

Results and discussion

Table 2 summarizes the total means of functionally different communicative acts shown at diverse ages, and the means and ranges of communicative acts related to different functional categories considered in the PICA interview. These categories, in order of complexity, are 'negotiations of attention' (5 different acts), 'expressions of emotions' (3 different acts), 'markings of events' (12 different acts), 'performances in games' (16 different acts), 'discussions' (24 different acts), 'negotiations of action' (25 different acts), and 'clarifications of communication' (2 different acts) (see Ninio & Goren, 1993; Ninio & Snow, 1996).

The mean numbers of different communicative acts increased consistently with age: at 7 months children showed 13 different non-verbal acts, and at 36 months, 77.8 different, mostly verbal acts. In the age range 6 to 18 months, monthly assessments showed a consistent month-by-month increment in the number of diverse communicative acts, such that this skill advanced at a different rate from lexical development. It appears that up to the age of 16–17 months,

Table 2. Mean numbers of total acts, and means and ranges of communicative acts referred to different categories and ages

Age (months)	n	Total mean	Attn neg (total = 5)	Exp emot (total = 3)	Mark event (total = 12)	Games perf (total = 16)	Discus (total = 24)	Act neg (total = 25)	Clarif (total = 2)
7	8	13	3.1	2.8	1.5	0.2	3.3	2.0	0
			[1 to 4]	[2 to 3]	[1 to 3]	[0 to 2]	[0 to 5]	[0 to 6]	
12	8	33	4.1	3	6.3	2.2	8.6	8.6	0
			[3 to 5]		[5 to 8]	[0 to 5]	[5 to 13]	[5 to 13]	
18	8	53	4.1	3	8.2	10.6	14.2	13.8	0
			[3 to 5]		[4 to 11]	[8 to 13]	[7 to 18]	[7 to 17]	0
24	8	61	4.7	3	8.6	10.8	17.2	15.5	0.8
			[3 to 5]		[6 to 11]	[3 to 15]	[7 to 22]	[9 to 21]	[0 to 2]
30	8	72	5	3	10.2	11.3	20.6	20.2	1.2
					[8 to 11]	[6 to 14]	[11 to 22]	[12 to 24]	[0 to 2]
36	4	78	5	3	10.2	12.2	23.7	22.5	1.0
					[9 to 11]	[8 to 13]	[22 to 24]	[20 to 24]	[0 to 2]

Values are means and [ranges].

communicative acts are mostly non-verbal, and afterwards they are mostly verbal, even if this was not the case for all functional categories examined.

At 2 years of age the mean total number of different acts in these children was 61, which is lower than in the two samples in my longitudinal study described above, and lower than the means of American and Israeli peers observed by Ninio & Snow (1996). Israeli children (n = 114) in particular seem more productive, since at age 2 they master from 70 to 90 different communicative acts (Ninio & Goren, 1993). All their acts were verbally produced, while Italian children show a range regarding verbally expressed acts from 82 per cent to 100 per cent of total produced acts. They show some non-verbally expressed acts, especially relating to the 'expressions of emotions' (37 per cent of produced acts belonging to this category) and to the 'performance in games' (50 per cent of produced acts belonging to this category). We may suppose that there is a trend to maintain some gestures even later, because at 36 months Italian children still show some non-verbal acts in these same two categories (25 per cent and 41 per cent of produced acts belonging to these categories, respectively). The verbal form of these acts seems to appear later in Italian children than in the American or Israeli children studied by Ninio & Snow (1996).

The development of acts that are used for 'markings of events' is similar in Italian and American or Israeli children; in 'performances in games', the Israeli sample seemed more precocious. 'Negotiations of action' is very important in communication; these acts increase dramatically, in the Italian sample, beginning at 18 months. Compared with the results of Ninio & Snow, some acts in the 'negotiations of action' seem to emerge later in Italian children.

Regarding the expression of different functional categories and sex differences, Italian girls show a slight advantage over boys in relation to 'negotiations of attention' acts, especially at ages 18 and 24 months. Girls and boys do not differ significantly with regard to 'expressions of emotions'. In development of acts that are used for 'markings of events' Italian girls have a slight advantage over Italian boys at 7 and 11 months.

Italian girls once again show a slight advantage over boys in 'performances in games', starting at 24 months, and the same is true of 'discussions' acts, especially at ages 18 and 24 months. The 'clarifications of communication' have a meta-communicative function, and these acts therefore begin to emerge only at age 24 months in all samples. Italian girls show a significant advantage over boys, as at age 24 months 75 per cent of girls produce these functional acts, compared with only 12 per cent of boys.

In conclusion, there are similarities and differences with regard to both sex and culture. Socio-economic factors, not considered here, may nevertheless be the most important.

References

Austin, J.L. (1962): *How to do things with words*. Oxford: Clarendon Press.

Bates, E. (2003): Natura e cultura nel linguaggio (On the nature and nurture of language). In: *Frontiere della biologia. Il cervello di Homo sapiens*, eds. E. Bizzi, P. Calissano & V. Volterra, pp. 241–265. Rome: Istituto dell'Enciclopedia Ital. Fondata da G. Treccani Spa.

Bonifacio, S. & Hvastja Stefani, L. (1998): *L'interazione comunicativa e linguistica nel bambino con ritardo di linguaggio*. Tirrenia (PI, Italy): Ediz. del Cerro.

Bonifacio, S. & Hvastja Stefani, L. (2004): *Modelli d'intervento precoce per il bambino Parlatore Tardivo: il modello INTERACT*. Tirrenia (PI, Italy): Ediz. del Cerro.

Bruner, J.S. (1990): *Acts of meaning*. Cambridge, MA: Harvard University Press.

Caldwell B.M. & Bradley R.H. (1984): *Home Observation for the Measurement of the Environment*. Little Rock, AR: University of Arkansas at Little Rock.

Camaioni, L. (2001): *Psicologia dello sviluppo del linguaggio*. Bologna: Il Mulino.

Camaioni, L., Volterra, V. & Bates, E. (1986): *La comunicazione nel primo anno di vita*. Torino: Boringhieri.

Caselli, M.C. & Casadio, P. (1995): *Il primo vocabolario del bambino. Guida all'uso del questionario MacArthur per la valutazione della comunicazione e del linguaggio nei primi anni di vita*. Milan: FrancoAngeli.

Green, G.M. (1989): *Pragmatics and natural language understanding*. Hillsdale, NJ: Lawrence Erlbaum.

Grice, H.P. (1989): *Studies in the way of words*. Cambridge, MA; London: Harvard University Press.

Hvastja Stefani, L. (1998): Lo sviluppo comunicativo – pragmatico nella prima infanzia. In: *L'interazione comunicativa e linguistica nel bambino con ritardo di linguaggio*, eds. S. Bonifacio & L. Hvastja Stefani, pp. 17–54. Tirrenia (PI, Italy): Ediz. del Cerro.

Hvastja Stefani, L. (2004): Lo sviluppo del linguaggio nel contesto: aspetti pragmatici e sociali. In: *Modelli d'intervento precoce per il bambino Parlatore Tardivo: il modello INTERACT*, eds. S. Bonifacio & L. Hvastja Stefani, pp. 52–77. Tirrenia (PI, Italy): Ediz. del Cerro.

Law, S.& Sivyer, J. (2003): Promoting the communication skills of primary school children excluded from school or at risk of exclusion: an intervention study. *Child Lang. Teaching Ther.* **19**, 1–25.

Ninio, A. & Goren, H. (1993): *PICA 100*. Jerusalem: Hebrew University.

Ninio, A. & Snow, C.E. (1996): *Pragmatic development*. London: Westview Press.

Ninio, A. & Snow, C.E. (1999): The development of pragmatics: learning to use language appropriately. In: *Handbook of child language acquisition*, eds. W.C. Ritchie & T.K. Bathia, pp. 347–383. London: Academic Press.

Ninio A., Snow, C.E., Pan, B.A. & Rollins P.R. (1994): Classifying communicative acts in children's interactions. *J. Commun. Disord.* **27**, 158–187.

Orsolini, M. (1995): L'acquisizione di competenze pragmatiche. In: *Manuale di neuropsicologia dell'età evolutiva*, ed. G. Sabbadini. Bologna: Zanichelli.

Paul, R., Hernandez, R., Taylor, L. & Johnson K. (1996): Narrative development in late talkers: early school age. *J. Speech Hearing Res.* **39**, 1295–1303.

Tomasello, M. (1999): Perceiving intentions and learning words in the second year of life. In: *Language development*, eds. M. Tomasello & E. Bates, pp. 111–128. Oxford: Blackwell.

Wells, G. (1985): *Language development in the preschool years*. New York: Cambridge University Press.

Language and neurofunctional correlates

Chapter 5

Auditory comprehension of language in young children

Madison M. Berl[*], Erin N. Moore[*], Chandan Vaidya[*,°], Gerard A. Gioia[*], Bernstein Ratner[§], and William Davis Gaillard[*,#]

[*] Department of Neurosciences, Children's National Medical Center, George Washington University School of Medicine, 111 Michigan Ave NW, Washington DC 20010, USA
[#] Clinical Epilepsy Section, NINDS, NIH, Bethesda, Maryland, USA
[°] Department of Psychology, Georgetown University, Washington DC, USA
[§] Department of Hearing and Speech Sciences, University of Maryland, College Park, Maryland
mberl@cnmc.org

Summary

Infant studies reveal left temporal activation when a child listens to a woman's voice but not to other auditory stimuli. In older children, when different aspects of language may be formally assessed, auditory processing paradigms identify activation along the superior temporal sulcus, with primary auditory processing in Heschl's gyrus. An increase in the burden and complexity of auditory stimuli is associated with increases in activation in the superior temporal sulcus posteriorly. The inferior temporal cortex may also be involved in auditory tasks; however, activation in this area may not be critical or unique to auditory processing. In contrast, reading paradigms consistently activate the posterior inferior temporal cortex and the middle temporal gyrus. In recent studies, healthy children ranging in age from 4 to 12 years completed a panel of functional magnetic resonance imaging tasks. These included listening to stories, categorizing words (modification of a verbal fluency task), and making a semantic decision. Group analyses showed that language areas are localized and lateralized by age 4. Differences in activation may be influenced by various issues including anatomical maturation, varying task demands, and different levels of task difficulty. Different auditory tasks engage frontal as well as temporal language areas. Frontal areas are involved in aspects of language processing such as semantic decision, working memory, and phonology.

Introduction

Since the 1800s, neuroscientists have debated whether language functions are localized to specific cortical areas. Seminal work by Paul Broca and Carl Wernicke support the hypothesis that language is localized to specific brain regions. In the traditional model of language processing, Broca's area – located in the frontal lobe – is critical for expressive language functions, while Wernicke's area – located in the temporal lobe – is critical for receptive language functions. Several studies since then have confirmed the importance of these regions in language processing. Furthermore, later studies established the neuroanatomical underpinnings of language processing. Various methods were used, including animal models

(Rauschecker et al., 1997; Romanski et al., 1999), cadaver lesion studies, anatomical imaging studies [computed tomography (CT) and magnetic resonance imaging (MRI)], as well as functional studies using evoked potential and metabolic and blood flow change techniques (Wise et al., 1991; Zatorre et al., 1992). More recently, functional magnetic resonance imaging (fMRI) has been developed as a non-invasive technique that provides insights into the development of language networks. In this chapter we will focus specifically on the contributions of fMRI studies to our understanding of the normal development of networks critical for auditory comprehension of language in children.

Background

Neuroanatomy

A brief review of the neuroanatomy relevant to language processing will be presented. Initially, sound is interpreted by receptors within the ear and translated to frequency maps. This information travels through the auditory nerve (CVIII) to the cochlear nuclei in the brain stem, on to the inferior colliculus in the midbrain, and then through the medial geniculate body before projecting to the primary auditory neocortex. Information enters the cortex either ventrally or dorsally. The ventral route terminates in Brodmann's area (BA 41) which is the primary auditory cortex, whereas the dorsal route terminates directly in the secondary auditory cortex (BA 41/42). In contrast to the visual system, the cortex receives both ipsilateral and contralateral input; however, a majority of the input is from the contralateral ear.

Once auditory information enters the cortex, several key areas comprise the language network. Initially, cortical activation occurs bilaterally within the primary auditory cortex, also known as Heschl's gyrus (BA 41), followed by second order processing of sound (for example, tone, pitch). Subsequently, there is processing of sound for language, which occurs in adjacent association cortical areas typically residing in the left temporal lobe. Akin to the visual system, auditory information follows either a dorsal or a ventral route of processing (Alain et al., 2001). The ventral route is proposed as the 'what' system because it is important for object identification, whereas the dorsal route is the 'where' system as it is important for object location. There is debate regarding the functional aspects of the dorsal route (Hickok & Poeppel, 2004); however, this paper emphasizes the ventral route as it is relevant to the 'what' system because of our focus on language comprehension.

Information that follows the ventral route is initially processed superiorly along the superior temporal gyrus, better known as Wernicke's area (BA 42/22) and may extend into the parietal areas including the supramarginal and angular gyri. The processing stream then involves areas ventrally along the superior temporal sulcus extending into middle temporal gyrus and sometimes into the inferior temporal gyrus. Another area that could be recruited is the fusiform gyrus, which is thought to be an association area involving the visual processing of information (Booth et al., 2001).

As mentioned previously, Broca's area in the frontal lobe is also activated during many language-processing tasks. Broca's area (BA 44/45) spans the inferior frontal gyrus and is clearly important for speech production in terms of planning and phonological processing; however, this area also has a major role in the comprehension of speech [see the chapter by Heim (p. 61) for further discussion on the role of Broca's and Wernicke's areas].

In summary, the cortex used during auditory comprehension of language involves a broad but well defined network of areas including the temporal (superior temporal gyrus, superior temporal sulcus, middle temporal gyrus, inferior temporal gyrus), parietal (angular and supramarginal gyri), and frontal (inferior frontal gyrus) areas.

Principles of fMRI

A brief review of the principles of fMRI is critical for an understanding of the capacity and limitations of functional imaging studies. Brain mapping techniques are founded upon the observation that increased neuronal activity is associated with local increases in blood flow (Roy & Sherrington, 1890; Fox & Raichle, 1986). Studies commonly use the blood oxygen-level-dependent (BOLD) technique, which is an indirect measure of brain activity. There is a haemodynamic response within specific cortical regions when there is a change in conditions – namely, increased neuronal activity – that creates different metabolic demands for that area. Thus fMRI measures the relative change in cerebral blood flow between two conditions for a cortical area. The measurement is based on the paramagnetic properties of haemoglobin, which vary according to oxygen binding. During increased neuronal activity, there is an initial increased extraction of oxygen followed by increased local blood flow, with concomitant over-abundance of oxygenated haemoglobin in the capillary and venous bed. Paradoxically, the ultimate result is that the ratio of oxygenated to deoxygenated haemoglobin is much greater during an active state compared with a resting or baseline state. The MR signal is based on this difference in ratios. The change in ratio is associated with a change in MR signal (Cohen *et al.*, 1994).

From these principles it is important to recognize that fMRI is a relative and not an absolute measure. In addition, the BOLD response is an epiphenomenon and only an indirect measure of neuronal activity. The temporal resolution of this technique is 4 to 8 seconds, which is the time for the haemodynamic response to peak. Therefore, a limitation of fMRI is that the results do not capture the millisecond back and forth timing of network processes. The spatial resolution for fMRI ranges from 3 to 10 mm. Spatial resolution varies according to technological factors as well as to the placement of the vasculature relative to the neural activity (Kinahan & Noll, 1999).

An experiment is specifically designed to maximize this relative change. A type that is often used is a block design where there are at least two conditions (rest and baseline). Presentation of each condition alternates for a block of time (for example, 30 seconds). Over multiple samplings, one is able to produce a different signal for each condition. Essentially, the activation that is common between two tasks cancels out. On the other hand, it is assumed that the areas of the brain that are active for one condition and not for the other are associated in some way for that cognitive process. This principle is important because later studies have become increasingly sophisticated in parsing apart different aspects of language processing.

Imaging language functions

The first fMRI studies investigating the neural networks of language were conducted with adults and involved passive listening to different conditions, including rest, white noise, pseudowords, single words, and passages (Binder *et al.*, 1994, 1995). These studies showed bilateral activation in primary and second order auditory cortex. The word-based tasks showed greater activation in the left temporal lobe than in the right, but it was difficult to isolate language as opposed to sound processing (for example, pitch, tone) *per se*. This difficulty was a result of the task design. Using rest as a baseline condition does not parse general audition from language processing (phonological, semantic, and so on). Subsequent comparisons that used reverse speech or tones as the baseline task separated language functions from audition. As a result, these later fMRI studies confirmed that auditory language processing is primarily a left-lateralized function (Binder et al., 1995; Binder et al., 1997; Binder et al., 2000). Moreover, extraction of meaning of words occurs posteriorly and inferiorly from Heschl's gyrus, along the superior temporal sulcus.

Results from fMRI studies are customarily presented as group maps, which are statistical maps that show only the areas that are significantly activated for the group as a whole. Examination of individual maps also yields important findings, and is essential for interpreting data from developmental or patient populations where heterogeneity of activation patterns for a task may confound traditional group analysis methods. For example, individuals with overall strongly left-lateralized language activation during verbal fluency tasks also show varying degrees of activation in homologous right frontal regions (Binder, 1997; Gaillard et al., 2003b). Children carrying out either an auditory-based naming to description task or a reading task show varying recruitment of the left inferior and mid-frontal gyrus (Balsamo et al., 2002; Gaillard et al., 2003a). The individual differences in weighting of activation within the broad neural networks that mediate language processing are not well understood but may indicate use of different strategies or an additional effort to complete the given task. These individual differences may occur as normal variants or, in children, as developmental variants.

In summary, these early adult studies of language functioning replicated and confirmed some important observations. First, primary and second order auditory processing is a bilateral function. Second, processing that occurs in adjacent association areas is strongly lateralized to the left hemisphere for the majority of people. The areas commonly activated on a group basis include frontal and temporal-parietal regions traditionally associated with language processing. However, the individual differences observed in activation maps may reveal important findings about the developmental aspects of language acquisition and consolidation.

Developmental studies of language

An extension of the early work with fMRI and language functions is to characterize the activation patterns in children. As children acquire and consolidate language functions, it is presumed that these patterns change over development; however, the age at which humans achieve a mature network for mediating language is unclear. Clinical studies indicate that in the setting of brain injury, children's brains have the capacity to reorganize language functions into late childhood and early adolescence (Muller et al., 1998; Hertz-Pannier et al., 2002).

Conducting studies with children poses several challenges. The child's brain is continuously maturing, undergoing significant anatomical and physiological changes. For example, the brain as a whole reaches a relatively stable volume by the age of 5 (Caviness et al., 1996; Giedd et al., 1996) but is marked by continued changes in cortical composition. The timing of these cortical changes is not uniform across brain regions (for example, temporal lobe, frontal lobe, association areas) resulting in greater variability for different regions at different ages (Huttenlocher & Dabholkar, 1997; Yakovlev & Lecours, 1967; Giedd, 2004; Gogtay et al., 2004). These changes have implications when interpreting functional imaging data. Relevant to our discussion, language processing tasks that involve the temporal lobe may reveal activation differences between children and adults. However, it is a challenge to determine whether the observed differences are influenced by any of the aforementioned structural changes.

Similarly, these anatomical differences may also affect image-analysis strategies. For example, a common processing step in order to compare individual results is to warp individual brains into standard stereotactic space (Friston *et al.*, 1995). Given that brains with different measurements may be warped more or less, group differences may reflect a bias introduced by the image analysis rather than true activation differences.

Paradigm design and assumptions are another challenge when studying developing populations. For example, the stimuli used in adult studies need to be modified to a child's conceptual level. Furthermore, it is important to have several levels of stimuli, as children's abilities are very diverse even within similar age groups. Moreover, situations such as a rest condition may not be ideal, as a child may be more easily distracted and have difficulty 'resting' their minds. Performance differences are a difficult confounding factor that also needs to be addressed when working with children. Imaging studies with children have evolved to account better for many of these issues; however, sometimes they cannot be adequately controlled for, and thus results are interpreted cautiously. This is particularly true for the initial language studies with children and in studies with younger children.

Auditory comprehension in children

A study with infants suggests that a lateralized network sensitive to passive listening of linguistic information is established early in life (Dehaene-Lambertz *et al.*, 2002). Twenty 3-month-old infants were imaged during three listening conditions: silence, forward speech of a female voice reading a children's book, and reverse speech of the female voice. Silence compared with forward speech revealed a left lateralized pattern in the superior temporal gyrus and the angular gyrus. Interestingly, the contrast between the forward and reverse conditions showed differences only in the angular gyrus. Thus the temporal lobe processing activated at this early age is probably not activation of a 'language' network but rather a more fundamental communication network which is later adapted and develops into a specialized language network.

The first language studies with children extended those previously conducted on adults (Ulualp *et al.*, 1998; Booth *et al.*, 1999; Balsamo *et al.*, 2002). These studies produced mixed evidence about whether children showed more bilateral activation than adults. However, these early studies often used rest as a baseline task, which probably accounted for some of the bilateral activation. In addition, some studies used the same stimuli for adults and children, which may have been a problem because later studies found evidence that task complexity can increase activation of homologous regions (Just *et al.*, 1996). Subsequent child studies that employed a reverse speech control task, stimuli that were matched for a child's ability, and larger sample sizes showed a strongly lateralized pattern for language tasks by the age of 5 (Ahmad *et al.*, 2003; Balsamo *et al.*, 2003). Moreover, these later studies suggest that children's activation maps for language tasks are fundamentally similar to those of adults. Currently, meaningful fMRI studies investigating auditory language processing in children younger than 4 or 5 years are precluded by imaging and cooperation constraints.

In addition to general patterns of language activation, these studies used different tasks; this allows for exploration into specific aspects of language processing because different tasks emphasize different cognitive demands. In the study by Balsamo and colleagues (2003), children were given a category (for example, animals) and then single words were presented a few seconds apart (dog, cat, shoe, bird...). Children were instructed to press the button if the word matched the category. In the study by Ahmad *et al.* (2003), children listened passively to stories adjusted for age. For both tasks, the baseline condition was reverse speech. The activation maps showed that each task burdens different regions within the language network to a greater or lesser extent. For the auditory category decision task, robust activation was seen in frontal areas, probably reflecting the active retrieval and decision making demands. The fusiform gyrus (BA37) is also strongly activated for this task, which is thought to represent a visual strategy where a child may be visualizing the features of the object to match it to the category. In contrast, the 'listening to stories' task produced strong temporal activation along the superior temporal sulcus back to the supramarginal gyrus (BA 37/39), which are the areas critical for comprehension of whole language. Thus the linguistic burden of each task is different, resulting in different patterns of activation. The auditory comprehension task (listening to stories) is rich in context and content and does not involve the frontal lobes to the same extent as the single word auditory decision task.

An important caveat when interpreting activation patterns is not to assume that because an area is not shown to be activated on a group map, that area is not involved in the task. Rather, it is just as likely that that area is not sufficiently burdened to reach threshold. Therefore, temporal regions are likely to be involved in the auditory decision task; however, comprehension of single words does not present the same temporal lobe load as comprehension of more linguistically complex stories that involve syntax, grammar, and semantic processing.

Recent studies have refined methods to begin answering more sophisticated questions about development and to specify what cortical areas are involved in different aspects of language processing (Schlaggar *et al.*, 2002; Gaillard *et al.*, 2003b). Some study refinements include matching performance between adult and child populations with performance data as a regressor, using a parametric task correlating test performance with activation, and using a panel of tasks. In the remainder of this chapter we discuss these aspects as they pertain to auditory comprehension. Extensive discussion of the issues in the context of single word lexical processing is to be found in the chapter by Schlaggar (p. 77).

A common issue in studies with children is to determine whether any differences in activation result from performance effects. In addition, if performance differences are evident, then identifying the areas of the brain that mediate these differences is important. In a study by Balsamo and colleagues, children carried out the auditory category decision task described above (Balsamo *et al.*, 2003). Accuracy of button press responses was correlated with activation. No correlation was found for temporal areas; however, greater middle frontal gyrus activation was significantly correlated with better performance. One hypothesis is that the middle frontal gyrus plays an integral role in mediating performance and may represent a specific cognitive process such as working memory. Although working memory may not be specific to language processing, it is inherent in better performance.

Our ongoing studies are designed to address further issues of performance and development. The preliminary data presented here represent two groups of children, a young group of 10 typically developing children (4 to 6 years old) and an older group of 10 children (10 to 12 years old). Results from three different language tasks with increasing linguistic complexity and demands are shown (Figs. 1a–1c). All tasks have reverse speech as the baseline condition. The first task is the auditory category decision task as described above. The second task is listening to stories. The modification for the story listening task is that children press a button when they hear a beep in the midst of listening to the story or reverse speech. This performance measure is an indication of attention to the task while in the scanner. The third task is an auditory description decision task where children listen to a description (for example, 'A long yellow fruit is a banana', 'Something you sit on is spaghetti') then press the button only if the description is accurate. There are several levels of difficulty for each of the three tasks and each volunteer is given the level that matches their ability as determined by a neuropsychological evaluation conducted before scanning.

Similar to observations from previous studies, the three tasks generate different patterns within the expected language network. Moreover, these patterns are generally similar for both older and younger children (see below for discussion of differences). The auditory category task which involves single words and a decision primarily activates the frontal regions and the fusiform gyrus, with limited temporal lobe activation (Fig. 1A). In contrast, listening to stories revealed extensive activation within the temporal lobe from the superior temporal sulcus into the middle temporal gyrus (Fig. 1B). Interestingly, the auditory description task appears to be intermediate between the category and story tasks by consistently activating both frontal and temporal regions (Fig. 1C). This task is linguistically complex, like the 'listening to stories' task (temporal activation), yet also has the decision and working memory components of the category task (frontal activation).

Several observations may be made when comparing the older children with the younger children. Both groups show lateralized patterns of activation; however, the younger children appear to have more bilateral activation – specifically for the tasks with a decision component. Although the tasks within each paradigm are matched for age to account for difficulty, younger children may still exert more effort to complete the task. It may be that, because frontal areas have protracted development (Bourgeois *et al.*, 1994), the bilateral activation represents a less consolidated network for younger children. Another observation is that older children show more extensive activation down the superior temporal sulcus and the middle temporal gyrus, which may be because their stimuli are more complex and have greater content. Another explanation for the developmental differences is that the younger group may be using a different strategy than the older group to complete the various tasks. Future analyses will elucidate the contributions of age and performance to these results.

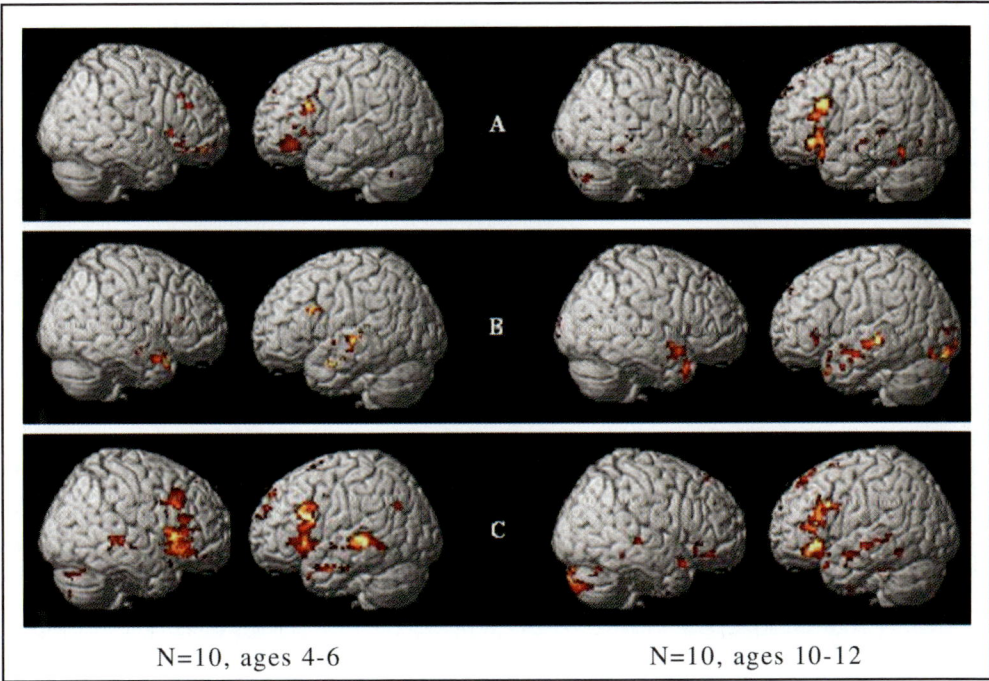

Fig. 1. SPM2 3-D renderings displayed in Talairach space showing activated regions with auditory category decision task (A), auditory listening to stories task (B), and auditory description decision task (C), using a random effect analysis in 20 (10 older, 10 younger) normal child volunteers (p<0.001).

Conclusions

Functional imaging studies contribute greatly to our understanding of auditory processing of language in children. There appears to be an innate capacity for processing linguistic information early in life. Overall, children and adults have more areas of activation in common than not in common. The cortical underpinnings of language involve a lateralized network of functional areas primarily within the left inferior and mid-frontal lobe and the left temporal lobe. The processing stream along the superior temporal sulcus extending into middle temporal gyrus is critical for extraction of meaning. The emphasis of activation in frontal *versus* temporal lobe language processing areas changes with task demands, yet activation patterns are fundamentally more similar than different across tasks and across development. Large population samples and thoughtful methods are required to detect differences attributable to performance or age. However, when differences are found, they tend to involve the association cortex, where higher order processing occurs and synaptic consolidation and myelination are known to continue. A homologous network exists and represents the substrate available for recruitment during more difficult tasks or reorganization because of injury.

Acknowledgments: Supported by NINDS R01 NS44280.

References

Ahmad, Z., Balsamo, L.M., Sachs, B.C., Xu, B. & Gaillard, W.D. (2003): Auditory comprehension of language in young children: neural networks identified with fMRI. *Neurology* **60**, 1598–1605.

Alain, C., Arnott, S.R., Hevenor, S., Graham, S. & Grady, C.L. (2001): 'What' and 'where' in the human auditory system. *Proc. Natl. Acad. Sci. USA* **98**, 12301–12306.

Balsamo, L.M., Xu, B., Grandin, C.B., Petrella, J.R., Braniecki, S.H., Elliott, T.K. & Gaillard, W.D. (2002): A functional magnetic resonance imaging study of left hemisphere language dominance in children. *Arch. Neurol.* **59**, 1168–1174.

Balsamo, L.M., Xu, B., Sachs, B. & Gaillard, W.D. (2003): Language networks underlying auditory based category decision in children identified with fMRI. *Ann. Neurol.* **54** (Suppl. 7), S105.

Binder, J.R. (1997): Neuroanatomy of language processing studied with functional MRI. *Clin. Neurosci.* **4**, 87–94.

Binder, J.R., Rao, S.M., Hammeke, T.A., Yetkin, F.Z., Jesmanowicz, A., Bandettini, P.A., Wong, E.C., Estkowski, L.D., Goldstein, M.D., Haughton, V.M., *et al.* (1994): Functional magnetic resonance imaging of human auditory cortex. *Ann. Neurol.* **35**, 662–672.

Binder, J., Rao, S., Hammeke, T., Frost, J.A., Bandettini, P., Jesmanowicz, A. & Hyde, J. (1995): Lateralized human brain language systems demonstrated by task subtraction functional magnetic resonance imaging. *Arch. Neurol.* **52**, 593–601.

Binder, J.R., Frost, J.A., Hammeke, T.A., Cox, R., Rao, S.M. & Prieto, T. (1997): Human brain language areas identified by functional magnetic resonance imaging. *J. Neurosci.* **17**, 353–362.

Binder, J.R., Frost, J.A., Hammeke, T.A., Bellgowan, P.S.F., Springer, J.A., Kaufman, J.N. & Possing, E.T. (2000): Human temporal lobe activation by speech and nonspeech sounds. *Cereb. Cortex* **10**, 512–528.

Booth, J.R., Macwhinney, B., Thulborn, K.R., Sacco, K., Voyvodic, J. & Feldman, H.M. (1999): Functional organization of activation patterns in children: whole brain fMRI imaging during three different cognitive tasks. *Prog. Neuropsychopharmacol. Biol. Psychiatry* **23**, 669–682.

Booth, J.R., Burman, D.D., Van Santen, F.W., Harasaki, Y., Gitelman, D.R., Parrish, T.B. & Marsel Mesulam, M.M. (2001): The development of specialized brain systems in reading and oral-language. *Neuropsychol. Dev. Cogn. Sect. C Child Neuropsychol.* **7**, 119–141.

Bourgeois, J.P., Goldman-Rakic, P.S. & Rakic, P. (1994): Synaptogenesis in the prefrontal cortex of rhesus monkeys. *Cereb. Cortex* **4**, 78–96.

Caviness, V.S., Kennedy, D.N., Richelme, C., Rademacher, J. & Filipek, P.A. (1996): The human brain age 7–11 years: a volumetric analysis based on magnetic resonance images. *Cereb. Cortex* **6**, 726–736.

Cohen, R.M., Gross, M., Semple, W.E., Nordahl, T.E. & Sunderland, T. (1994): The metabolic brain pattern of young subjects given scopolamine. *Exp. Brain Res.* **100**, 133–143.

Dehaene-Lambertz, G., Dehaene, S. & Hertz-Pannier, L. (2002): Functional neuroimaging of speech perception in infants. *Science* **298**, 2013–2015.

Fox, P.T. & Raichle, M.E. (1986): Focal physiological uncoupling of cerebral blood flow and oxidative metabolism during somatosensory stimulation of human subjects. *Proc. Natl. Acad. Sci. USA* **323**, 806–809.

Friston, K.J., Holmes, A., Worsley, K.J., Poline, J.B., Frith, C.D. & Frackowiak, R.S. (1995): Statistical parametric maps in functional imaging: a general linear approach. *Hum. Brain Mapp.* **2**, 189–210.

Gaillard, W.D., Balsamo, L.M., Ibrahim, Z., Sachs, B.C. & Xu, B. (2003a): fMRI identifies regional specialization of neural networks for reading in young children. *Neurology* **60**, 94–100.

Gaillard, W.D., Sachs, B.C., Whitnah, J.R., Ahmad, Z., Balsamo, L.M., Petrella, J.R., Braniecki, S.H., McKinney, C.M., Hunter, K., Xu, B. & Grandin, C.B. (2003b): Developmental aspects of language processing: fMRI of verbal fluency in children and adults. *Hum. Brain Mapp.* **18**, 176–185.

Giedd, J.N. (2004): Structural magnetic resonance imaging of the adolescent brain. *Ann. N.Y. Acad. Sci.* **1021**, 77–85.

Giedd, J.N., Snell, J.W., Lange, N., Rajapakse, J.C., Casey, B.J., Kozuch, P.L., Vaituzis, A.C., Vauss, Y.C., Hamburger, S.D., Kaysen, D. & Rapoport, J.L. (1996): Quantitative magnetic resonance imaging of human brain development: ages 4–18. *Cereb. Cortex* **6**, 551–560.

Gogtay, N., Giedd, J.N., Lusk, L., Hayashi, K.M., Greenstein, D., Vaituzis, A.C., Nugent, T.F., Herman, D.H., Clasen, L.S., Toga, A.W., Rapoport, J.L. & Thompson, P.M. (2004): Dynamic mapping of human cortical development during childhood through early adulthood. *Proc. Natl. Acad. Sci. USA* **101**, 8174–8179.

Hertz-Pannier, L., Chiron, C., Jambaque, I., Renaux-Kieffer, V., Van de Moortele, P.F., Delalande, O., Fohlen, M., Brunelle, F. & Le Bihan, D. (2002): Late plasticity for language in a child's non-dominant hemisphere: a pre- and post-surgery fMRI study. *Brain* **125**, 361–372.

Hickok, G. & Poeppel, D. (2004): Dorsal and ventral streams: a framework for understanding the aspects of the functional anatomy of language. *Cognition* **92**, 67–99.

Huttenlocher, P.R. & Dabholkar, A.S. (1997): Regional differences in synaptogenesis in human cerebral cortex. *J. Comp. Neurol.* **387**, 167–178.

Just, M.A., Carpenter, P.A., Keller, T.A., Eddy, W.F. & Thulborn, K.R. (1996): Brain activity modulated by sentence comprehension. *Science* **274**, 114–116.

Kinahan, P. & Noll, D.C. (1999): A direct comparison between whole-brain pet and bold fMRI measurements of single-subject activation response. *Neuroimage* **9**, 430–438.

Muller, R.A., Rothermel, R.D., Behen, M.E., Muzik, O., Mangner, T.J., Chakraborty, P.K. & Chugani, H.T. (1998): Brain organization of language after early unilateral lesion: a PET study. *Brain. Lang.* **62**, 422–451.

Rauschecker, J.P., Tian, B., Pons, T. & Mishkin, M. (1997): Serial and parallel processing in rhesus monkey auditory cortex. *J. Comp. Neurol.* **382**, 89–103.

Romanski, L.M., Tian, B., Fritz, J., Mishkin, M., Goldman-Rakic, P.S. & Rauschecker, J.P. (1999): Dual streams of auditory afferents target multiple domains in the primate prefrontal cortex. *Nat. Neurosci.* **2**, 1131–1136.

Roy, C.S. & Sherrington, C.S. (1890): On the regulation of blood flow to the brain. *J. Physiol. (Lond)* **11**, 85–108.

Schlaggar, B.L., Brown, T.T., Lugar, H.M., Visscher, K.M., Miezin, F.M. & Petersen, S.E. (2002): Functional neuroanatomical differences between adults and school-age children in the processing of single words. *Science* **296**, 1476–1479.

Ulualp, S.O., Biswal, B.B., Yetkin, F.Z. & Kidder, T.M. (1998): Functional magnetic resonance imaging of auditory cortex in children. *Laryngoscope* **108**, 1782–1786.

Wise, R., Chollet, F., Hadar, U., Friston, K., Hoffner, E. & Frackowiak, R. (1991): Distribution of cortical neural networks involved in word comprehension and word retrieval. *Brain* **114**, 1803–1817.

Yakovlev, P.I. & Lecours, A.R. (1967). The myelogenic cycles of regional maturation of the brain. In: *Regional development of the brain in early life*, ed. A. Minkowski, pp. 3–70. Oxford: Blackwell Scientific Publications.

Zatorre, R.J., Evans, A.C., Meyer, E. & Gjedde, A. (1992): Lateralization of phonetic and pitch discrimination in speech processing. *Science* **256**, 846–849.

Chapter 6

The language production-comprehension network in functional imaging

Stefan Heim

Research Centre Jülich, Institute of Medicine, D-52425 Jülich, Germany
s.heim@fz-juelich.de

Summary

This chapter reviews current neuroimaging evidence for the processing of language with a particular focus on the relation between production and comprehension. The neural correlates of semantic, phonological, and syntactic processing are reviewed. For semantics and phonology, there appear to be different fronto-temporal networks which are shared in production and comprehension. The results for the processing of syntactic information are not entirely conclusive but suggest at least partly overlapping networks. Moreover, the data show that phonological strategies may be used in syntactic tasks. This finding opens the discussion of alternative, phonology-based strategies for language processing. Such strategies are accounted for by dual route models featuring one direct and one indirect route.

Introduction

During the past 150 years, there have increasingly been attempts to identify the neural systems underlying human linguistic abilities. First evidence for a localist approach to mapping different aspects of language to distinct brain regions was reported in the late 19th century by Paul Broca (1861) and Carl Wernicke (1874) on the basis of single case studies. The patient Leborgne described by Broca suffered from a severe production deficit, allowing him only to utter the syllable 'tan' – though with variable prosody related to the intended meaning. Broca examined the patient's brain postmortem and detected a profound lesion in the left inferior frontal region, covering approximately Brodmann's area (BA) 44 and BA 45 in the left inferior frontal gyrus (IFG), the deep left frontal operculum, and parts of the left insula. From these findings, Broca concluded that the lesion site (which later was named *Broca's area* in honour of its discoverer) was somehow related to language production. Thirteen years later, Wernicke presented results from a different patient who, after acquiring a lesion in the superior temporal lobe (later referred to as *Wernicke's area*), developed severe problems in understanding normal speech. Interestingly, his own speaking ability was preserved in the sense that his verbal fluency was unaffected; however, his utterances were meaningless, as the content words were chosen inappropriately. On the basis of this double dissociation, the so-called *neurological model* of language processing was formulated by Wernicke and revised by

Geschwind (1970), attributing language production to the motor-related frontal areas and comprehension to Wernicke's area, located in the posterior portion of the superior temporal gyrus (pSTG). Additional neural structures such as the angular gyrus and the arcuate fasciculus connecting the two regions were included in the model, which for a long time was the principal reference for neurologists dealing with language disorders.

With the advent of functional neuroimaging techniques, however, there was evidence available from healthy subjects providing insight into the regular functions of the brain regions associated with language processing. These data, in turn, led (at least partially) to dramatic changes in the perception of the brain's functionality. Some of the neuroimaging evidence will be presented in this chapter. As the focus of the chapter is on the question of whether language production and comprehension share a common neural network, their relation in psycholinguistic approaches will be sketched briefly first.

The functional relation of production and comprehension

Most psycholinguistic models only concentrate on one aspect of communication (that is, production or comprehension) while neglecting the other. In the Levelt model of language production (Levelt et al., 1999), a self-monitoring mechanism relates language production to comprehension. By controlling the phonological output, errors in the syllabification progress can be detected and corrected. Levelt and colleagues assume that production and comprehension share the same systems from the lemma stratum (where lexico-semantic and syntactical information is represented) upwards; however, they state explicitly that the phonological system underlying comprehension and the self-monitoring system are different systems. Evidence for this comes from a study by Pickering et al. (2000), who found syntactic priming at the sentence level not only from production to production, but also from production to comprehension. However, the results of Jacobsen (1999) suggest some caution in assuming identical lemma levels for production and comprehension. In that study, in German, subjects had to name pictures or read words. Using a paradigm in which a sentence fragment did or did not prime the grammatical gender picture or word target, Jacobsen observed facilitation and inhibition in the picture-naming task relative to gender-neutral primes for gender-congruent and gender-incongruent primes, respectively. However, in the reading task, there were only inhibition effects. On the basis of these results, one might conclude that production and comprehension (as operationalized by word reading) only share partly overlapping lemma levels.

In line with the arguments of Levelt et al. (1999) in favour of partly distinct systems for production and comprehension are the results of Nickels & Howard (1995). They compared the performance of aphasic patients and showed that the input and output deficits differed. They concluded that this must mean that there are separate phonological systems for production and comprehension (on the theoretical as well as the neural level). However, in a review considering the theoretical implications of several proposed mechanisms for self-monitoring, Postma (2000) pointed out that a single central comprehension-based monitor which is supported by some automatic production-based modules provides the best solution for a self-monitoring mechanism. Considering the role of the production network for language comprehension and *vice versa* on the basis of numerous results, Garrett (2000) argued that comprehension may support error-free production, while (as assumed by the motor theory by Liberman et al., 1967) production could serve as an auxiliary for comprehension:

'[...] production systems should be viewed as having a functionally similar role with respect to comprehension, namely, that they provide a continual error control mechanism via the

production monitoring of partial products of the recognition system. A somewhat broader way of putting this point is to think of the production system as a filter on the generation of multiple analyses by the recognition system.' (Garrett (2000), pp. 48–49).

This point is party supported by a recent imaging study by Wilson *et al.* (2004). These investigators found overlapping activation in motor and premotor areas dedicated to speech production when subjects listened passively to meaningless monosyllables.

To conclude, the exact relation between the production system and the perception system remains subject to further research. This research can take two different forms. First, behavioural studies may reveal further similarities and dissimilarities of the architecture of the two domains. Moreover, electrophysiological time-sensitive measures, especially EEG and magnetoencephalography (MEG), may provide new insights into the temporal aspects of the subprocesses of production and comprehension. Second, functional neuroimaging studies using functional magnetic resonance imaging (fMRI) or positron emission tomography (PET) are most likely to reveal insights into the neural systems in the brain which support semantic, syntactic, phonological, and other linguistic processes in the two domains, and in particular the extent to which these systems are identical for both production and comprehension. Such evidence may, in turn, feed back to the discussion on the psycholinguistic level.

Some remarks on anatomical issues

One aspect of any discussion of the various functions associated with different cortical regions needs reviewing. In most papers, anatomical terms such as 'BA 44' or 'BA 45' are used to describe the localization of brain activations. These terms suggest a high degree of accuracy of the localization – that is, localization with respect to microstructurally defined cortical areas (such as the ones identified by Brodmann in 1909). It is therefore tempting to speculate about different functions associated with distinct microanatomical regions such as Brodmann's areas. However, this anatomical precision is in most cases not justified. There is a substantial amount of intersubject variability in the localization of cytoarchitectonic borders of BA 44 and BA 45, which do not necessarily coincide with macroanatomical landmarks such as gyri or sulci (Amunts *et al.*, 1999; Amunts *et al.*, 2004). Moreover, the Talairach atlas (Talairach & Tournoux, 1988), from which the locations of Brodmann's areas are commonly derived, only provides rather rough information, as the areas are reported according to the macroanatomical landmarks of one hemisphere of a 60 year old woman's brain, and no exact borders are specified. Owing to the considerable intersubject variability in size, shape, and location of BA 44 and BA 45, they cannot be distinguished reliably.

At present, a possible alternative for determining the localization of brain activation with a higher degree of specificity is to superimpose the functional data on probability maps, which are based on an observer-independent analysis of the cytoarchitecture in a sample of 10 post-mortem brains (Amunts *et al.*, 1999; Schleicher *et al.*, 1999; Zilles *et al.*, 2002; Amunts *et al.*, 2004). These probability maps provide information about the location and variability of cortical regions in a standard reference space (the MNI space). The maps can be combined into a single summary map by using the maximum probability map approach (Eickhoff *et al.*, 2004). In the resulting maximum probability map (MPM), each voxel in the brain is assigned to the cytoarchitectonical area which is most likely to be found at that position. The advantage of this method in comparison with methods for the automated anatomical labelling of functional activations based on the Talairach & Tournoux atlas (for example, Maldijan *et al.*, 2003) is that functions identified with imaging techniques can be related to brain structures with much greater accuracy and validity. Moreover, the probability of false classification within this system can be estimated.

Thus, when referring to localizations based on, for example, the Talairach atlas, a more cautious labelling (such as '~BA' indicating the approximate Brodmann's area) should be used. In this chapter, I will stick to this cautious nomenclature and will only use the label 'BA' when referring to data identified on the basis of cytoarchitectonic probability maps. I also try to apply the common anatomical abbreviations.

Semantic processing

Of the different subdomains of language, semantics is among the most commonly investigated in neuroimaging studies. Accordingly, there is a extensive knowledge of the neural networks supporting semantic processing. Since the results presented by Wernicke (1874), there have been hints of the contribution of the temporal lobe to semantic knowledge.

Production

In language production, the temporal lobe appears to play an important role in semantic processing. In a picture-naming experiment with healthy subjects, Damasio et al. (1996) replicated the activations in the middle and inferior temporal lobe. In a baseline task, subjects had to indicate whether unknown faces were presented upright or upside down by saying 'up' or 'down'. The investigators were able to show category-specific activations in distinct regions within these regions. While pictures of animals activated the inferior temporal gyrus (ITG), pictures of tools required activation in the posterior aspects of the temporal lobe. Pictures of faces of famous persons evoked activation in the vicinity of the temporal pole. Moreover, pictures of all three categories required activation of the left IFG (~BA 45). In a parallel experiment, the investigators showed that patients with lesions in these regions had selective naming deficits for pictures belonging to the categories shown to activate the lesioned area.

Further evidence for the specialisation of certain regions to the processing of items of a particular semantic class comes from a study by Martin et al. (1996). In a silent naming task, subjects were presented with pictures of tools, animals, or non-objects. While both tools and animals (as compared to non-objects) activated the left insula as well as the fusiform gyri bilaterally, there was specific activation for tools in prefrontal areas (~BA 44/6), whereas pictures of animals additionally activated the visual cortices. These results were replicated by Chao & Martin (2000) (experiment 2).

Comprehension

In language comprehension, comparable results were reported with respect to the distinction between natural and man-made objects (for example, Kapur et al., 1994; Miceli et al., 2002; Noesselt et al., 2003). Kapur et al. compared a semantic task ('living or non-living') using written words with a task they called 'lexical' decision (detecting the letter 'a') and found activation in left inferior frontal regions (~BA 45, ~BA 46, ~BA 47, and ~BA 10). Similarly, Miceli et al. reported the involvement of the left IFG (~BA 47) and middle frontal gyrus (MFG) (~BA 9 and ~BA 9/46) in an animateness decision task on written stimuli relative to silently read pseudo-words. Noesselt et al. also found activation in the ventral IFG (~BA 47) when subjects decided whether a spoken word denoted an animal or not.

Besides the decision between animals and artefacts, the decision whether a given word is abstract or concrete has been widely used as a semantic decision task (for example, Desmond *et al.*, 1995; Gabrieli *et al.*, 1996; Poldrack *et al.*, 1999; Friederici *et al.*, 2000b). There is again unequivocal evidence for the involvement of the IFG in semantic decision-making. Desmond *et al.* (1995) conducted an fMRI study with a case-judgment task (upper or lower case?) as a baseline. These investigators obtained activation in the left ~BA 45, ~BA 46, and ~BA 47 for the semantic decision relative to baseline. With the same design, the results were replicated by Gabrieli *et al.* (1996) and by Wagner *et al.* (1997), who also reported activation in the left ~BA 44, ~BA 45, ~BA 46, ~BA 47, and ~BA 9, as well as in the right ~BA 44, ~BA 45, and ~BA 9. Using nouns and prepositions as stimuli, Friederici *et al.* (2000b) also found activation in ~BA 45 as well as in temporal areas (posterior portion of the left MTG, ~BA 21/37; posterior portion of the left STG, ~BA 22) relative to a baseline task in which subjects decided whether a consonant letter string was presented with wide or narrow spacing.

Are there 'semantic maps'?

As reported so far, there is compelling evidence that semantic processing in both production and comprehension relies on the contribution of (at least partially) specialized regions within the temporal lobe. In order to test whether the same temporal regions are activated for the processing of semantic information during both production and comprehension, Vandenberghe *et al.* (1996) presented subjects with triplets of items (pictures of objects or their written names) in a PET study. In three tasks, subjects had to make judgements either about the semantic relatedness of the objects, or about their natural size, or about the physical size of the items on the computer screen. In the semantic relatedness decision task, the investigators observed activation for both words (comprehension) and pictures (production) in the left MTG (~BA 21), the left ITG (~BA 20), the left fusiform gyrus (~BA 21/37), the left parieto-occipital junction (~BA 19/39), the left SOG (~BA 19), the left hippocampus, the vermis, and the right cerebellum. Moreover, there was frontal activation in the left IFG (~BA 45 and ~BA 11/47). These findings were corroborated by Chee *et al.* (2000), who used the same design as Vandenberghe *et al.* (1996). These investigators reported a common semantic network for English words, pictures, and Chinese characters (Kanji) that comprised the left IFG (~BA 44 and 45), MFG (~BA 9), the left fusiform gyrus, and the left posterior temporal regions. This network was activated when subjects decided which of two objects or characters was semantically more closely related to a probe. A perceptual size judgement served as a baseline task.

These data might suggest that the temporal lobe regions responsible for the processing of semantic information are parcelled so that in each single region one particular class of semantic information (such as animals, or dogs, or even terriers) is stored. However, in their meta-analysis of studies claiming to provide evidence for the existence of semantic maps, Devlin *et al.* (2002) concluded that the only valid distinction between semantic classes that results in a distinct activation pattern is that between natural objects (medial anterior temporal poles) and man-made objects (left posterior MTG).

A common network for production and comprehension

From the studies discussed so far, it becomes obvious that frontal areas (in particular, inferior) and temporal areas (particularly middle and inferior) are involved in semantic processing. Moreover, it appears that frontal areas are more often recruited whenever a semantic decision has to be made, while declarative knowledge (such as semantic categories) is stored in the temporal lobe. This assumption was confirmed by an fMRI study by Thompson-Shill et al. (1997) for both production and comprehension. These investigators applied a design consisting of a combination of three tasks [word generation (production), classification, and comparison (written words = comprehension)] by three conditions (baseline, 'low selection', and 'high selection'). In the low-selection condition, the semantic information was easily accessible, whereas in the high-selection condition, specific information (such as the price of an object or its weight) had to be retrieved. In all three tasks, the investigators obtained evidence that the activation in the inferior frontal gyrus (~BA 44 and ~BA 45) varied as a function of the semantic information that had to be accessed in order to perform the task correctly. In other words, the greater the need for selection of particular bits of information, the more pronounced is the inferior frontal activation. In line with these data, another fMRI study by Thompson-Schill and colleagues (Thompson-Schill et al., 1999) provided evidence that, relative to an unprimed word generation task, 'correct' priming (that is, producing the target word in two successive trials) led to a decrease in activation in the IFG (~BA 44), while incorrect priming (producing different target words in successive trials) increased the inferior frontal activation. In contrast, activation in temporal regions (roughly the medial fusiform gyrus) decreased whenever a prime occurred before the target, whether it be identical to or different from the target. As a conclusion drawn from both studies, Thompson-Schill et al. state that there appears to be functional differentiation between the temporal and the frontal areas in processing semantic information, with the temporal areas being involved in access to semantic information in general, while activation of inferior frontal regions is required in particular when the need for selection of detailed information increases (see the study by Burton et al., 2000, for comparable results from phonological processing during comprehension). This notion was further supported by a recent study carried out by Amunts et al. (2004), who investigated semantic processing in a verbal fluency task. Compared with an undemanding task (for example, continuously repeating familiar items such as the months of the year or the days of the week), higher semantic demands (generating examples of semantic categories such as furniture or flowers) elicited activation in the cytoarchitectonically defined BA 45. It should be noted, however, that Swick & Knight (1996) found that patients with lesions in the prefrontal regions (~BAs 6, 8, 9, 10, 44, 45, and 46) were hardly or not at all affected in a cued recall task or in concreteness judgements.

Summary

Resuming the results from studies of semantic processing reported here, the following pattern emerges. First, middle and inferior temporal regions (~BA 20, 21, 37, and 38) appear to house the semantic aspects of the mental lexicon, to some extent showing specialisation in the processing of distinct classes of information (for example, artefacts and animals). Second, left inferior frontal areas (~BA 45 and 47) may be required for selecting specific semantic information from the lexicon. Third, language production (as operationalized, for example, by picture naming or word generation) and language comprehension (concreteness or animateness judgements on words) involve activation of the same frontal and temporal areas. As Gernsbacher & Kaschak (2003) put it: 'These findings are consistent with studies that argue for a common semantic system across modalities'. On the basis of this pattern of evidence, it may be presumed that the same holds true for syntactic and phonological processing. These issues are discussed in the following sections.

Phonological processing

Comprehension

Focusing on activity in the temporal lobe, recent studies of phonological processing in patients and healthy subjects can demonstrate the contribution of the pSTG (that is, Wernicke's area) in language comprehension (see Burton *et al.*, 2000). With respect to the frontal regions, there is consistent activation in the superior posterior portion of Broca's area (~BA 44) when subjects perform phonological decision tasks such as phoneme monitoring, phoneme discrimination, or phoneme sequencing (Démonet *et al.*, 1992; Zatorre *et al.*, 1992; Fiez *et al.*, 1995; Zatorre *et al.*, 1996; Fiez & Petersen, 1998; Poldrack *et al.*, 1999; Burton *et al.*, 2000). A recent meta-analysis by Bookheimer (2002) nicely summarizes many of the available data.

Production

In production, a similar pattern was observed with respect to pSTG activation (Anderson *et al.*, 1999; Benson *et al.*, 2001; Buchsbaum *et al.*, 2001). However, the situation is somewhat different for frontal activation, as there is high variability in the reported data. Price *et al.* (1997) sought to investigate phonological processes during production in particular. They had subjects undertake different naming task (objects, colours, letters, and words) together with an articulatory baseline task. The investigators calculated the contrasts of each task against baseline and conducted conjunction analyses for pairs of contrasts. As a result, activations related to the processes common to both contrasts in each conjunction analysis showed up. In the conjunction analysis explicitly stated to track phonological processing (experiment 5: naming objects and colours), no activation of ~BA 44 but activation of ~BA 46 was reported. Phonological processing was again the only cognitive component of interest that was measured by the conjunction analysis in experiment 4 (although this was not explicitly mentioned by the authors). Again, Price *et al.* did not report any activation of Broca's area. Two of the picture naming studies – the one by Levelt *et al.* (1998) using MEG and the one by Murtha *et al.* (1999) using PET – reported activation of Broca's area that was related to phonological processes. Chao & Martin (2000) presented subjects with pictures of real objects (experimental conditions) or scrambled objects (baseline). When subjects simply looked at the objects, there was no inferior frontal activation (experiment 1); however, if they had to name these objects silently, this evoked additional activation in Broca's area (experiment 2). The latter results are corroborated by the data of Crosson *et al.* (2001) and Thompson-Schill *et al.* (1997), who reported activation of ~BA 44 in word generation tasks in which subjects have to produce a semantically appropriate verb in response to a noun. The study by Lurito *et al.* (2000) employed a rhyming task and a 'fluency' task, in which subjects had to generate words starting with a particular phoneme, and found practically identical activation foci in Broca's area in both tasks.

A common network for production and comprehension?

The reported results do not allow final conclusions to be drawn about the neural correlates of phonological processing during language production (for reviews, see Fiez, 1997; Fiez & Petersen, 1998; Poldrack *et al.*, 1999; Indefrey & Levelt, 2000). This may reflect the different paradigms used in the different studies. Thus, in order to investigate the direct relation between the neural correlates of phonological processing during language production and during comprehension, it is advisable to apply comparable paradigms. The above mentioned studies of phonological processing during language comprehension employed decision tasks on phonological properties of target words or syllables. In the domain of language production, similar paradigms (for example, van Turennout et al., 1997) are well established but so far have not been used in studies investigating the neural correlates of language production.

On this basis, we conducted an fMRI study investigating the neural correlates of language production (Heim et al., 2003b). We used two phonological decision tasks that were carried out on the initial phonemes of German picture names (PHON1: Does the picture name begin with the phoneme /b/ or not? PHON2: Does the picture name begin with a vowel or not?). Subjects indicated their answers by pressing one of two buttons. In line with the production model by Levelt et al. (1999), a semantic decision task (SEM: Is the presented object natural or man-made?) served as the baseline condition (for the use of these and similar tasks, compare van Turennout et al., 1997; van Turennout et al., 1998; Abdel-Rahman & Sommer, 2000; Schmitt et al., 2000; Szatkowska et al., 2000; Rodriguez-Fornells et al., 2002). In a second baseline condition (BASE), the subjects were required to make a target decision. In all contrasts (PHON1–SEM; PHON2–SEM; PHON1–BASE; PHON2–BASE) and in the conjunction analyses yielding the common (that is, task-independent) activation caused by phonological processing, we observed foci in the superior portion of ~BA 44 (Broca's area) and in the pSTG. Thus our data showed that the same network activated in phonological processing during language comprehension also contributes to phonological processing during production.

Syntactic processing

Comprehension

On the basis of neuropsychological studies (see Grodzinsky, 2000) and experiments on healthy subjects using neuroimaging methods, it appears that Broca's area is involved in processing syntactic information during language comprehension. At the sentence level, there is a positive relation between an increase in syntactic complexity of a sentence and the amount of regional cerebral blood flow in regions supposed to be part of Broca's area (including ~BA 44, ~BA 45, and even ~BA 47) (Just et al., 1996; Stromswold et al., 1996; Caplan et al., 1998; Caplan et al., 1999; Caplan et al., 2000). The mid-portion of ~BA 44 was shown to be activated, in particular, as a function of the syntactic memory required to process syntactically complex sentences rather than as a function of syntactic complexity as such (Fiebach et al., 2001; Cooke et al., 2002). Friederici et al. (2000a) varied the semantic and syntactic content of sentences independently and found the opercular part of Broca's area (~BA 44) to be activated only in the condition in which the syntactic structure of the sentence was preserved but all content words had been replaced by pseudo-words. A similar region in the deep ~BA 44 was observed for pseudo-word sentences containing syntactic and morphosyntactic information (Moro et al., 2001). In the domain of single word syntax, Broca's area was involved in the processing of verbs but not nouns in a lexical decision task (Perani et al., 1999). The left ~BA 44/6 was activated for function words (prepositions) but not for content words (nouns) when subjects performed a detection task on subsequent synonyms (Nobre et al., 1997). As function words tend to be more abstract than content words, the investigators concluded that abstract entries are harder to access and need an extra 'motor' representation in the premotor cortex. However, this difference between processing function words and content words disappears if concreteness is counterbalanced between the word categories (Friederici et al., 2000b). In this latter study, subjects were presented with nouns and prepositions. Half the items of either category were concrete, the other half abstract. In a syntactic task, subjects made a word category decision; in the semantic task they judged the word's concreteness. The result indicated that task requirements rather than word class determined activation differences in the inferior frontal cortex as a function of task: the semantic task (abstract *vs.* concrete) activated ~BA 45, whereas the syntactic task (noun *vs.* preposition) activated ~BA 44. This finding implies that Broca's area is not the cortical localization site of a particular word class (that is, function words) but rather supports the underlying processes of word category decision and assignment (for somatotopic activations along the motor strip for action words related to face, arm, or leg, see Hauk *et al.*, 2004).

If it is syntactic task or processing requirements that characterize the role of the inferior tip of ~BA 44, one may further speculate that not only word category information but any kind of syntactic information is processed here. A language like German, which offers different types of syntactic information (namely, word category and gender), is an ideal testing ground for this hypothesis. According to syntax-first models of comprehension, only word category information such as noun, verb, article is processed during an initial phase of phrase structure building, while lexically bound verb argument structure information and syntactic gender information are processed in a second phase. While word category information is an essential part of every language, this is not true of grammatical gender. Some languages (such as German and French) make use of gender information; others (like English or Japanese) do not. Within the group of languages that implement grammatical gender, the gender of the same word may differ among the languages (for example, the car: el[masc] coche [Spanish] *vs.* la[fem] voiture [French] *vs.* das[neut] Auto [German]). This indicates that syntactic gender, in contrast to natural gender (s/he) is an idiosyncratic part of the lexical entry for a given noun in a given language.

We directly compared the processing of word category information (SYN1) and grammatical gender information (SYN2) in German (Heim *et al.*, 2003a). A non-lexical task in which subjects had to decide whether consonant letter strings were written with wide or narrow spacing served as the baseline (see also Friederici *et al.*, 2000b). In each single contrast (SYN1–BASE; SYN2–BASE) and in the conjunction analysis, we observed activation in the inferior tip of ~BA 44. In addition, there were task-specific activations in other parts of the left inferior frontal gyrus. This result suggests that the lower portion of Broca's area as part of different networks plays an important role in the processing of several types of syntactic information.

Production

In the field of language production, there is much less knowledge about neural systems supporting syntactic processing. Indefrey *et al.* (2001) set out to bridge this gap. Having subjects describe scenarios in which coloured objects moved towards and away from one another in different formats, Indefrey *et al.* (2001) obtained PET evidence for the involvement of Broca's area in syntactic processing. In one condition, subjects had to produce complete sentences (for example, 'Das rote Dreieck jagt den blauen Kreis' – The[neut] red triangle is chasing the[masc] blue[masc] circle). In the second condition, they had to indicate the elements by gender-marked adjective–noun phrases and the action by the infinitive (for example, 'rotes Dreieck, blauer Kreis, jagen' – red[neut] triangle, blue[masc] circle, to chase), while in the third condition, word lists had to be produced – that is, the objects were named – and the adjectives as well as the action was referred to in the basic form ('Dreieck, rot, Kreis, blau, jagen' – triangle, red, circle, blue, to chase). Thus syntactic information in the utterance was varied parametrically, with the sentences containing the full syntactic information (sentential structure information, phrase structure information, gender marking, subject-object differentiation, and so on), the adjective-noun phrases having phrase structure information and gender marking, and the word lists containing no syntactic information. Indefrey and colleagues reported activation in Broca's area and, predominantly, in the Rolandic operculum (dorsally adjacent to the inferior part of BA 44) that co-varied with the amount of syntactic information required. A replication of their study (Indefrey & Levelt, 2004) yielded comparable results, with slightly more anterior activation (that is, in the inferior portion of ~BA 44). In sum, it appears that the inferior portion of Broca's area plays an important role in the explicit and implicit processing of syntactic information.

A common network for production and comprehension?

The evidence reported here may be taken to support the view that, as for semantic and phonological processing, there are shared networks in the brain for syntactic processing as well. As was demonstrated above, the inferior tip of ~BA 44 was consistently involved in a number of experiments investigating syntactic processing. However, there is other evidence suggesting caution in the interpretation. The study by Indefrey & Levelt (2004) also included a second part in which subjects did not describe the animated scenes but listened to descriptions of the scenes while watching them. In this condition, the brain activity in ~BA 44 was not modulated by the syntactic complexity. Finally, as the review by Kaan & Swaab (2002) demonstrates, there is a high variability in the locations of activations related to syntactic processing, even if these are grouped with respect to task demands and stimulus characteristics. Thus the answer to the question of a common network for production and comprehension in syntactic processing could be a tentative 'Yes'.

Phonological processing in non-phonological tasks

Verbalisation in syntactic tasks

When investigating grammatical gender processing in German, we observed a somewhat surprising effect, as reported by Heim (2003) (experiment 2) and by Heim *et al.* (2005a). Our sample actually consisted of two subgroups that used different strategies for the gender-decision task. While one group had direct access to the gender information, the other group used a verbalisation strategy – that is, they produced the definite determiner of the word in order to undertake the judgement. Interestingly, Miceli *et al.* (2002) reported that the same strategy was employed by their subjects. Verbalisers and non-verbalisers differed significantly in their reaction times (verbalisers being faster) and showed different patterns of brain activation. The non-verbalisers showed the same activation in the inferior tip of ~BA 44 as was observed in the word category decision. The verbalisers, however, displayed activation in other cortical areas, among them the more anterior parts of the left inferior frontal gyrus and the superior portion of ~BA 44 (similar to that observed in phonological processing, and to that reported by Miceli *et al.* (2002) in their verbalising sample). These data are in line with dual route models of access to grammatical gender featuring a direct, implicit, lexically-based route and an indirect, explicit, form-based route (Gollan & Frost, 2001; Friedmann & Biran, 2003). Moreover, Schiller *et al.* (2003) obtained electrophysiological and behavioural facilitation effects in a gender decision task when the stimuli were phonologically marked.

There are some additional data from language production that should also be considered here. In one fMRI study (Heim *et al.*, 2006 in press) (experiment 1), subjects had to indicate by button pressing if the grammatical gender of the German name of a picture was masculine or feminine. Again, many subjects managed this task by silently generating the definite determiner of the picture name before responding. As in the comprehension study (Heim *et al.*, 2005a), this group showed activation in the superior portion of Broca's area, resembling the pattern observed in phonological processing.

We therefore conducted an event-related fMRI experiment where in one task the subjects were explicitly instructed to produce overtly the definite determiner of a picture name, while in a control condition, they simply named the picture (Heim *et al.*, 2002). Our results showed that the production of the determiner selectively involved the most superior portion of Broca's area. This activation very much resembles that observed by Heim *et al.* (2005a; 2006 in press) (experiments 1 and 2), when the definite determiner was silently produced in a production or comprehension task, respectively. Most interestingly, this activation is in a region comparable to that activated in phonological tasks – that is, the superior portion of ~BA 44. Moreover, the verbalisation strategy draws upon phonological information. Thus the question arises as to what extent the access to the word form (the phonological code) mediates the performance in linguistic contexts (Miceli *et al.*, 2002; Heim *et al.*, 2005a; 2006 in press; Schiller *et al.*, 2003). I will focus on this issue in the following section.

Dual route models of visual word recognition

As Frost (1994) reported, subjects reading Hebrew characters tended to wait until the vowel marks were presented (with some delay) (prelexical phonology) although the Hebrew characters would have provided enough cues for the words to be read (lexical phonology). Unsworth & Pexman (2003) investigated the relation between reading skill and three phonological effects (homophone, homograph, and regularity effects). Unskilled but not skilled readers showed regularity effects in a lexical decision task and a phonological task. The investigators concluded that the skilled readers made more efficient use of phonological knowledge. Ziegler *et al.* (2000) undertook a reading study in Chinese, where the characters can be associated with meaning without access to the phonological form. Their results showed, however, that reading times were faster for characters with higher phonological frequencies but not with higher orthographical frequencies. They suggest an automatic phonological mechanism involved in reading. In contrast, Hanley & McDonnell (1997) reported the case of patient PS, who had a good understanding of written language but could not access the second meaning of a written homophone (AIR/HEIR); thus they argued that phonological processing can be regarded as helpful but not obligatory in the understanding of written language.

The facilitative effect of phonological processing has been observed in several contexts by various researchers, often as dissociations between spared and impaired performance of patients but also in neuroimaging studies. As a result, models have been proposed that share the label 'dual route model'. As mentioned above, dual route models for access to grammatical gender information were formulated by Friedmann & Biran (2003) and by Gollan & Frost (2001).

Other dual route models focus on written language comprehension (for example, Coltheart *et al.*, 2001). They have in common one direct route and another indirect pathway which is form-related or phonologically mediated. In the direct, fast route, orthographic percepts are mapped onto stored word form representations (addressed phonology), whereas in the indirect non-lexical pathway, graphemic input is translated to phonological information ('assembled phonology', 'grapheme-to-phoneme conversion') (for an outline of the dual route model of reading, see Coltheart *et al.*, 2001).

In the literature, there are some imaging studies in agreement with a dual route account (Rumsey *et al.*, 1997; Fiez *et al.*, 1999; Fiebach *et al.*, 2002; Ischebeck *et al.*, 2004; and see Mechelli *et al.*, 2003, for a review). Fiez *et al.* (1999) applied a word-naming paradigm and observed activation in

~BA 44 for low frequency words with inconsistent spelling-to-sound mapping, as well as for non-words. As this region had been shown to be involved in phonological processing, Fiez and colleagues interpreted their result as demonstrating rule-based phonological processes in accessing these infrequent and irregular words. Similarly, when investigating the effects of word frequency with fMRI, Fiebach et al. (2002) observed activation for pseudo-words and low frequency words compared with high frequency words in ~BA 44 (but see Chen et al., 2002). Fiebach et al. suggested that this posterior part of Broca's area might support the rule based grapheme-to-phoneme conversion. The same region was also observed in a study tapping the reversed process – that is, phoneme-to-grapheme conversion (Omura et al., 2004). However, as all these interpretations were *ex post facto*, further imaging studies are necessary to directly demonstrate the relation of activation in ~BA 44 with the processes hypothesized by dual route models.

We conducted one such study (Heim et al., 2005b). In this fMRI study, we investigated the influence of task (lexical decision, LEX; phonological decision, PHON) and experimental design (blocked *vs.* event-related) on activation in Broca's region (left ~BA 44 and 45) during the reading of words and pseudo-words. In both designs, reaction times were slower for pseudo-words than for words in LEX but did not differ in PHON. By combining the fMRI data with cytoarchitectonic anatomical probability maps, we demonstrated that the left BA 44 and BA 45 were more strongly activated for pseudo-words than for words. Separate analyses for LEX and PHON revealed that the left BA 44 was activated in both tasks, whereas left BA 45 was only involved in LEX. The results were interpreted within a dual route model of reading with the left BA 44 being involved in grapheme-to-phoneme conversion (non-lexical route), and the left BA 45 being related to lexical search. In reading, both a direct (lexical) and an indirect (non-lexical) route work in parallel. The indirect route starts the grapheme-to-phoneme conversion for each letter, while the lexical route begins to search the mental lexicon. For highly frequent words, the lexical route may successfully retrieve the word even before the last grapheme is converted to a phoneme by the non-lexical route. In contrast, for low frequency words, pseudo-words, or non-words, the lexical search finishes later or times out. Meanwhile, more or even all letters are converted to sounds by the indirect route. This 'more' is reflected by the stronger activation in BA 44 for NOWO>WO independent of task, whereas the explicitly required lexical search in LEX results in stronger activation for NOWO>WO in BA 45. This interpretation is in line with published reports suggesting the involvement of BA 44 in phonological processing and of BA 45 in lexical-semantic processing.

Conclusions

The data presented in this chapter demonstrate two major points. First, in general – and despite of some substantial variability (see for example Seghier et al., 2004) – the neural systems supporting different types of linguistic information are anatomically distinguishable. This may be exemplified by the activation in the left IFG. Processing of semantic information recruits the anterior portion (~BA 45 and 47), whereas phonological information is processed in the posterior part (superior portion of ~BA 44) (Bookheimer, 2002; Miceli et al., 2002; Matthews et al., 2003; Seghier et al., 2004). Second, these distinguishable networks are in large part overlapping for production and comprehension. Finally, it should be mentioned that different processing strategies (as demonstrated for the dual route approaches) may result in different brain activation patterns for the processing of identical information. This aspect is encouraging for patients with acquired brain lesions: It implies a potential to process information even in the absence of the originally relevant brain regions (see Grodzinksy, 2000).

Acknowledgments: This manuscript is an updated excerpt from the lecture 'The structure and dynamics of language processing' (Heim, 2005). Free reprints of this lecture may be requested from the author via email (s.heim@fz-juelich.de).

References

Abdel-Rahman, R. & Sommer, W. (2000): Parallel access to semantics and phonology in object recognition? *Journal of Psychophysiology (Suppl.)* **14**, 124.

Amunts, K., Schleicher, A., Bürgel, U., Mohlberg, H., Uylings, H.B.M. & Zilles, K. (1999): Broca's regions revisited: cytoarchitecture and intersubject variability. *J. Comp. Neurol.* **412**, 319–341.

Amunts, K., Weiss, P.H., Mohlber, H., Pieperhoff, P., Eickhoff, S., Gurd, J.M., Marshall, J.C., Shah, N.J., Fink, G.J. & Zilles, K. (2004): Analysis of neural mechanisms underlying verbal fluency in cytoarchitectonically defined stereotaxic space – the roles of Brodmann areas 44 and 45. *Neuroimage* **22**, 42–56.

Anderson, J.M., Gilmore, R., Roper, S., Crosson, B., Bauer, R.M., Nadeau, S., Beversdorf, D.Q., Cibula, J., Rogish, M., Kortenkamp, S., Hughes, J.D., Gonzalez Rothi, L.J. & Heilman, K.M. (1999): Conduction aphasia and the arcuate fasciculus: a reexamination of the Wernicke-Geschwind model. *Brain Lang.* **70**, 1–12.

Benson, R.R., Whalen, D.H., Richardson, M., Swainson, B., Clark, V.P., Lai, S. & Liberman, A.M. (2001): Parametrically dissociating speech and nonspeech perception in the brain using fMRI. *Brain Lang.* **78**, 364–396.

Bookheimer, S. (2002): Functional MRI of language: new approaches to understanding the cortical organization of semantic processing. *Annu. Rev. Neurosci.* **25**, 151–188.

Broca, P. (1861): Remarques sur le siège de la faculté de langage articulé, suivies d'une observation d'aphemie. *Bulletin des Societés Anatomiques de Paris* **2**, 330–357.

Brodmann, K. (1909): Beiträge zur histologischen Lokalisation der Grosshirnrinde. VI. Die Cortexgliederung des Menschen. *Journal für Psychologie und Neurologie* **10**, 231–246

Buchsbaum, B.R., Hickok, G. & Humphreys, C. (2001): Role of left posterior superior temporal gyrus in phonological processing for speech perception and production. *Cogn. Sci.* **25**, 663–678.

Burton, M.W., Small, S.L. & Blumstein, S.E. (2000): The role of segmentation in phonological processing: an fMRI investigation. *J. Cogn. Neurosci.* **12**, 679–690.

Caplan, D., Alpert, N. & Waters, G. (1998): Effects of syntactic structure and propositional number on patterns of regional cerebral blood flow. *J. Cogn. Neurosci.* **10**, 541–552.

Caplan, D., Alpert, N. & Waters, G. (1999): PET studies of syntactic processing with auditory sentence presentation. *Neuroimage* **9**, 343–351.

Caplan, D., Alpert, N., Waters, G. & Olivieri, A. (2000): Activation of Broca's area by syntactic processing under conditions of concurrent articulation. *Hum. Brain Mapp.* **9**, 65–71.

Chao, L.L. & Martin, A. (2000): Representation of manipulable man-made objects in the dorsal stream. *Neuroimage* **12**, 478–484.

Chee, M.W.L., Weekes, B., Lee, K.M., Soon, C.S., Schreiber, A., Hoon, J.J. & Chee, M. (2000): Overlap and dissociation of semantic processing of Chinese characters, English words, and pictures: evidence from fMRI. *Neuroimage* **12**, 392–403.

Chen, Y., Fu, S., Iversen, S.D., Smith, S.M & Matthews, P M (2002): Testing for dual brain processing routes in reading: a direct contrast of chinese character and pinyin in reading using fMRI. *J. Cogn. Neurosci.* **14**, 1088–1098.

Coltheart, M., Rastle, K., Perry, C., Langdon, R. & Ziegler, J. (2001): DRC: a dual route cascaded model of visual word recognition and reading aloud. *Psychol. Rev.* **108**, 204–256.

Cooke, A., Zurif, E.B., DeVita, C., Alsop, D., Koenig, P., Detre, J., Gee, J., Pinango, M. Balogh, J. & Grossman, M. (2002): Neural basis for sentence comprehension: grammatical and short-term memory components. *Hum. Brain Mapp.* **15**, 80–94.

Crosson, B., Sadek, J.R., Maron, L., Gokcay, D., Mohr, C.M., Auerbach, E.J., Freeman, A.J., Leonard, S.M. & Briggs, R.W. (2001): Relative shift in activity from medial to lateral frontal cortex during internally vs. externally guided word generation. *J. Cogn. Neurosci.* **15**, 272–283.

Damasio, H., Grabowski, T.J., Tranel, D., Hichwa, R.D. & Damasio, A.R. (1996): A neural basis for lexical retrieval. *Nature* **380**, 499–505.

Démonet, J.-F., Chollet, F., Ramsay, S., Cardebat, D., Nespoulous, J.-L., Wise, R., Rascol, A. & Frackowiak, R. (1992): The anatomy of phonological and semantic processing in normal subjects. *Brain* **115**, 1753–1768.

Desmond, J.E., Sum, J.M., Wagner, A.D., Demb, J.B., Shear, P.K., Glover, G.H., Gabrieli, J.D.E. & Morrell, M.J. (1995): Functional MRI measurement of language lateralization in Wada-tested patients. *Brain* **118**, 1411–1419.

Devlin, J.T., Moore, C.J., Mummery, C.J., Gorno-Tempini, M.L., Phillips, J.A., Noppeney, U., Frackowiak, R.J.S., Friston, K.J. & Price, C.J. (2002): Anatomic constraints on cognitive theories of category specifity. *Neuroimage* **15**, 675–685.

Eickhoff, S., Mohlberg, H., Stephan, K.E., Fink, G.R., Zilles, K. & Amunts, K. (2004): A new SPM toolbox for the combined analysis of fMRI data and probabilistic cytoarchitectonic maps. Poster presented at the 10th Annual Meeting of the Organization for Human Brain Mapping, 13–17 June, Budapest, Hungary.

Fiebach, C.J., Schlesewsky, M. & Friederici, A.D. (2001): Syntactic working memory and the establishment of filler-gap dependencies: Insights from ERPs and fMRI. *J. Psycholinguist. Res.* **30**, 321–338.

Fiebach, C.J., Friederici, A.D., Müller, K. & von Cramon, D.Y. (2002): fMRI evidence for dual routes to the mental lexicon in visual word recognition. *J. Cogn. Neurosci.* **14**, 11–23.

Fiez, J.A. & Petersen, S.E. (1998): Neuroimaging studies of word reading. *Proc. Natl. Acad. Sci. USA* **95**, 914–921.

Fiez, J.A. (1997): Phonology, semantics, and the role of the left inferior prefrontal cortex. *Hum. Brain Mapp.* **5**, 79–83.

Fiez, J.A., Raichle, M.E., Miezin, F.M., Petersen, S.E., Tallal, P. & Katz, W.F. (1995): PET studies of auditory and phonological processing: effects of stimulus characteristics and task demands. *J. Cogn. Neurosci.* **7**, 357–375.

Fiez, J.A., Balota, D.A., Raichle, M.E. & Petersen, S.E. (1999): Effects of lexicality, frequency, and spelling-to-sound consistency on the functional anatomy of reading. *Neuron* **24**, 205–218.

Friederici, A.D., Meyer, M. & von Cramon, D.Y. (2000a): Auditory language comprehension: an event-related fMRI study on the processing of syntactic and lexical information. *Brain Lang.* **74**, 289–300.

Friederici, A.D., Opitz, B. & von Cramon, D.Y. (2000b): Segregating semantic and syntactic aspects of processing in the human brain: an fMRI investigation of different word types. *Cereb. Cortex* **10**, 698–705.

Friederici, A.D., Wang, Y., Herrmann, C.S., Maess, B. & Oertel, U. (2000c): Localization of early syntactic processes in frontal and temporal cortical areas: a magnetoencephalographic study. *Hum. Brain Mapp.* **11**, 1–11.

Friedmann, N. & Biran, M. (2003): When is gender accessed? A study of paraphasias in Hebrew anomia. *Cortex* **39**, 441–463.

Frost, R. (1994): Prelexical and postlexical strategies in reading: evidence from a deep and shallow orthography. *J. Exp. Psychol. Learn. Mem. Cognit.* **20**, 116–129.

Gabrieli, J.D.E., Desmond, J.E., Demb, J.B., Wagner, A.D., Stone, M.V., Vaidya, C.J. & Glover, G.H. (1996): Functional magnetic resonance imaging of semantic memory processes in the frontal lobes. *Psychol. Sci.* **7**, 278–283.

Garrett, M.F. (2000): Remarks on the architecture of language processing systems. In: *Language and the brain*, eds. Y. Grodzinsky, L.P. Shapiro & D. Swinney, San Diego, CA: Academic Press.

Gernsbacher, M.A. & Kaschak, M.P. (2003): Neuroimaging studies of language production and comprehension. *Annu. Rev. Psychol.* **54**, 16.1–16.24.

Geschwind, N. (1970): Organization of language in the brain. *Science* **170**, 940–944.

Gollan, T.H. & Frost, R. (2001): Two routes to grammatical gender: evidence from Hebrew. *J. Psycholinguist. Res.* **30**, 627–651.

Grodzinsky, Y. (2000): The neurology of syntax: language use without Broca's area. *Behav. Brain Sci.* **23**, 1–71.

Hauk, O., Johnsrude, I. & Pulvermüller, F. (2004): Somatotopic representation of action words in human motor and premotor cortex. *Neuron* **41**, 301–307.

Heim, S., Eickhoff, S.B., Opitz, B. & Friederici, A.D. (2006, in press): Broca's region supports grammatical gender decisions in language production. *Neuroreport*.

Heim, S. (2005): The structure and dynamics of normal language processing: insights from neuroimaging. *Acta Neurobiol. Exp. (Wars.)* **65**, 95–116.

Heim, S., Opitz, B. & Friederici, A.D. (2002): Broca's area in the human brain is involved in the selection of grammatical gender for language production: evidence from functional magnetic resonance imaging. *Neurosci. Lett.* **328**, 101–104.

Heim, S., Opitz, B., Müller, K. & Friederici, A.D. (2003b): Phonological processing during language production: fMRI evidence for a shared production-comprehension network. *Cogn. Brain Res.* **16**, 285–296.

Heim, S., Opitz, B. & Friederici, A.D. (2003a): Distributed cortical networks for syntax processing: Broca's area as the common denominator. *Brain Lang.* **85**, 402–408.

Heim, S., Alter, K., Ischebeck, A.K., Amunts, K., Eickhoff, S., Mohlberg, H., Zilles, K., von Cramon, D.Y. & Friederici, A.D. (2005b): The role of the left Brodmann's Areas 44 and 45 in reading words and pseudowords. *Cognitive Brain Research* **25**, 982–993.

Heim, S., Alter, K. & Friederici, A.D. (2005a): A dual-route account for access to grammatical gender: evidence from functional MRI. *Anatomy and Embryology* **210**, 473–483.

Indefrey, P. & Levelt, W.J.M. (2000): The neural correlates of language production. In: *The cognitive neurosciences*, 2nd edition, ed. M. Gazzaniga, pp. 845–865: Cambridge, MA: MIT.

Indefrey, P. & Levelt, W.J.M. (2004): The spatial and temporal signatures of word production components. *Cognition* **92**, 101–144.

Indefrey, P., Brown, C.M., Hellwig, F., Amunts, K., Herzog, H., Seitz, R.J. & Hagoort, P. (2001): A neural correlate of syntactic encoding during speech production. *Proc. Natl. Acad. Sci. USA* **98**, 5933–5936.

Ischebeck, A., Indefrey, P., Usui, N., Nose, I., Hellwig, F. & Taira, M. (2004): Reading in a regular orthography: an fMRI study investigating the role of visual familiarity. *J. Cogn. Neurosci.* **16**, 727–741.

Jacobsen, T. (1999): Effects of grammatical gender on picture and word naming: evidence from German. *Journal of Psycholinguistic Research* **28**, 499–514.

Just, M.A., Carpenter, P.A., Keller, T.A., Eddy, W.F. & Thulborn, K.R. (1996): Brain activation modulated by sentence comprehension. *Science* **274**, 114–116.

Kaan, E. & Swaab, T.Y. (2002): The brain circuitry of syntactic comprehension. *Trends Cogn. Sci.* **6**, 350–356.

Kapur, S., Rose, R., Liddle, P. f., Zipursky, R.B., Brown, M.G., Stuss, D., Houle, S. & Tulving, E. (1994): The role of the left prefrontal cortex in verbal processing: semantic processing or willed action? *Neuroreport* **5**, 2193–2196.

Levelt, W.J.M., Praamstra, P., Meyer, A.S., Helenius, P. & Salmelin, R. (1998): A MEG study of picture naming. *Journal of Cognitive Neuroscience* **10**, 533–567.

Levelt, W.J.M., Roelofs, A. & Meyer, A.S. (1999): A theory of lexical access in speech production. *Behav. Brain Sci.* **22**, 1–75.

Liberman, A.M., Cooper, F.S., Shankweiler, D.S. & Studdert-Kennedy, M. (1967): Perception of the speech code. *Psychological Review* **74**, 431–461.

Lurito, J.T., Kareken, D.A., Lowe, M.J., Chen, S.H.A. & Mathews, V.P. (2000): Comparison of rhyming and word generation with FMRI. *Hum. Brain Mapp.* **10**, 99–106.

Maldjian, J.A., Laurienti, P.J., Kraft, R.A. & Burdette, J.H. (2003) An automated method for neuroanatomic and cytoarchitectonic atlas-based interrogation of fMRI data sets. *Neuroimage* **19**, 1233–1239.

Martin, A., Wiggs, C.L., Ungerleider, L.G. & Haxby, J.V. (1996): Neural correlates of category-specific knowledge. *Nature* **379**, 649–652.

Matthews, P.M., Adcock, J., Chen, Y., Fu, S., Devlin, J.T., Rushworth, M.F.S., Smith, S., Beckmann, C. & Iversen, S. (2003): Towards understanding language organisation in the brain using fMRI. *Hum. Brain Mapp.* **18**, 239–247.

Mechelli, A., Gorno-Tempini, M.L. & Price, C.J. (2003) Neuroimaging studies of words and pseudoword reading: consistencies, inconsistencies, and limitations. *J. Cogn. Neurosci.* **15**, 260–271.

Miceli, G., Turriziani, P., Caltagirone, C., Capasso, R., Tomaiuolo, F. & Caramazza, A. (2002): The neural correlates of grammatical gender: an fMRI investigation. *J. Cogn. Neurosci.* **14**, 618–628.

Moro, A., Tettamanti, M., Perani, D., Donati, C., Cappa, S.F. & Fazio, F. (2001): Syntax and the brain: disentangling grammar by selective anomalies. *Neuroimage* **13**, 110–118.

Murtha, S., Chertkow, H., Beauregard, M. & Evans, A. (1999): The neural substrate of picture naming. *J. Cogn. Neurosci.* **11**, 399–423.

Nickels, L. & Howard, D. (1995): Phonological errors in aphasic naming: comprehension, monitoring and lexicality. *Cortex* **31**, 209–237.

Nobre, A.C., Price, C.J., Turner, R. & Friston, K. (1997): Selective processing of nouns and functions words in the human brain. *Neuroimage* **5**, 53.

Noesselt, T., Shah, N.J. & Jäncke, L. (2003): Top-down and bottom-up modulation of language-related areas – an fMRI study. *BMC Neurosci.* **4**, 13.

Omura, K., Tsukamoto, T., Kotani, Y., Ohgami, Y. & Yoshikawa, K. (2004): Neural correlates of phoneme-to-grapheme conversion. *Neuroreport* **15**, 949–953.

Perani, D., Cappa, S., Schnur, T., Tettamanti, M., Colina, S., Rosa, M.M. & Fazio, F. (1999): The neural correlates of verb and noun processing. A PET study. *Brain* **122**, 2337–2344.

Pickering, M.J., Branigan, H.P., Cleland, A.A. & Steward, A.J. (2000): Activation of syntactic information during language production. *Journal of Psycholinguistic Research* **29**, 205–216.

Poldrack, R.A., Wagner, A.D., Prull, M.W., Desmond, J.E., Glover, G.H. & Gabrieli, J.D.E. (1999): Functional specialization for semantic and phonological processing in the left inferior prefrontal cortex. *Neuroimage* **10**, 15–35.

Postma, A. (2000): Detection of errors during speech production: a review of speech monitoring models. *Cognition* **77**, 97–131.

Price, C.J., Moore, C.J. & Friston, K.J. (1997): Subtractions, conjunctions, and interactions in experimental design of activation studies. *Hum. Brain Mapp.* **5**, 264–272.

Rodriguez-Fornells, A., Schmitt, B.M., Kutas, M. & Münte, T.F. (2002): Electrophysiological estimates of the time course of semantic and phonological encoding during listening and naming. *Neuropsychologia* **40**, 778–787.

Rumsey, J.M., Horwitz, B., Donohue, B.C., Nace, K., Maisog, J.M. & Andreason, P. (1997) Phonological and orthographic components of word recognition. *Brain* **120**, 739–759.

Schiller, N.O., Münte, T.F., Horemans, I. & Jansma, B.M. (2003): The influence of semantic and phonological factors on syntactic decisions: an event-related brain potential study. *Psychophysiology* **40**, 869–877.

Schleicher, A., Amunts, K., Geyer, S., Morosan, P. & Zilles, K. (1999) Observer-independent method for microstructural parcellation of cerebral cortex: a quantitative approach to cytoarchitectonics *Neuroimage* **9**, 165–177.

Schmitt, B.M., Münte, T.F. & Kutas, M. (2000): Electrophysiological estimates of the time course of semantic and phonological encoding during implicit picture naming. *Psychophysiology* **37**, 473–484.

Seghier, M.L., Lazeyras, F., Pegna, A.J., Annoni, J.M., Zimine, I., Mayer, E., Michel, C.M. & Khateb, A. (2004): Variability of fMRI activation during a phonological and semantic language task in healthy subjects. *Hum. Brain Mapp.* **23**, 140–155.

Stromswold, K., Caplan, D., Alpert, N. & Rauch, S. (1996): Localization of syntactic comprehension by positron emission tomography. *Brain Lang.* **52**, 452–473.

Swick, D. & Knight, R.T. (1996): Is prefrontal cortex involved in cued recall? A neuropsychological test of PET findings. *Neuropsychologia* **34**, 1019–1028.

Szatkowska, I., Grabowska, A. & Szymańska, O. (2000): Phonological and semantic fluencies are mediated by different regions of the prefrontal cortex. *Acta Neurobiol. Exp. (Wars)* **60**, 503–508.

Talairach, J. & Tournoux, P. (1988): *Co-planar stereotaxic atlas of the human brain*. Stuttgart: Thieme.

Thompson-Schill, S.L., D'Esposito, M. & Kan, I.P. (1999): Effects of repetition and competition on activity in left prefrontal cortex during word generation. *Neuron* **23**, 513–522.

Thompson-Schill, S.L., D'Esposito, M., Aguirre, G.K. & Farah, M.J. (1997): Role of left inferior prefrontal cortex in retrieval of semantic knowledge: a reevaluation. *Proc. Natl. Acad. Sci. USA* **94**, 14792–14797.

Unsworth, S.J. & Pexman, P.M. (2003): The impact of reader skill on phonological processing in visual word recognition. *Q. J. Exp. Psychol. Sect. A* **56**, 63–81.

van Turennout, M., Hagoort, P. & Brown, C.M. (1997): Electrophysiological evidence on the time course of semantic and phonological processes in speech production. *J. Exp. Psychol. Learn. Mem. Cogn.* **23**, 787–806.

van Turennout, M., Hagoort, P. & Brown, C.M. (1998): Brain activity during speaking: from syntax to phonology in 40 milliseconds. *Science* **280**, 572–574.

Vandenberghe, R., Price, C., Wise, R., Josephs, O. & Frackowiak, R.S.J. (1996): Functional anatomy of a common semantic system for words and pictures. *Nature* **383**, 254–256.

Wagner, A.D., Desmond, J.E., Demb, J.B., Glover, G.H. & Gabrieli, J.D.E. (1997): Semantic repetition priming for verbal and pictorial knowledge: a functional MRI study of left inferior prefrontal cortex. *J. Cogn. Neurosci.* **9**, 714–726.

Wernicke, C. (1874): *Der Aphasische Symptomenkomplex*. Breslau: Cohn & Weigart.

Wilson, S.M., Saygin, A.P., Sereno, M.I. & Iacoboni, M. (2004): Listening to speech activates motor areas involved in speech production. *Nat. Neurosci.* **7**, 701–702.

Zatorre, R.J., Evans, A.C., Meyer, E. & Gjedde, A. (1992): Lateralization of phonetic and pitch discrimination in speech processing. *Science* **256**, 846–849.

Zatorre, R.J., Meyer, E., Gjedde, A. & Evans, A.C. (1996): PET studies of phonetic processing in speech: Review, replication, and reanalysis. *Cereb. Cortex* **6**, 21–30.

Ziegler, J.C., Tan, L.H., Perry, C. & Montant, M. (2000): Phonology matters: the phonological frequency effect in written Chinese. *Psychol. Sci.* **11**, 234–238.

Zilles, K., Schleicher, A., Palomero-Gallagher, N. & Amunts, K. (2002) Quantitative analysis of cyto- and receptor architecture of the human brain. In: *Brain mapping, the methods*, 2nd edition, ed. J. Mazziotta & A. Toga, pp. 573–602. San Diego: Academic Press.

Chapter 7

Developmental changes in human cerebral functional organization for word generation

Timothy T. Brown[1,2], Heather M. Lugar[2,3], Rebecca S. Coalson[2,3], Fran M. Miezin[2], Steven E. Petersen[1,2,3,4] and Bradley L. Schlaggar[2,3,4,5]

[1] Department of Psychology; [2] Department of Neurology;
[3] Department of Radiology; [4] Department of Anatomy and Neurobiology;
[5] Department of Pediatrics, Washington University School of Medicine, 660 S. Euclid, Box 8111,
St Louis, MO 63110, USA
schlaggarb@neuro.wustl.edu

Timothy T. Brown, Heather M. Lugar, Rebecca S. Coalson, Fran M. Miezin, Steven E. Petersen & Bradley L. Schlaggar (2005): 'Developmental Changes in Human Cerebral Functional Organization for Word Generation', *Cerebral Cortex* 15 (3), 275-290 (originally published online on August 5, 2004).
Cerebral Cortex V 15 N 3 © Oxford University Press 2004; Reproduced with permission from Oxford University Press.

Summary

A fundamental issue in cognitive neuroscience is the nature of developmental changes in human cerebral functional organization for higher cognitive functions. Event-related functional magnetic resonance imaging was used to measure developmental changes in the functional neuroanatomy subserving controlled lexical association. First, brain regions showing significant differences in activity between school-age children and young adults, despite equivalent task performance, were identified. Then, activity in these regions was more fully characterized in individuals spanning the ages of 7–32 years old. Cross-sectional and regression analyses showed systematic increases and decreases in levels of activity over age, by region. Age-related increases in activity were primarily newly recruited, later-stage processing regions, such as in left frontal and left parietal cortex. Decreases, on the other hand, were all positive activations that attenuated with age and were found across a wider neuroanatomical range, including earlier processing regions such as bilateral extrastriate cortex. The haemodynamic magnitude, neuroanatomical location and maturational timecourse of these progressive and regressive changes have implications for models of the developing specialization in human cerebral functional organization.

Introduction

The human brain likely undergoes dramatic changes in its functional organization in relation to cognitive development. The nature of these changes is a fundamental issue in cognitive neuroscience. A better understanding of maturational changes in human cerebral functional organization might inform our view of cognitive development, give insight into the mature organization, and could potentially lead to new ways of identifying, remedying and possibly preventing developmental cognitive disorders.

Theories of the relationship between brain maturation and cognitive development have emphasized both progressive and regressive neural mechanisms of change – i.e. regions of the brain becoming increasingly or decreasingly involved in cognitive tasks with age. Scientists have proposed competing views that either regressive or progressive neurobiological changes are the principal mechanism underlying cognitive growth. Often referred to as 'selectionist' and 'constructivist' traditions, several such models have been outlined in detail (e.g. Hebb, 1949; Jerne, 1967; Changeux & Danchin, 1976; Gottlieb, 1976; Mehler, 1985; Edelman, 1987; Greenough et al., 1987; Quartz & Sejnowski, 1997; Bourgeois, 2001; see also Thelen & Smith, 1994; Elman et al., 1996).

For example, according to the selective stabilization hypothesis proposed by Changeux and Danchin (1976), cortical connectivity progresses from greater to fewer connections by way of regressive phenomena. Mechanisms that are largely intrinsic control the initial formation of large pools of synaptic contacts. Extrinsic, evoked activity largely determines the subsequent stabilization of the most active synapses and the elimination of the less active ones. In the 'constructivist manifesto' proposed by Quartz and Sejnowski (1997), on the other hand, connectivity progresses from fewer to greater connections. According to this model, spontaneous activity and patterns of evoked activity cause the formation of new synapses (through dendritic and axonal arborization and other mechanisms) and bias elaboration of the structural organization. The losses of neurons and synapses, in their view, are simply epiphenomenal. These theories, though often highly specified in terms of purported underlying mechanisms, have not drawn heavily on human developmental evidence that links brain measures with behavior.

Studies of human neuroanatomical growth have also focused on both progressive and regressive changes and have provided evidence that different brain structures mature at different rates. Although limited in humans, available evidence suggests frontal brain regions develop more slowly than other regions, maturing even into late adolescence. For example, measures of myelination (Yakovlev & Lecours, 1967; Dobbing & Sands, 1973; Klingberg et al., 1999), synaptic density and pruning (Huttenlocher & Dabholkar, 1997), and gray to white matter proportions (Jernigan et al., 1991; Pfefferbaum et al., 1994; Giedd et al., 1999; Sowell et al., 2003) all show protracted development of frontal cortex.

There is still relatively little empirical evidence demonstrating developmental changes in human cerebral functional organization. Positron emission tomographic (PET) studies have corroborated structural evidence, showing delayed maturation of frontal resting metabolic rates relative to other cortical regions (Chugani et al., 1987). Functional magnetic resonance imaging (fMRI) studies comparing healthy school-age children and young adults during controlled processing tasks have largely confirmed the general belief that frontal maturation is involved (Casey et al., 1995, 1997, 2002; Thomas et al., 1999; Gaillard et al., 2000, 2003; Holland et al., 2001; Luna et al., 2001; Bunge et al., 2002; Klingberg et al., 2002; Kwon et al., 2002; Schlaggar et al., 2002b; Tamm et al., 2002; Booth et al., 2003). These studies, to varying degrees, have found both progressive and regressive changes in the developing functional neuroanatomy. Nevertheless, they have not concentrated on a functional distinction between these two kinds of change.

Regardless of the specific underlying mechanisms, fMRI can be used to characterize and compare progressive and regressive changes over development in several ways. Haemodynamic response timecourses can be used to distinguish different kinds of involvement among brain regions that change over development. For example, among regions that show increases with age in levels of activity for the same tasks, regions that are not activated by children but activated by adults would be interpreted to play a different functional role than regions that are deactivated by children and not activated by adults. Likewise, information on differences between progressive and regressive developmental changes in neuroanatomical location and in developmental timing (i.e. the rate at which activity matures) would help to develop a functional distinction between them.

The purpose of the present study was to explore this functional distinction by providing an empirical characterization of progressive and regressive developmental changes in the functional brain organization underlying controlled lexical association. Because of their simplicity and flexibility for use in a variety of experimental paradigms, controlled lexical association or word generation tasks have been commonly used with healthy subjects and diverse clinical groups, across many ages (e.g. Petersen *et al.*, 1988, 1990; Posner *et al.*, 1988; Wise *et al.*, 1991; McCarthy *et al.*, 1993; Petersen & Fiez, 1993; Raichle *et al.*, 1994; Buckner *et al.*, 1995; Passingham, 1996; Seger *et al.*, 1997; Thompson-Schill *et al.*, 1998; Barch *et al.*, 2000; Holland *et al.*, 2001; Ojemann *et al.*, 2002; Schlaggar *et al.*, 2002b; Burton *et al.*, 2003; Corina *et al.*, 2003; Gaillard *et al.*, 2003). These tasks are among the most frequently studied and perhaps best characterized in functional neuroimaging. They, therefore, provide a particularly reliable context in which to build developmental theory.

In order to test for effects in a way that allows distinctions to be made among various types of developmental change, we combined several conceptual and methodological features. First, levels of brain activity were measured and analyzed as haemodynamic response timecourses in an event-related design, not as relative differences between children and adults. This provided a check for the physiological plausibility of observed effects and allowed for the dissociation of regions that are activated, not activated or deactivated across age – distinctions that are key to the current purpose. Second, we tested for effects that were statistically reliable across several related tasks, allowing for the identification of developmental changes that are general to these controlled lexical task types. The focus of this report is not on differences among these tasks but rather in their functional neuroanatomical and developmental commonalities. Third, we employed an approach for exploring the potentially confounding effects of task performance discrepancy during imaging, thereby increasing the confidence with which we could interpret differences across age as being related to changes in functional brain organization. Finally, we used both cross-sectional and regression analysis approaches in a rather large sample size, providing measures of the rates of functional maturation for all developing regions. By investigating developmental changes in the functional neuroanatomy of word generation in this way, we hoped to advance the current understanding of the functional brain changes associated with the development of controlled cognition.

Materials and methods

General methods

Subjects

Ninety-five healthy individuals 7–32 years old served as participants in the study. All were right-handed native English speakers. All adult subjects gave informed consent, and subjects under the age of 18 gave assent with parental informed consent. Individuals with metal implants, heart arrhythmias, claustrophobia or a history of head trauma, neurological or psychiatric illness, including the use of psychotropic medications, were excluded. Adult subjects were screened by interview and questionnaire. Minor subjects were examined by a pediatric neurologist (BLS) and screened for neurological, psychiatric and medical problems that may impact on development. To document intellectual level, minor participants were administered the Wechsler Abbreviated Scale of Intelligence (Wechsler, 1999) by a neuropsychologist at St

Louis Children's Hospital. Adult participants were college students and graduates, graduate and medical students, and one postdoctoral fellow, mostly from Washington University. Adult intellectual levels were calculated using established full-scale IQ estimates based on educational attainment (Matarazzo, 1972). Children were acclimated to the MRI environment through the use of a mock scanner several days prior to the experiment. The study was approved by the Washington University Human Studies Committee and all subjects were reimbursed for their participation.

Word generation tasks

All subjects were scanned while performing three controlled lexical association tasks: (1) verb generation in response to a noun (e.g. stimulus: 'CAR', a correct response: 'drive'); (2) opposite generation (e.g. stimulus: 'UP', a correct response: 'down'); and (3) rhyme generation (e.g. stimulus: 'HAT', a correct response: 'cat'). These tasks were chosen because they are similar to those previously employed in many adult studies, and the neural substrates underlying these tasks are thought to undergo significant development across the ages we studied here.

While in the scanner, stimuli for the three tasks were presented to participants in both visual and auditory modalities. Therefore, all participants completed a total of six task runs. Subjects were asked to generate single word responses aloud to stimulus words that either appeared on a screen or were heard through headphones. They were instructed to give each response as quickly and accurately as possible and to minimize head movement, even while speaking. Subjects' overt verbal responses were recorded during scanning, allowing reaction times and accuracy to be measured, as previously described (Nelles *et al.*, 2003). Each word was presented every second, third or fourth MR frame (T_R = 3.08 s; average interstimulus interval = 9.24 s) in pseudo-random fashion. This jittering allowed the event-related timecourse of the response to be extracted (Miezin *et al.*, 2000).

Visual stimulus duration was relatively prolonged to aid reading (1.37 s) and auditory stimuli varied by word length. Each run lasted 3 min 39 s and consisted of 21 stimulus trials (i.e. 21 words were presented), followed by ~90 s of rest between runs. Each run included only one task type with words presented only in one sensory modality. Task runs were presented in a pseudo-randomized order across subjects. Words were white on black, and each letter subtended ~0.5°. A fixation crosshair was presented in the center of the screen at the beginning of each run and remained on the screen for the duration of the run, except when replaced by a visual stimulus word. For auditory tasks, the crosshair remained on the screen. Subjects were asked to maintain visual fixation on the crosshair. Word lists were counterbalanced for syllables, and words were presented in random order. Stimulus words were derived from available lists of US children's first-encountered reading words.

Imaging data acquisition and preprocessing

Functional and structural neuroimaging data were collected on a Siemens 1.5 Tesla MAGNETOM Vision system (Erlangen, Germany) as previously described (Miezin *et al.*, 2000). Rapid three-dimensional high-resolution structural images were acquired using a sagittal magnetization-prepared rapid gradient echo (MP-RAGE) sequence (slice T_E = 4 ms, T_R = 9.7 ms, T_I = 300 ms, flip angle = 12°, 128 slices, 1.25 × 1 × 1 mm voxels). Functional data were collected parallel to the anterior commissure–posterior commissure plane using an asymmetric spin-echo echo-planar pulse sequence sensitive to blood oxygenation level-dependent (BOLD) contrast (T_R = 3.08 s, T_2^* evolution time = 50 ms, flip angle = 90°). During each scan, 73 frames of 16 contiguous interleaved 8 mm axial slices were acquired (3.75 × 3.75 mm in-plane resolution), allowing complete brain coverage. Steady state was assumed after three frames (~9 s). Thus, acquisition of functional imaging data began with the fourth frame of each run.

Preliminary automated image data processing was carried out in order to remove noise and artifacts (see Miezin *et al.*, 2000, for detailed procedures). This preprocessing included removal of a single pixel spike caused by signal offset, whole-brain normalization of signal intensity across MR frames, correction for subject movement within and across runs, and slice-by-slice normalization to correct for changes in signal intensity introduced by the acquisition of interleaved slices.

Prior to statistical analysis, functional (BOLD) data were registered to the structural (MP-RAGE) data for a given subject. Importantly, data for all subjects were transformed into the same standard stereotactic space (based on Talairach & Tournoux, 1988), allowing direct voxel-wise statistical comparisons to be made. It has been assumed that the variability in children's structural and functional neuroanatomy and brain size is sufficient to preclude direct statistical comparisons with adults within the same stereotactic space. Recent empirical studies demonstrate, however, that these differences are below a level that would adversely affect results in most current fMRI experiments (Muzik *et al.*, 2000; Burgund *et al.*, 2002; Schlaggar *et al.*, 2002b; Kang *et al.*, 2003).

To encourage minimal movement, subjects were positioned in the scanner using a thermoplastic mask individually fitted to the face and attached to the head coil. Subject motion was corrected and quantified using an analysis of head position based on rigid body translation and rotation. The data derived from the adjustments needed to realign head movement on a frame-by-frame basis were calculated as root mean square (RMS) values for translation and rotation in the x, y and z planes in millimeters. Total RMS values were calculated on a run-by-run basis for each subject derived from deviations from the initial position for each run. For each subject, a median RMS was calculated for the six runs. Median RMS values ranged from 0.19 to 1.37 mm, with an average of 0.47 mm of movement over all tasks and subjects. Median RMS was negatively correlated with age, showing that head motion decreased with increasing subject age ($r = -0.57$, $P < 0.001$).

Imaging data analyses

Statistical analyses of event-related fMRI data were based on the general linear model (GLM) as previously described (Miezin *et al.*, 2000; Schlaggar *et al.*, 2002b), conducted using in-house software programmed in the Interactive Data Language (IDL; Research Systems, Inc., Boulder, CO). The purpose of the present study was to identify common functional neuroanatomical and developmental aspects of controlled lexical association across the three task types and across visual and auditory stimulus modalities. Studies in adults comparing lexical tasks requiring phonological *versus* semantic association have shown considerable overlap in their patterns of activation (Klein *et al.*, 1995; Duncan & Owen, 2000; McDermott *et al.*, 2003). Likewise, in direct comparisons among verb-, opposite- and rhyme-generation tasks, we have found similarities in recruited regions across these tasks for both children and adults (Schlaggar *et al.*, 2002b). In addition, preliminary studies have yielded very few regions that show stimulus modality effects in these tasks. In a brain-wide direct statistical comparison, only four regions showed modality specificity – all in extrastriate cortex (Schlaggar *et al.*, 2002a). So, although important for future studies, a characterization of individual task and modality effects is orthogonal to the scope of the current inquiry. Therefore, for the present purposes, we combined imaging data for each subject across verb-, opposite- and rhyme-generation tasks, and across visual and auditory stimuli. Importantly, all analyses for all subjects included functional imaging data only for trials in which correct behavioral responses were made. In this way, all comparisons included only brain responses reflecting successful task performance.

The GLM design included time as a seven-level factor, made up of the seven MR frames following presentation of the stimulus. Since no assumptions were made regarding the shape of the haemodynamic response function (HRF), this allowed detection of a BOLD response with any shape over time. The HRF (% BOLD signal change as a function of time) was modeled over a period of ~21 s (7 frames, 3.08 s per frame). For all analyses, timecourse values were entered into an ANOVA using a random effects model. A significant effect of time indicated that the detected haemodynamic response was not a flat line across the seven frames.

Timecourses for all subjects across all regions were screened for highly aberrant values, blind to age. Outlier timecourses were defined as those showing any time point with greater than 2 per cent signal change. Regions containing 10 or more outlying timecourses across subjects were removed from subsequent analyses. All regions removed in this way were at or near the edges of brain space. Regions showing fewer than 10 outlying timecourses were retained, but data from those particular subjects were removed for analyses of that region. Regions that showed effects but were determined by close inspection of the group anatomical average to be squarely within white matter or ventricle were also removed.

For all voxel-wise analyses, a correction based on Monte Carlo simulation was implemented to guard against false positives that may result from conducting a large number of statistical comparisons over many images (Forman *et al.*, 1995; McAvoy *et al.*, 2001). To achieve $P < 0.05$ corrected for voxel clusters, we used a threshold of 24 contiguous voxels with a z-value > 3.5. For all region-wise analyses, Box's sphericity correction was used, adjusting for temporal autocorrelation and possible inhomogeneity of variance over the repeated measure (i.e. time).

Analysis step 1: Identification of brain regions showing age/performance-independent, performance-related and age-related effects using endpoint age groups

Subjects

In order to identify brain regions showing different functional relation-ships between childhood and adulthood, we began with two 'endpoint' age groups made up of only our youngest and oldest subjects. Twenty-six adults (13 male, 13 female; aged 18–32, mean age 24.9) and 32 children (14 male, 18 female; aged 7–10, mean age 9.3) were included. Using an approach similar to that of Schlaggar *et al.* (2002b), we used performance matching in order to identify regions showing three different kinds of responses: (i) age/performance-independent effects; (ii) performance-related effects; and (iii) age-related effects.

In regions showing age/performance-independent effects, children and adults show statistically comparable responses regardless of differences in levels of task performance (as measured by reaction time and accuracy). Regions showing performance-related effects are those where children and adults show differences in activity only in subjects who show statistically differing task performance. In other words, these brain regions appear to be used similarly by children and adults when they perform similarly. Performance-related regions are those where differences, if performance matching were not done, would likely be mistakenly attributed to maturational differences in functional organization. Brain regions showing age-related effects, on the other hand, are regions where children and adults show significant differences in activity even when they exhibit statistically indistinguishable behavioral performance. Voxel-level analyses were used to test brain-wide for candidate regions showing these three effect types, and region-level analyses were used to extract precise timecourses of activity and to verify the specific functional relations.

Identification of age/performance-independent effects

In order to identify brain regions that show statistically equivalent activation between children and adults, we first tested for a main effect of time in the ANOVA model. The most highly significant main effects of time constitute timecourses that are likely to be (but are not necessarily) statistically similar between the two age groups. So, a voxel-wise main effect of time image was created. A peak-finding and region-defining algorithm was then used to obtain center of mass and cluster coordinates for statistically significant voxels in the time image. Peaks were identified using a 4 mm hard sphere preblur and a statistical threshold of $z > 11.0$. Regions were then defined beginning with a radius of 10 mm, searching for significant voxel clusters around the peaks that surpassed the Monte Carlo correction, and then consolidating regions with extremes closer than 10 mm. Regions smaller than 24 voxels (the size of the Monte Carlo correction) were eliminated from further analysis. Negative-going main effects of time were also eliminated; for the present report, we sought regions where children and adults showed equivalent positive activations only. A region-wise ANOVA was then conducted on brain activity within the remaining regions of interest, comparing the endpoint child and adult groups. If there was no statistical difference between the adult and child timecourses, the region was considered to be age/performance independent.

Identification of performance-related and age-related effects

In order to test for overall group differences, age group was included as a between-subjects factor in the GLM. Thus, an age group (2 levels: child/adult) × time (7 levels: BOLD measures every ~3 s for ~21 s) ANOVA model was used. An activation difference between children and adults was expressed, by region, as a significant group × time interaction. In other words, regions where adults and children differed were those in which the haemodynamic response over time differed across the two age groups. Peaks were identified and regions were defined in the age group × time image using the same algorithm and parameters applied to the main effect of time image, this time with a statistical threshold of $z > 3.0$.

We next sought to distinguish regions that differed across age regardless of performance (age-related regions) from regions that showed age differences related to performance discrepancy (performance-related regions). Although the child and adult groups differed on average in their task performance as measured by percent correct (% cor) and reaction time (RT) ($t = 7.10$, $P < 0.001$; $t = 5.60$, $P < 0.001$, respectively), some subjects from each age group did not differ. From the original two groups, we selected a subset of 10 adults and 10 children who, during spontaneous task performance, were statistically equivalent in both % cor and RT, creating four total groups – performance-matched children and adults and non-matched children and adults (see Table 1).

It is important to note that we did not conduct performance matching at the trial level – i.e. choosing trials from across individuals where performance was the best and comparing it to trials in which performance was the worst. Rather, we simply capitalized on the spontaneous clustering of children and adults whose overall accuracy and reaction times during scanning were statistically indistinguishable and, therefore, suggested similar levels of ability and effort at the time of the study.

A region-wise ANOVA was then conducted to examine, in performance-matched and non-matched children and adults, task-related brain activity in the regions identified as showing

Table 1. Demographic and task performance characteristics of the 'endpoint' groups

	Children, ages 7–10		Adults, ages 18–32	
	Non-matched	Matched	Matched	Non-matched
n	22	10	10	16
Gender	12 F/10 M	6 F/4 M	5 F/5 M	8 F/8 M
Age (years)	9.4 (0.9)	9.2 (1.2)	22.7 (1.8)	26.3 (3.6)
% correct	69.1 (11.7)	76.2[a] (8.6)	82.7[a] (5.1)	92.6 (3.0)
RT (ms)	2236 (478)	1661[a] (257)	1556[a] (265)	1390[a] (236)
Verbal IQ	121[a] (12)	123[a] (15)	–	–
Perf IQ	109[a] (12)	114[a] (17)	–	–
Full Scale IQ	117[a] (11)	121[a] (17)	116[a] (13)	118[a] (12)

[a] Statistically equivalent across groups by ANOVA, $P \setminus 0.05$.

significant group differences overall. This investigation of performance allowed us to classify these brain regions as showing effects that were likely driven by either age group or performance. Performance-related regions were identified as those that showed an age difference for performance non-matched groups but showed no significant difference when performance was matched. In other words, performance, not age, appeared to be driving the differences in these regions. Age-related regions, on the other hand, were defined as those regions that exhibited a difference between children and adults for both matched and non-matched groups. These regions showed statistically robust differences in brain activity even in children and adults who showed statistically equivalent task performance.

Analysis Step 2: Characterization of brain activity in age-related regions over development using cross-sectional and regression analyses

Subjects

In order to explore how task-related brain activity in the 40 age-related regions of interest changes over maturation, we then conducted analyses using BOLD data from all 95 subjects across all ages, filling in the age range between our endpoint groups. Using both cross-sectional and regression analysis approaches by age, we sought a more complete characterization of the developing functional neuroanatomy for controlled lexical association.

Cross-sectional analysis by age group

The 95 participants were divided into six groups of similar size based on age: (1) 7–8 year olds; (2) 9–10 year olds; (3) 11–13 year olds; (4) 14–15 year olds; (5) 16–22 year olds; and (6) 23–32 year olds (see Table 2). These six groupings allowed the measurement of finer developmental changes at younger ages and were statistically balanced for gender ($\chi^2 = 4.65$, $P = 0.46$) and IQ (ANOVA, VIQ $P = 0.14$; PIQ $P = 0.07$; FSIQ $P = 0.30$).

We then performed region-wise ANOVAs across all 40 age-related regions of interest and extracted average timecourses of brain activity for each of the six age groups. All of the regions were characterized according to the specific changes they exhibited in the direction and hemodynamic shape of their BOLD responses over development. Using a combination of statistical reliability and a measure of signal magnitude, we classified the responses at each region for each age group as statistically positive, negative or flat over time. In order for a group's regional timecourse to be considered an activation or deactivation, it was required that activity show a significant effect over time (by ANOVA, corrected for multiple tests and nonsphericity), and

Table 2. Forty-three brain regions showing age/performance-independent effects in children and adults

x	y	z	Size (cm³)	Location	Approx. Brodmann area
Left					
−44	6	26	3.91	frontal	9
−40	−4	34	3.63	frontal	6
−39	16	−2	3.42	frontal	13
−29	41	26	3.75	frontal	10
−25	30	23	3.81	frontal	9
−1	10	41	4.22	med. front./ant. cing.	32
−40	−39	26	3.68	parietal	40
−19	−35	54	4.14	parietal	3
−28	−57	43	3.72	parietal	7
0	−45	41	3.71	med. par./post. cing.	31
−9	−70	−11	3.70	med. occip./med. temp.	18
−9	−45	−4	3.44	med. occip./med. temp.	30
−6	−76	5	3.55	med. occip./med. temp.	18
−54	−22	3	4.22	occipital/temporal	41
−52	−41	9	4.02	occipital/temporal	22
−49	8	1	3.88	occipital/temporal	22
−38	−35	11	3.87	occipital/temporal	41
−36	−59	−21	3.90	occipital/temporal	37
−22	−89	−10	3.88	occipital/temporal	18
−14	−58	−9	3.55	occipital/temporal	19
−31	−18	13	3.74	subcortical	−
−27	−23	0	3.71	subcortical	−
−22	−10	5	3.20	subcortical	−
−15	6	13	3.68	subcortical	−
−9	−24	2	4.07	subcortical	−
Right					
39	−3	33	3.72	frontal	6
33	−41	25	4.00	frontal	13
52	−10	25	3.95	parietal	43
26	−56	45	3.77	parietal	7
16	−35	52	3.93	parietal	5
6	−47	8	3.41	med. par./post. cing.	29
3	−34	45	3.48	med. par./post. cing.	7
8	−68	6	4.06	med. occip./med. temp.	18
7	−39	1	3.29	med. occip./med. temp.	30
2	−77	19	3.35	med. occip./med. temp.	18
55	−35	5	3.29	occipital/temporal	42
52	−24	0	3.34	occipital/temporal	41
47	−33	−8	3.14	occipital/temporal	22
24	−85	−2	3.30	occipital/temporal	18
30	−16	8	4.02	subcortical	−
19	−3	29	3.99	subcortical	−
17	−1	6	4.18	subcortical	−
9	−21		4.14	subcortical	−

that the timecourse exhibit a peak > 0.1 or < -0.1 percent signal change. Group timecourses not meeting both of these criteria were deemed to be statistically flat over time.

Across all subjects and all age-related regions, time point three (representing BOLD signal within the period from 6.17 to 9.24 s) showed the greatest variability and was almost invariably the point of peak magnitude for the BOLD response. Therefore, we used time point three to explore changes in peak brain activity and variability over age. Using Levene's test of equality of variance across the six age groups, we tested whether the variability in peak activity changes significantly over development.

Regression analysis by age

In order to fully utilize the information provided by this large sample size in the service of characterizing developmental changes, we also used regression analysis with curve fitting to show trends in regional brain activity over maturation. Data from all 95 subjects were entered into a regression model for each of the 40 age-related regions. Peak BOLD activity was modeled as a function of age to tenths of a year. Two nonlinear regression functions were found to optimally explain the data (maximize the coefficients of determination) without being over-parameterized (i.e. no dependencies equaled 1.0). For regions showing systematic increases in activity over age, a three-parameter, single-exponent rise to max function was used: $[y = y_0 + a(1 - e^{-bx})]$. For regions showing age-related decreases in activity, a complementary three-parameter, single-exponent decay function was used: $[y = y_0 + ae^{-bx}]$. Curves for these functions were fitted to the data, showing maturational trends in brain activity for each of the 40 developing regions.

These fitted curves also permitted a calculation of the rate at which brain activity becomes 'adult-like' within each of the maturing regions. Using the regression model for each region, we determined the ages at which peak activity became 50 per cent adult-like (i.e. reached a level that is 50 per cent of the total range observed over the youngest and oldest subjects) and 75 per cent adult-like.

Results

Analysis step 1

Our approach successfully identified and dissociated brain regions showing statistically reliable age/performance-independent effects, performance-related effects and age-related effects (see Fig. 1). Forty-three regions showed similar activation by children and adults, regardless of performance. These age/performance-independent regions were evident throughout the brain, in cortical and subcortical locations bilaterally (see Fig. 2). Using both inspection of the group-averaged anatomy and the Talairach Daemon atlas (Lancaster *et al.*, 2000), we classified the 43 regions according to their broad neuroanatomical locations and approximate Brodmann areas (see Table 2). Age/performance-independent effects were seen mostly in left and right frontal cortex, anterior and posterior cingulate, left, right and medial occipital and temporal cortex, and thalamus.

Seventy-seven brain regions showed statistically significant differences between children and adults. Of these, 37 regions showed differences between children and adults that were driven by performance (see Fig. 3 and Table 3). Performance-related regions were found predominantly in right and medial frontal cortex, medial parietal cortex, posterior cingulate, and left and right occipital cortex.

Forty brain regions were classified as showing age-related effects. These regions were divided according to whether adults or children showed greater activity (see Fig. 4 and Table 4). In other words, they could be classified according to whether brain activity 'grew up' or 'grew down'. The majority of regions – 30 out of 40 (75 per cent) – showed decreases in activity over age. These developmentally decreasing regions were distributed bilaterally and were evident most prominently in medial frontal and anterior cingulate cortex, right frontal cortex, medial parietal and posterior cingulate cortex, and bilateral occipito-parietal cortex. On the other hand, 10 of the 40 age-related brain regions (25 per cent) exhibited increases in activity over age. The majority of regions that showed significant developmental increases were found in left lateral and medial dorsal frontal cortex and left parietal cortex, including supramarginal gyrus.

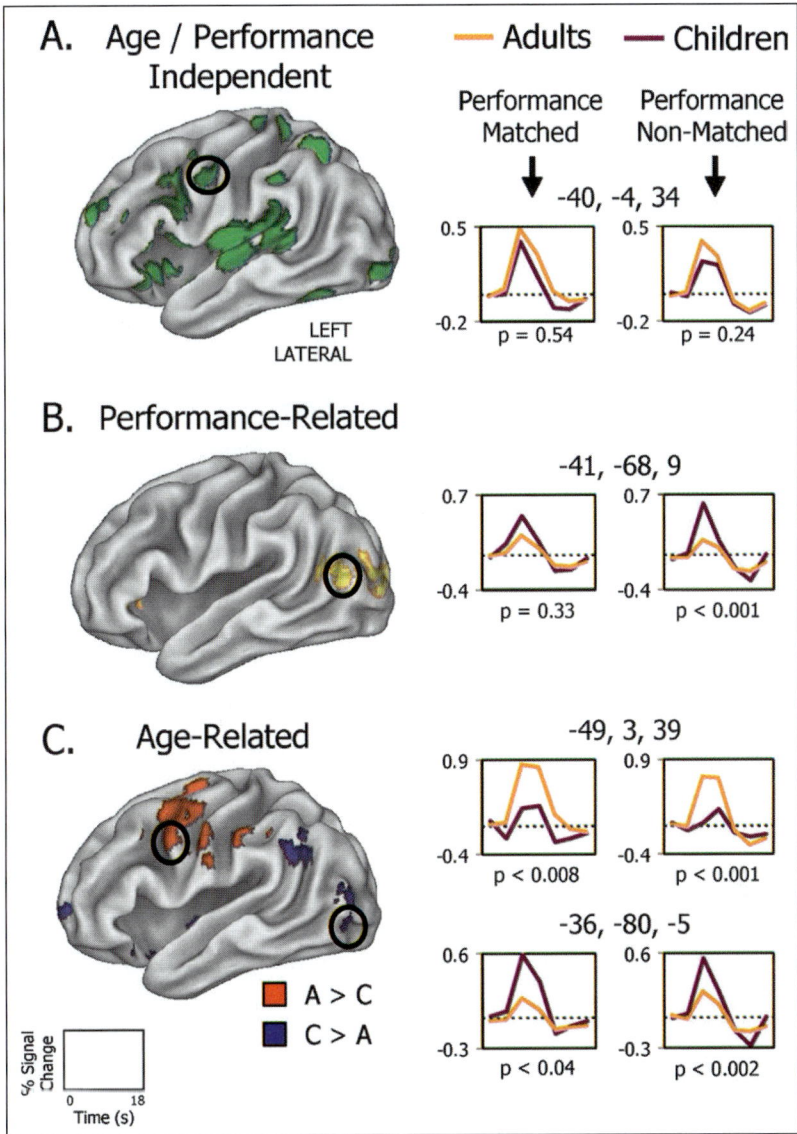

Figure 1. Three developmental functional relationships. The haemodynamic response function time-courses for performance matched and non-matched adults and children and the P-values derived from the group 3 time interactions are shown for four example regions derived from the ANOVA. Three of the regions are derived from the interaction image and one region is derived from the main effect of time image. The percentage of MR signal change is plotted against time in seconds (see legend icon in lower left). The numeric coordinates (e.g. −49, 3, 39) indicate the location of the center of mass of the region in standard atlas space. *(A)* Age/performance-independent effects. Regions that exhibited age/performance-independent effects are shown in green. The example region is indicated with an oval. *(B)* Performance-related effects. Regions that exhibited performance-related effects are shown in yellow, with the example region indicated by an oval. *(C)* Age-related regions. Regions that exhibited age-related effects are shown in red and blue. Red indicates regions where adults showed greater levels of activity than children and blue indicates regions where children showed greater activity than adults. One of each region type is indicated by ovals. All surface-rendered images were created using CARET software and surface-based atlases (Van Essen et al., 2001; Van Essen, 2002).

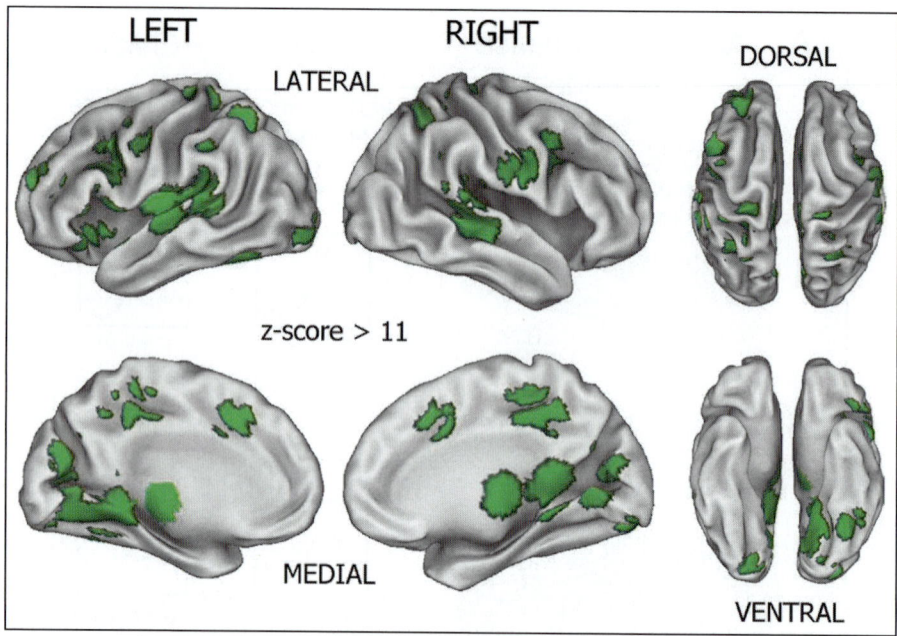

Figure 2. Age/performance-independent effects. Regions that exhibited positive age/performance-independent effects are shown in green (43 regions). These regions were activated by children and adults to a statistically equivalent degree, regardless of performance. All effects shown surpassed a z-statistic of 11.0, and negative-going timecourses (deactivations) were excluded.

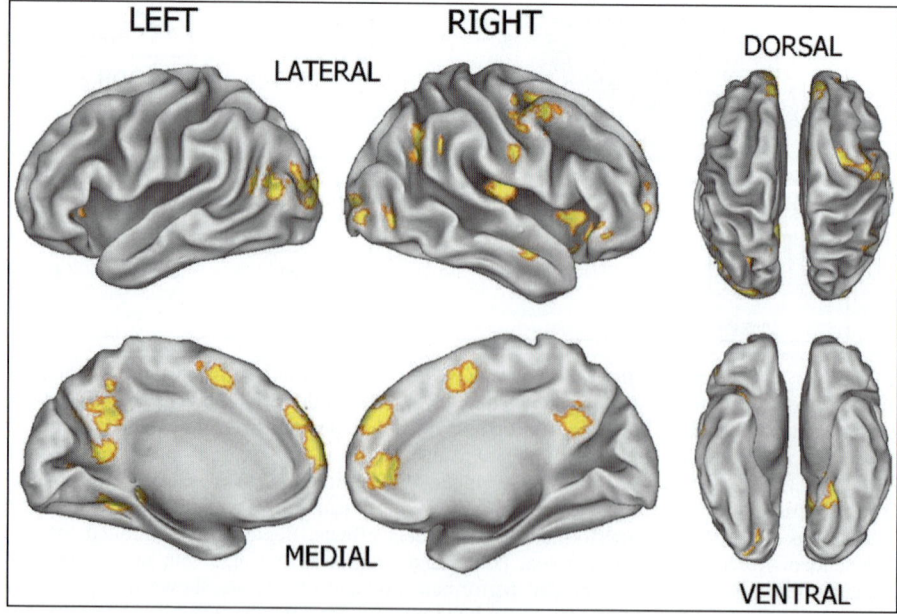

Figure 3. Performance-related effects. Regions that exhibited performance-related effects are shown in yellow (37 regions). These regions showed statistically significant differences in activity between performance non-matched children and adults, but not between matched children and adults (corrected ANOVAs, $P < 0.05$).

Table 3. Thirty-seven brain regions showing performance-related differences in children and adults

x	y	z	Size (cm³)	Location	Approx. Brodmann area
Left					
−32	22	5	0.23	frontal	13
−8	44	40	1.72	med. front./ant. cing.	8
−6	56	21	2.99	med. front./ant. cing.	9
−1	0	52	2.73	med. front./ant. cing.	6
−22	−62	27	0.44	parietal	7
−9	−56	40	0.56	med. par./post. cing.	7
−8	−62	29	0.98	med. par./post. cing.	31
−6	−52	29	1.40	med. par./post. cing.	31
−5	−55	12	1.00	med. par./post. cing.	29
−29	−58	9	1.06	med. occip./med. temp.	30
−28	−70	8	0.99	med. occip./med. temp.	30
−41	−68	9	1.51	occipital/temporal	19
−33	−82	15	0.34	occipital/temporal	19
−32	−93	2	0.62	occipital/temporal	18
−24	−44	−5	1.98	occipital/temporal	37
−20	−84	7	1.16	occipital/temporal	17
−18	−55	−7	0.44	occipital/temporal	19
−17	−98	8	1.17	occipital/temporal	18
Right					
51	−13	31	0.61	frontal	6
50	27	−2	0.21	frontal	47
44	4	49	0.97	frontal	6
41	−16	44	0.25	frontal	4
37	11	−13	0.22	frontal	13
33	−21	15	0.91	frontal	13
26	−5	49	1.31	frontal	6
19	49	11	1.45	frontal	10
7	48	39	2.74	med. front./ant. cing.	8
10	40	9	2.53	med. front./ant. cing.	32
43	−56	30	1.55	parietal	39
5	−54	29	1.18	med. par./post. cing.	31
61	−6	−14	0.42	occipital/temporal	21
38	−69	−4	0.51	occipital/temporal	19
31	−91	−2	1.45	occipital/temporal	18
22	−77	−4	0.31	occipital/temporal	18
31	8	0	1.74	subcortical	−
27	4	20	0.86	subcortical	−
24	16	3	1.78	subcortical	−

In order to ensure that a difference in power was not artificially driving the distinction between age-related and performance-related regions, we conducted an analysis of peak BOLD response magnitudes. For all of the regions showing the three different kinds of effects, we calculated the difference in peak BOLD signal magnitude between non-matched children and adults and subtracted from it the difference in peak BOLD signal magnitude between matched children and adults as follows: non-matched children − non-matched adults − Matched children − Matched adults. This index captures, for all regions, the degree to which the age difference in BOLD signal magnitude changes with performance. If our statistical classification is working reasonably well (i.e. is capturing haemodynamic differences as opposed to being driven merely by power differences), age-related regions should show a stable BOLD magnitude relationship across performance, and performance-related regions should show BOLD magnitude differences across levels of performance.

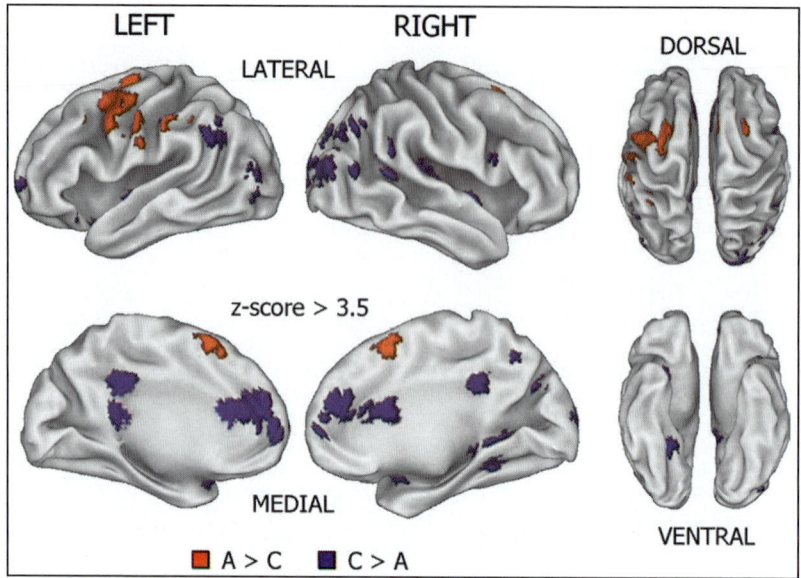

Figure 4. Age-related effects. Regions that exhibited age-related effects are shown in red and blue (40 regions). Red indicates regions where adults showed greater levels of activity than children and blue indicates regions where children showed greater activity than adults. In all regions, performance-non-matched children and adults as well as matched children and adults showed statistically significant differences in activity that surpassed a z-statistic of 3.5.

Indeed, age- and performance-related regions showed precisely this relationship (see online Supplementary Material). The index of magnitude difference for age-related regions centered on a value near zero. Performance-related regions, in contrast, showed an index of magnitude difference that centers around 0.2% BOLD signal change, differing significantly from both age-related and age/performance-independent regions, which did not differ significantly from each other.

Analysis step 2

Cross-sectional analysis by age group

Age-related regions showed notable regularity in the specific patterns of change they exhibited over maturation (see Table 4 and Fig. 5). Among the regions decreasing over age, the most common pattern of change was activity that went from statistically positive in the youngest age group to significantly lower but still positive in the oldest age group (e.g. -36, -80, -5, left extrastriate cortex, ~BA 19). Fourteen of the 30 decreasing regions (47 per cent) demonstrated this pattern over age. The next most common pattern of developmental change in decreasing regions was activity that, again, began as significantly activated in the youngest children but diminished over age into a statistically flat line (e.g. –44, –55, 27, left occipital-temporal-parietal cortex, ~BA 39). These two developmental patterns – positive to smaller positive

Chapter 7 Developmental changes in human cerebral functional organization for word generation

Table 4. Forty brain regions showing age-related differences in children and adults

x	y	z	Size (cm³)	Location	Approximate Brodmann area	Activity 'grows'	Pattern of change (7–8 → 23–32)	Levene's statistic	P	Regression F	Regression P	Regression R²	Age adult-like 50%	Age adult-like 75%
Left														
−53	−12	40	1.70	frontal	4	up	pos → POS	1.1	0.365	20.2	\0.0001	0.31	12.5	15.5
−49	3	39	1.47	frontal	6	up	flat → POS	0.8	0.540	16.4	\0.0001	0.26	11.8	15.6
−41	−13	−2	0.36	frontal	13	down	POS → flat	0.9	0.484	9.9	\0.0001	0.18	11.6	14.3
−39	−4	48	2.66	frontal	6	up	NEG → POS	3.3	0.010	29.2	\0.0001	0.39	10.4	12.6
−25	3	50	2.24	frontal	6	up	NEG → POS	4.1	0.002	29.6	\0.0001	0.39	10.2	12.3
−24	−12	56	1.65	frontal	6	up	flat → POS	2.9	0.018	17.6	\0.0001	0.28	11.1	13.5
−18	55	8	1.84	frontal	10	down	POS → NEG	1.1	0.384	14.5	\0.0001	0.25	11.8	14.7
−10	32	20	2.55	med. front./ant. cing.	32	down	POS → pos	2.3	0.051	23.3	\0.0001	0.34	11.9	15.4
−8	43	24	2.99	med. front./ant. cing.	9	down	POS → pos	2.2	0.060	21.9	\0.0001	0.32	11.3	14.6
−5	23	19	2.43	med. front./ant. cing.	24	down	POS → pos	2.4	0.045	17.2	\0.0001	0.27	13.3	17.3
−3	52	11	3.06	med. front./ant. cing.	10	down	POS → NEG	1.1	0.342	13.0	\0.0001	0.22	10.6	12.8
0	12	56	2.56	med. front./ant. cing.	6	up	NEG → POS	0.7	0.626	14.0	\0.0001	0.24	10.3	12.0
−60	−21	33	0.94	parietal	2	up	flat → POS	2.6	0.032	6.4	0.0026	0.12	14.8	20.5
−57	−27	41	1.26	parietal	2	up	flat → POS	3.8	0.004	11.3	\0.0001	0.20	16.1	19.8
−37	−44	37	0.42	parietal	40	up	pos → POS	2.3	0.048	3.4	0.0372	0.07	11.8	14.4
−35	−32	30	0.32	parietal	2	up	POS → flat	4.3	0.002	12.0	\0.0001	0.21	9.8	11.2
−12	−42	12	1.58	med. par./post. cing.	29	down	POS → flat	4.0	0.003	18.4	\0.0001	0.29	12.1	15.6
−5	−41	29	1.50	med. par./post. cing.	31	down	POS → pos	3.2	0.010	6.7	0.0020	0.13	14.4	18.5
−44	−55	27	1.80	occipital/temporal	39	down	POS → flat	1.8	0.125	10.3	\0.0001	0.18	13.5	17.5
−41	−85	7	0.89	occipital/temporal	19	down	POS → NEG	2.0	0.091	14.0	\0.0001	0.23	17.0	21.3
−37	7	−18	1.58	occipital/temporal	38	down	POS → NEG	0.8	0.579	27.0	\0.0001	0.37	11.2	14.2
−36	−80	−5	0.36	occipital/temporal	19	down	POS → pos	2.6	0.031	5.1	0.0078	0.10	13.6	18.5
Right														
50	6	20	0.32	frontal	44	down	POS → pos	5.0	\0.001	14.2	\0.0001	0.24	11.2	14.6
43	−43	15	1.66	frontal	13	down	POS → pos	2.0	0.080	13.2	\0.0001	0.22	16.0	20.1
40	−12	0	1.25	frontal	13	down	POS → flat	2.3	0.056	19.4	\0.0001	0.30	12.1	15.8
26	7	52	1.02	frontal	6	up	NEG → flat	2.7	0.024	19.6	\0.0001	0.30	10.0	11.9
10	38	23	3.42	med. front./ant. cing.	32	down	POS → pos	4.1	0.002	22.7	\0.0001	0.33	11.8	15.4
9	11	20	2.04	med. front./ant. cing.	33	down	POS → flat	2.3	0.054	16.7	\0.0001	0.27	13.7	18.2
40	−69	31	1.44	parietal	39	down	POS → flat	2.8	0.021	13.8	\0.0001	0.23	12.0	15.2
19	−72	27	0.50	med par/pcst cing	31	down	POS → pos	2.9	0.019	14.0	\0.0001	0.23	11.8	15.6
14	−39	30	1.35	med. par./post. cing.	31	down	POS → flat	3.5	0.007	10.4	\0.0001	0.18	13.2	17.4
11	−61	45	0.45	med. par./post. cing.	7	down	POS → pos	1.9	0.097	4.0	0.0213	0.08	15.3	19.6
52	−66	9	0.58	occipital/temporal	37	down	POS → flat	0.4	0.838	9.2	0.0002	0.17	11.6	16.4
37	−85	9	1.74	occipital/temporal	19	down	POS → flat	1.1	0.388	16.3	\0.0001	0.26	13.7	18.3
36	−32	12	0.81	occipital/temporal	41	down	POS → pos	2.5	0.036	14.2	\0.0001	0.24	10.8	13.1
28	2	−14	0.68	occipital/temporal	34	down	POS → flat	1.0	0.404	11.9	\0.0001	0.21	10.9	13.3
26	−82	26	0.66	occipital/temporal	19	down	POS → pos	3.1	0.014	19.6	\0.0001	0.30	14.3	19.4
26	−52	10	1.50	occipital/temporal	30	down	POS → flat	5.0	\0.001	11.7	\0.0001	0.20	12.4	16.2
26	−43	−5	2.23	occipital/temporal	19	down	POS → pos	5.6	\0.001	14.3	\0.0001	0.24	14.3	18.2
23	−95	7	2.26	occipital/temporal	18	down	POS → NEG	0.4	0.834	15.3	\0.0001	0.25	15.5	20.8

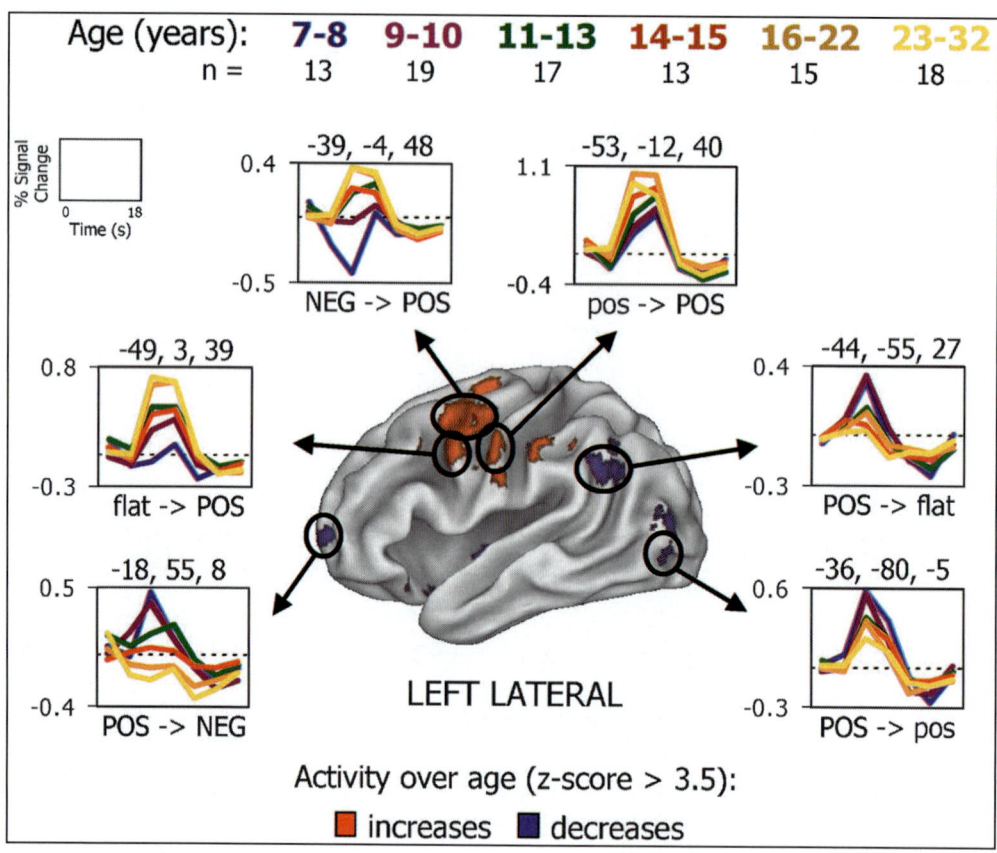

Figure 5. Age-related patterns of change in activity over development. Age-related effects took the form of several different patterns of change in the haemodynamic response function timecourses over development. Six example regions are shown, with the numeric coordinates (e.g. –49,3,39) indicating the location of the center of mass of the region in standard atlas space. For each region, timecourses of activity are shown for all six age groups (blue = 7–8 year olds, purple = 9–10, green = 11–13, red = 14–15, orange = 16–22, and yellow = 23–32). The percentage of MR signal change is plotted against time in seconds. Using a combination of statistical reliability and signal magnitude, the timecourse for each age group was characterized as showing significant positive change (activation), negative change (deactivation), or no change (a 'flat' line) over time. Regions are labelled according to the changes in activity that were observed between the youngest and oldeststage groups (7–8 and 23–32 year olds, respectively). These include activation becoming deactivation (POS → NEG), no activation becoming activation (flat → POS), deactivation becoming activation (NEG → POS), activation becoming significantly more activated (pos → POS), activation becoming no activation (POS → flat), and activation becoming significantly less activated (POS → pos) over maturation.

(POS → pos) and positive to flat (POS → flat) – together accounted for 25 (or 83 per cent) of the regions showing decreases in activity over maturation. The five remaining regions 'growing down' over age began as statistically positive activations in the youngest group and were deactivations in the oldest group (POS → NEG).

Among regions showing developmental increases, the most common pattern of change was activity that began in the youngest subjects as a statistically flat timecourse (i.e. not reliably activated during the tasks) and incremented over age into a significant positive activation for the oldest subjects (e.g. –49, 3, 39, left frontal cortex, ~BA 6). Four regions (out of 10 increasing over age) showed this maturational pattern (flat → POS). Three of the increasing regions changed over age from statistically negative-going activity to positive-going activity (NEG/POS, e.g. −39, −4, 48, left dorsal frontal cortex, ~BA 6). Two regions began as activations that grew up with age (pos → POS), and one region showed a change in its pattern of activity that began as negative and matured into no change from baseline (NEG/flat).

Left frontal cortex showed the most age-related increases in brain activity for these word generation tasks (see Fig. 6). Five of the seven left frontal regions showed significantly increasing involvement. In contrast, right frontal cortex showed mostly decreased involvement over the ages studied here. Only one right frontal region exhibited a reliable age-related increase in activity relative to baseline. This region, however, was not positively activated by any age group; it began as a deactivation and matured into a flat response. Medial frontal cortex and anterior cingulate mostly showed age-related decreases for these tasks. Only one medial frontal region showed increases in activity with age.

In brain regions outside frontal cortex, the majority of developmental changes took the form of age-related decreases in activity. Out of all non-frontal regions that showed age-related effects for controlled lexical processing, only three exhibited increases over development. All three of these regions were found in left parietal locations. The remaining regions all showed significant decreases in levels of activity over maturation.

The variability of peak activity within many but not all brain regions changed significantly over age (see Table 4). Using Levene's test, a test of homogeneity of variance across groups, 47 per cent of decreasing age-related regions and 70 per cent of increasing age-related regions showed statistically significant differences across the six age groups in BOLD signal variability ($P < 0.05$). Generally, brain activity showed the greatest variability in the youngest age group and variability decreased over development.

Regression analysis by age

For all 40 regions showing age-related differences, the nonlinear regression functions explained a statistically significant proportion of the variance in peak brain activity over development (see Table 5 and Fig. 7). Coefficients of determination (R^2) ranged from 0.08 to 0.39 across all regions. Regions growing up and regions growing down showed evidence of becoming adult-like at different ages. Activity in decreasing age-related regions on average became 50 per cent adult-like at age 12.8 and 75 per cent adult like at age 16.5. Regions showing maturational increases, on the other hand, matured somewhat earlier showing peak activity that became 50 per cent adult-like by the age of 11.9 and 75 per cent adult-like by the age of 14.8.

According to these measures, brain activity in frontal age-related regions matured at a faster rate than regions outside frontal cortex. Peak brain activity approached adult-like levels at systematically older ages, going generally from polar and dorsal frontal cortex to anterior and posterior cingulate, to temporal and parietal cortex, and then extrastriate cortex (see Fig. 8). Across all 40 regions showing age-related effects, there was a statistically significant relationship between measures of the age at which brain activity within a region matured and its neuroanatomical location in the posterior-anterior dimension. The ages at which activity became 50 per cent adult-like and 75 per cent adult-like were both significantly negatively correlated with region position along the horizontal axis ($r = -0.40$, $P < 0.01$ and $r = -0.44$, $P < 0.004$, respectively), indicating that, generally speaking, frontal regions were the earliest to reach mature levels of activity for these tasks.

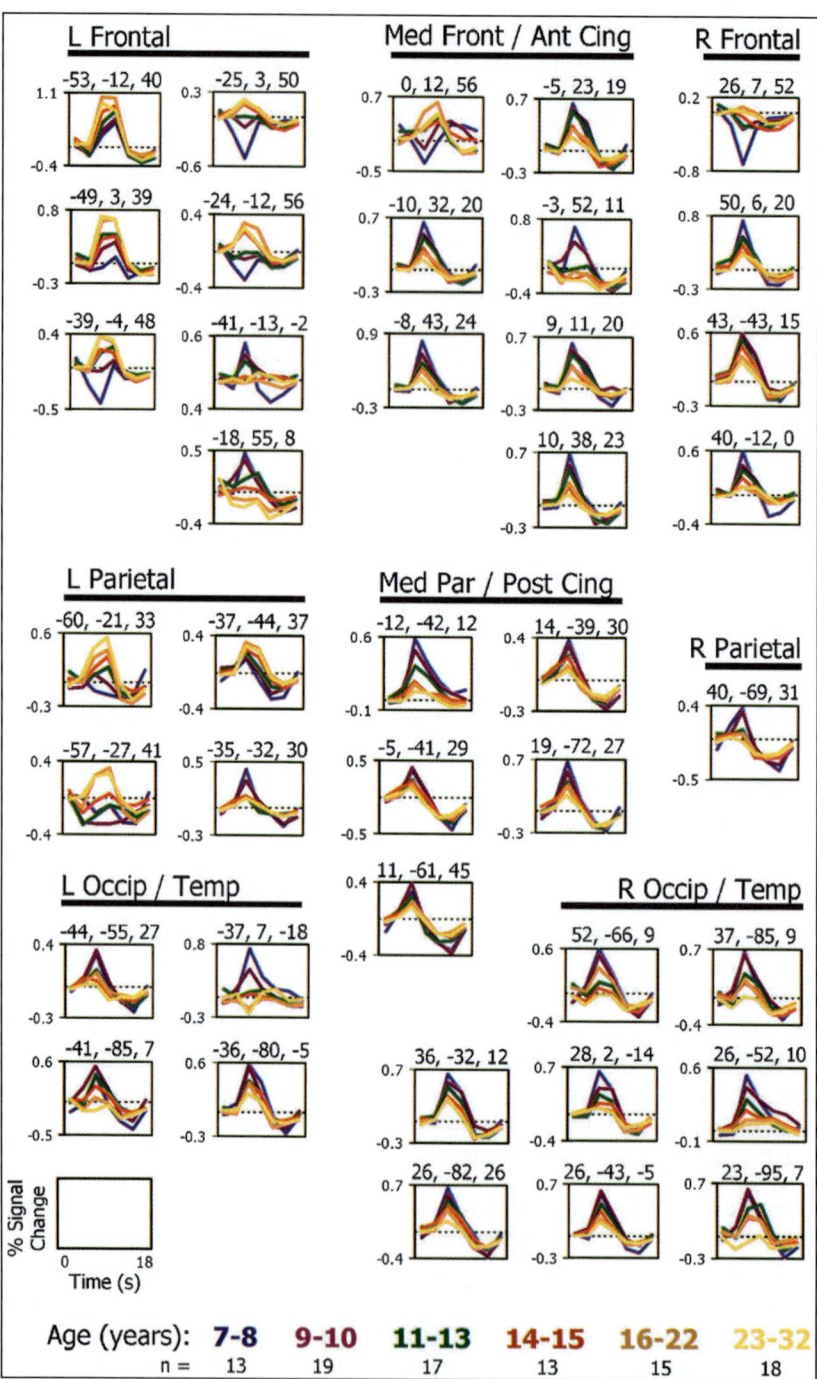

Figure 6. Timecourses by age group in 40 age-related regions. For all 40 regions showing age-related effects, haemodynamic response function timecourses are shown for each of the six cross-sectional age groups (blue = 7–8 year olds, purple = 9–10, green = 11–13, red = 14–15, orange = 16–22, and yellow = 23–32). Numeric coordinates (e.g. –49,3, 39) indicate the location of the center of mass of the region in standard atlas space. The percentage of MR signal change is plotted against time in seconds.

Table 5. Demographic and task performance characteristics of the six cross-sectional groups

	Age in years					
	7–8	9–10	11–13	14–15	16–22	23–32
n	13	19	17	13	15	18
Gender	8 F/5 M	10 F/9 M	10 F/7 M	5 F/8 M	11 F/4 M	8 F/10 M
Age (years)	8.3 (0.5)	10.1 (0.5)	12.4 (1.0)	15.1 (0.3)	19.4 (2.4)	26.6 (2.8)
% correct	70.9[a] (11.3)	71.6[a] (11.4)	80.2[a,b] (9.9)	85.1[b] (5.1)	87.3[b] (4.3)	89.9[b] (6.7)
RT (ms)	2089[a] (455)	2034[a,b] (535)	1806[a,b,c] (328)	1617[b,c] (277)	1551c (310)	1441[c] (259)
Verbal IQ	125[a] (20)	120[a] (8)	113[a] (7)	112[a] (11)	118[a] (6)	–
Perf IQ	118[a] (14)	107[a] (12)	117[a] (8)	115[a] (9)	117[a] (7)	–
Full Scale IW	125[a] (18)	115[a] (9)	117[a] (7)	116[a] (10)	120[a] (6)	118[a] (5)

[a,b,c] Statistically equivalent across groups by ANOVA, $P < 0.05$.

Discussion

The purpose of this study was to provide a detailed test and empirical characterization of maturational changes in human cerebral functional organization, focusing on a distinction between progressive and regressive developmental changes underlying controlled cognition. Regions 'growing up' and regions 'growing down' showed neuroanatomical segregation, different developmental changes in the magnitude of the haemodynamic response, and evidence of differences in maturational timing. The pattern of results we found suggests that progressive and regressive changes in the functional neuroanatomy may relate to two different kinds of developmental specialization: the recruitment of top-down control mechanisms and the tuning of lower-level mechanisms.

Progressive developmental changes were found exclusively in frontal and parietal cortex, including regions reliably demonstrated in adults to be involved in top-down cognitive control (Luria, 1966/1980; Stuss & Benson, 1984; Posner & Petersen, 1990; Kolb & Whishaw, 1996; Miller & Cohen, 2001; Corbetta & Shulman, 2002). In addition, these developmental increases in activity primarily began as statistically 'flat' responses in children (i.e. were not activated) and 'grew up' into robust activations in adults. This finding suggests that regions showing age-related increases in activity for these tasks are mostly 'new recruits' in the maturing functional organization.

Regressive developmental changes in activity, on the other hand, were more frequent and were found across a wider range of locations. Showing clear neuroanatomical dissociation from progressive effects, regressive changes were found mostly outside lateral frontal cortex and included earlier processing regions such as bilateral occipital and temporal cortex. All regions showing significant developmental decreases began as positively activated in children. The large majority declined over age into either smaller but still positive activation or into statistically flat responses (i.e. were not activated by adults). This finding suggests that the maturing functional organization also includes regions or sets of regions that become more selectively activated with age.

Evidence from functional neuroimaging studies of adults supports the notion that 'new' regions of the brain can be recruited over the course of learning, practice, and skill acquisition to support specialized control systems. Raichle et al. (1994) found that regions of the brain most

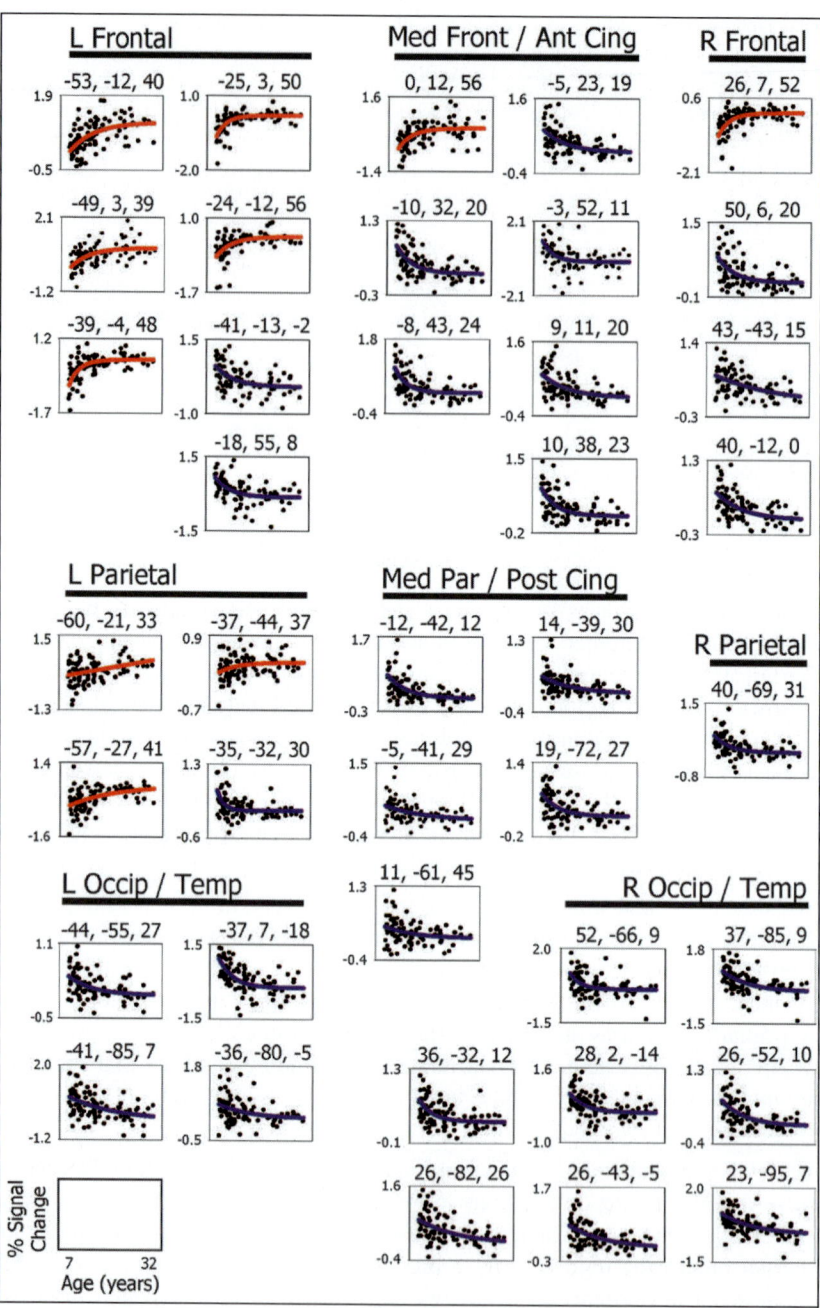

Figure 7. Peak brain activity as a function of age in 40 age-related regions. For all 40 regions showing age-related effects, fitted nonlinear regression curves are shown. For each region, peak brain activity in percentage of MR signal change is plotted as a function of age to tenths of a year for all 95 subjects. Regions showing increasing activity over age were modeled using a three-parameter, single-exponent rise to max function $[y = y_0 + a(1 - e^{-bx})]$ and are shown as red curves. Regions showing decreasing activity over age were modeled using a complementary three-parameter, single-exponent decay function $[y = y_0 + ae^{-bx}]$ and are shown as blue curves. Numeric coordinates (e.g. –49,3,39) indicate the location of the center of mass of the region in standard atlas space.

Chapter 7 Developmental changes in human cerebral functional organization for word generation

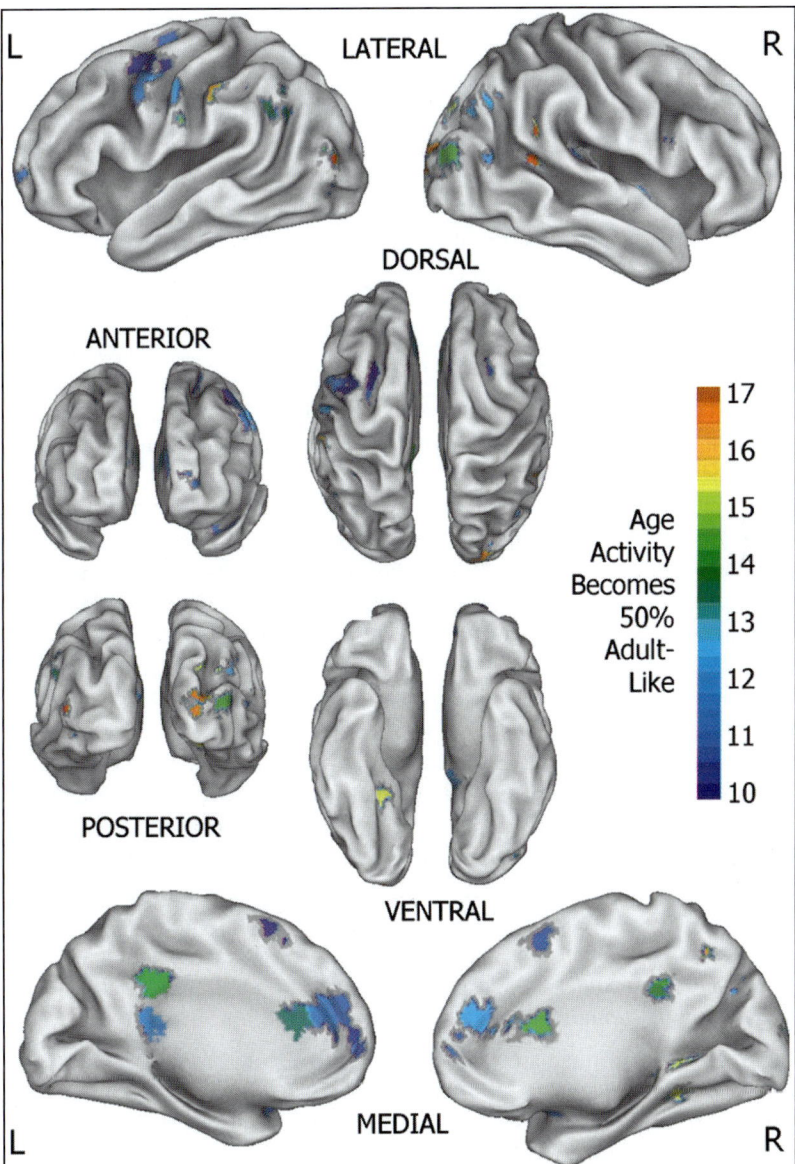

Figure 8. Maturation rates of 40 age-related regions. All 40 regions that exhibited age-related effects are shown with region color varying by the age at which brain activity became 50 per cent 'adult-like' (i.e. the age at which brain activity in that region equals 50 percent of the total range of activity exhibited across the youngest and oldest subjects).

active during initial performance of a verb-generation task (anterior cingulate, left prefrontal and left posterior temporal cortex, and the right cerebellar hemisphere), compared to reading nouns, were all significantly less active during practiced performance. These changes, however, were accompanied by increases in activation of the insular cortex bilaterally and left medial extrastriate cortex. Petersen et al. (1998) found similar changes in functional organization related to the practice of verb generation and maze tracing. For both tasks, practice induced a shift of activity away from regions in frontal cortex, anterior cingulate and cerebellum to greater activity in insular cortex and superior medial frontal cortex respectively, including newly recruited regions.

There is also evidence that specialization can take the form of 'tuning' brain regions – i.e. regions or sets of regions of the brain become more selectively activated over age for the same tasks (see Johnson, 2000). Using event-related potentials (ERPs), several studies have demonstrated that electrophysiological components sensitive to the processing of faces change significantly between the ages of 3 and 12 months old (de Haan, 1998; Johnson, 2001; Halit et al., 2003). The developmental changes in topography and amplitude that have been found suggest that the regions adults use for processing faces are selected from an initially larger set and may respond to a wider range of stimuli at younger ages. Similar tuning effects have been observed in studies of infant speech perception. For instance, ERPs were measured while infants (13–20 months old) listened to words they understood, words they did not understand and words spoken backwards (Mills et al., 1997). Differences between known and unknown words showed a wide spatial distribution of activity before the age of 17 months, evoking responses in broad bilateral anterior and posterior regions. In contrast, these effects were much more spatially limited in 20-month olds and were found only in temporal and parietal regions of the left hemisphere. All of these findings are consistent with the general notion that the input domain for cognitive and perceptual systems generally narrows over the course of development (Gauthier & Nelson, 2001). We found that activity in frontal regions approached adult-like levels at relatively younger ages than activity in other regions. In fact, there was a significant relationship between the age at which brain activity within a region became adult-like and its neuroanatomical location in the posterior-anterior dimension, with brain regions generally showing adult-like activity in anterior regions first with more posterior regions becoming adult-like at older ages. These results, though counterintuitive to a simple caudal-to-rostral maturational view of functional brain development, are in accord with other perspectives.

One alternative view of how the mature functional neuroanatomy for a particular cognitive task might emerge is by the use of a 'progressive neural scaffolding'. This view is similar to that which has been suggested for changes that accompany the acquisition of skilled task performance in adults (Petersen et al., 1998). In such a scenario, 'immature' performance might be carried out by a relatively large set of lower level brain regions recruited to cope with novel task demands; this set of regions may sustain task performance at early developmental levels. Then, higher-level control mechanisms (potentially in frontal and parietal cortex) might be recruited to provide top-down support, and to guide the selection of the lower-level mechanisms for specific task performance.

Our results are also strikingly consistent with predictions made by the interactive specialization framework of functional brain development articulated by Johnson and his colleagues (Johnson, 2000, 2001; Johnson et al., 2002). The specific kinds of progressive and regressive changes we have seen support the notions that generally more pathways are recruited at younger ages for the same tasks, that there are significant changes in functional localization during development, and that some prefrontal regions show precocious task involvement.

Several conceptual and methodological aspects of the current study warrant further discussion. The changes we observed in functional organization over development for these controlled lexical tasks could presumably be associated with age-related changes in the specific information-processing operations that are employed for task performance. For example, children might accomplish these tasks by using a general object recognition and manipulation approach. These operations may transition into more specialized lexical processing in adulthood. Such a change would be consistent with the decreasing reliance on extrastriate regions and the increasing reliance on left frontal regions over development that we found. Our study does not address these cognitive strategy differences that may exist between children and adults. Our study also does not provide evidence that speaks to the relative contributions of biological maturation versus individual task experience *per se*. This issue is of great interest in functional brain development and could be addressed by research that closely tracks and manipulates variables such as task exposure and practice and explores their relation to age.

Approximately half of the brain regions we found to show differences between children and adults showed differences in activity that were related to task performance discrepancy. These regions appeared to be functionally similar across age in that levels of activity were equivalent in adults and children who performed the tasks at the same level of proficiency. This observation demonstrates the importance of measuring and accounting for behavioral performance levels in functional neuroimaging studies. Indeed, this issue is not unique to child studies; it applies with equal importance to virtually any study that aims to compare two groups where one performs generally better than the other on cognitive tasks (e.g. see Weinberger & Berman, 1998, regarding similar issues in functional neuroimaging research on schizophrenia). For developmental studies, there are clear implications. Without some way of addressing performance differences, the differences in brain activity between children and adults could be misinterpreted as maturational differences in functional neuroanatomy. Although regions showing performance-related effects are interesting in their own right, they maintain an important functional distinction from regions showing effects that appear to be driven by age.

It is noteworthy that the youngest and oldest participants in our study showed statistically equivalent activation of much of the brain for these controlled lexical tasks. Similar activation was found in expected regions such as primary visual, auditory and motor cortex, but also in regions such as prefrontal cortex. Although we found age-related effects in left dorsal and posterior frontal regions for word generation, comparable brain regions have shown functional similarities between similarly aged adults and children for other tasks, such as visuospatial working memory (Klingberg *et al.*, 2002). It would appear, then, that there is no simple mapping of maturational effects onto broad brain regions, such as the mere 'coming online' of left frontal cortex. Instead, task-specific developmental changes appear to occur in a complex functional mosaic.

Because we set out to explore only regions that show reliable differences between our youngest and oldest subjects, it is possible that we have missed regions that show other kinds of nonlinear developmental effects over this age range. For example, this approach would fail to identify brain regions exhibiting 'U-' and 'inverted U-' shaped effects over age, where brain activity is the same in the endpoint age groups but shows significant differences at ages in between. Human cognition and behavior has long been known to exhibit changes of these types over development (e.g. Mehler, 1982a; Mehler, 1982b). Recent functional imaging studies suggest that some brain regions show these effects for certain tasks as well (Luna *et al.*, 2001).

Regression analysis approaches are increasingly being used to characterize the rate and course of changes in regional brain activity over development (e.g. Kwon *et al.*, 2002; Shaywitz *et* al., 2002; Turkeltaub et al., 2003). Our results provide evidence that these changes may be largely nonlinear and heteroscedastic, and may, therefore, require statistical methods that do not assume linearity and homogeneity of variance.

With increasing sophistication in conceptual and methodological approaches, functional neuroimaging holds promise for moving beyond a confirmatory role for existing knowledge about development. The accumulation of more empirical data on developmental changes in cerebral functional organization should create a richer theoretical context and lead to greater insight into the neural underpinnings of human cognitive development.

Supplementary material

Supplementary material can be found at: http://www.cercor.oupjournals.org/.

Notes

The authors gratefully thank the children, teens and adults who participated in this study; Mark McAvoy and Avi Snyder for neuroimaging application development; David Van Essen and his colleagues for the use of CARET; the Petersen and Schlaggar groups and other members of the NeuroImaging Laboratories at Washington University for thoughtful comments and suggestions. This work was supported in part by a National Science Foundation Graduate Research Fellowship to Tim Brown and by NIH NSADA (B.L.S.), NS32979 (S.E.P.), NS41255 (S.E.P.), NS46424 (S.E.P.), The McDonnell Center for Higher Brain Function (S.E.P., B.L.S.) and The Charles A. Dana Foundation (B.L.S.). Brad Schlaggar is a Scholar of the Child Health Research Center of Excellence in Developmental Biology at Washington University School of Medicine (HD01487). Portions of this work were presented at the 9th Annual Meeting of the Cognitive Neuroscience Society, San Francisco, CA and the 32nd Annual Meeting of the Society for Neuroscience, Orlando, FL.

References

Barch, D.M., Braver, T.S., Sabb, F.W. & Noll, D.C. (2000): Anterior cingulate and the monitoring of response conflict: evidence from an fMRI study of overt verb generation. *J. Cogn. Neurosci.* **12**, 298–309.

Booth, J.R., Burman, D.D., Meyer, J.R., Lei, Z., Trommer, B.L., Davenport, N.D., Li, W., Parrish, T.B., Gitelman, D.R. & Mesulam, M.M. (2003): Neural development of selective attention and response inhibition. *Neuroimage* **20**, 737–751.

Bourgeois, J.P. (2001): Synaptogenesis in the neocortex of the newborn: the ultimate frontier for individuation? In: *Handbook of developmental cognitive neuroscience*, eds. C. Nelson & M. Luciana, pp. 23–34. Cambridge, MA: MIT Press.

Buckner, R.L., Raichle, M.E. & Petersen, S.E. (1995): Dissociation of human prefrontal cortical areas across different speech production tasks and gender groups. *J. Neurophysiol.* **74**, 2163–2173.

Bunge, S.A., Dudukovic, N.M., Thomason, M.E., Vaidya, C.J. & Gabrieli, J.D. (2002): Immature frontal lobe contributions to cognitive control in children: evidence from fMRI. *Neuron* **33**, 301–311.

Burgund, E.D., Kang, H.-S.C., Kelly, J.E., Buckner, R.L., Snyder, A.Z., Petersen, S.E. & Schlaggar, B.L. (2002): The feasibility of a common stereotactic space for children and adults in fMRI studies of development. *Neuroimage* **17**, 184–200.

Burton, H., Diamond, J.B. & McDermott, K.B. (2003): Dissociating cortical regions activated by semantic and phonological tasks: a fMRI study in blind and sighted people. *J. Neurophysiol.* **90**, 1965–1082.

Casey, B.J., Cohen, J.D., Jezzard, P., Turner, R., Noll, D.C., Trainor, R.J., Giedd, J., Kaysen, D., Hertz-Pannier, L. & Rapoport, J.L. (1995): Activation of prefrontal cortex in children during a nonspatial working memory task with functional MRI. *Neuroimage* **2**, 221–229.

Casey, B.J., Trainor, R.J., Orendi, J.L., Schubert, A.B., Nystrom, L.E., Giedd, J.N., Castellanos, F.X., Haxby, J.V., Noll, D.C., Cohen, J.D., Forman, S.D., Dahl, R.E. & Rapoport, J.L. (1997): A developmental functional MRI study of prefrontal activation during performance of a go-no-go task. *J. Cogn. Neurosci.* **9**, 835–847.

Casey, B.J., Thomas, K.M., Davidson, M.C., Kunz, K. & Franzen, P.L. (2002): Dissociating striatal and hippocampal function developmentally with a stimulus-response compatibility task. *J. Neurosci.* **22**, 8647–8652.

Changeux, J.P. & Danchin, A. (1976): Selective stabilization of developing synapses as a mechanism for the specification of neuronal networks. *Nature* **264**, 705–712.

Chugani, H.T., Phelps, M.E. & Mazziotta, J.C. (1987): Positron emission tomography study of human brain functional development. *Ann. Neurol.* **22**, 487–497.

Corbetta, M. & Shulman, G.L. (2002): Control of goal-directed and stimulus-driven attention in the brain. *Nat. Rev. Neurosci.* **3**, 201–215.

Corina, D.P., San Jose-Robertson, L., Guillemin, A., High, J. & Braun, A.R. (2003): Language lateralization in a bimanual language. *J. Cogn. Neurosci.* **15**, 718–730.

de Haan, M. (1998): Electrophysiological correlates of face processing by adults and 6-month-old infants. *J. Cogn. Neurosci.* (Ann. Meeting Suppl.) **36**.

Dobbing, J. & Sands, J. (1973): Quantitative growth and development of human brain. *Arch. Dis. Child.* **48**, 757–767.

Duncan, J. & Owen, A.M. (2000): Common regions of the human frontal lobe recruited by diverse cognitive demands. *Trends Neurosci.* **23**, 475–483.

Edelman, G.M. (1987): *Neural Darwinism.* New York: Basic Books.

Elman, J.L., Bates, E.A., Johnson, M.H., Karmiloff-Smith, A., Parisi, D. & Plunkett, K. (1996): Rethinking innateness: a connectionist perspective on development. Cambridge, MA: MIT Press.

Forman, S.D., Cohen, J.D., Fitzgerald, M., Eddy, W.F., Mintun, M.A. & Noll, D.C. (1995): Improved assessment of significant activation in functional magnetic resonance imaging (fMRI): use of a cluster-size threshold. *Magn. Reson. Med.* **33**, 636–647.

Gaillard, W.D., Hertz-Pannier, L., Mott, S.H., Barnett, A.S., LeBihan, D. & Theodore, W.H. (2000): Functional anatomy of cognitive development: fMRI of verbal fluency in children and adults. *Neurology* **54**, 180–185.

Gaillard, W.D., Sachs, B.C., Whitnah, J.R., Ahmad, Z., Balsamo, L.M., Petrella, J.R., Braniecki, S.H., McKinney, C.M., Hunter, K., Xu, B. & Grandin, C.B. (2003): Developmental aspects of language processing: fMRI of verbal fluency in children and adults. *Hum. Brain Mapp.* **18**, 176–185.

Gauthier, I. & Nelson, C.A. (2001): The development of face expertise. *Curr. Opin. Neurobiol.* **11**, 219–224.

Giedd, J.N., Blumenthal, J., Jeffries, N.O., Castellanos, F.X., Liu, H., Zijdenbos, A., Paus, T., Evans, A.C. & Rapoport, J.L. (1999): Brain development during childhood and adolescence: a longitudinal MRI study. *Nat. Neurosci.* **2**, 861–863.

Gottlieb, G. (1976): The role of experience in the development of behavior and the nervous system. In: *Neural and behavioral specificity*, ed. G. Gottlieb. New York: Academic Press.

Greenough, W.T., Black, J.E. & Wallace, C.S. (1987): Experience and brain development. *Child Dev.* **58**, 539–559.

Halit, H., de Haan, M. & Johnson, M.H. (2003): Cortical specialization for face processing: face-sensitive event-related potential components in 3- and 12-month-old infants. *Neuroimage* **19**, 1180–1193.

Hebb, D.O. (1949): *The organization of behavior.* New York: John Wiley

Holland, S.K., Plante, E., Weber Byars, A., Strawsburg, R.H., Schmithorst, V.J. & Ball, W.S. Jr. (2001): Normal fMRI brain activation patterns in children performing a verb generation task. *Neuroimage* **14**, 837–843.

Huttenlocher, P.R. & Dabholkar, A.S. (1997): Regional differences in synaptogenesis in human cerebral cortex. *J. Comp. Neurol.* **387**, 167–178.

Jerne, N.K. (1967): Antibodies and learning: selection *versus* instruction. In: *The neurosciences*, eds. G. Quarton, T. Melnechuk & F. Schmitt, pp. 200–205. New York: The Rockefeller University Press.

Jernigan, T., Hesselink, J., Sowell, E. & Tallal, P. (1991): Cerebral structure of magnetic resonance imaging in language- and learning-impaired children. *Arch. Neurol.* **48**, 539–545.

Johnson, M.H. (2000): Functional brain development in infants: elements of an interactive specialization framework. *Child Dev.* **71**, 75–81.

Johnson, M.H. (2001): Functional brain development in humans. *Nat. Rev. Neurosci.* **2**, 475–483.

Johnson, M.H., Halit, H., Grice, S.J. & Karmiloff-Smith, A. (2002): Neuroimaging of typical and atypical development: a perspective from multiple levels of analysis. *Dev. Psychopathol.* **14**, 521–536.

Kang, H.-S.C., Burgund, E.D., Lugar, H.M., Petersen, S.E. & Schlaggar, B.L. (2003): Comparison of functional activation foci in children and adults using a common stereotactic space. *Neuroimage* **19**, 16–28.

Klein, D., Milner, B., Zatorre, R.J., Meyer, E. & Evans, A.C. (1995): The neural substrates underlying word generation: a bilingual functional-imaging study. *Proc. Natl. Acad. Sci. USA* **92**, 2899–2903.

Klingberg, T., Vaidya, C.J., Gabrieli, J.D., Moseley, M.E. & Hedehus, M. (1999): Myelination and organization of the frontal white matter in children: a diffusion tensor MRI study. *Neuroreport* **10**, 2817–2821.

Klingberg, T., Forssberg, H. & Westerberg, H. (2002): Increased brain activity in frontal and parietal cortex underlies the development of visuo-spatial working memory capacity during childhood. *J. Cogn. Neurosci.* **14**, 1–10.

Kolb, B. & Whishaw, I.Q. (1996): *Fundamentals of human neuropsychology*. New York: W.H. Freeman.

Kwon, H., Reiss, A.L. & Menon, V. (2002): Neural basis of protracted developmental changes in visuo-spatial working memory. *Proc. Natl. Acad. Sci. USA* **99**, 13336–13341.

Lancaster, J.L., Woldorff, M.G., Parsons, L.M., Liotti, M., Freitas, C.S., Rainey, L., Kochunov, P.V., Nickerson, D., Mikiten, S.A. & Fox, P.T. (2000): Automated Talairach atlas labels for functional brain mapping. *Hum. Brain Mapp.* **10**, 120–131.

Luna, B., Thulborn, K.R., Munoz, D.P., Merriam, E.P., Garver, K.E., Minshew, N.J., Keshavan, M.S., Genovese, C.R., Eddy, W.F. & Sweeney, J.A. (2001): Maturation of widely distributed brain function subserves cognitive development. *Neuroimage* **13**, 786–793.

Luria, A.R. (1966/1980): *Higher cortical functions in man*. New York: Basic Books.

Matarazzo, J.D. (1972): *Wechsler's measurement and appraisal of adult intelligence*. Baltimore: Williams & Wilkins.

McAvoy, M.P., Ollinger, J.M. & Buckner, R.L. (2001): Cluster size thresholds for assessment of significant activation in fMRI. *Neuroimage* **13**, S198.

McCarthy, G., Blamire, A.M., Rothman, D.L., Gruetter, R. & Shulman, R.G. (1993): Echo-planar magnetic resonance imaging studies of frontal cortex activation during word generation in humans. *Proc. Natl. Acad. Sci. USA* **90**, 4952–4956.

McDermott, K.B., Petersen, S.E., Watson, J.M. & Ojemann, J.G. (2003): A procedure for identifying regions preferentially activated by attention to semantic and phonological relations using functional magnetic resonance imaging. *Neuropsychologia* **41**, 293–303.

Mehler, J. (1982a): Studies in the development of cognitive processes. In: *U-shaped behavioral growth*, ed. S. Strauss, pp. 271–293. New York: Academic Press.

Mehler, J. (1982b): Unlearning: dips and drops – a theory of cognitive development. In: *Regressions in development: basic phenomena and theoretical alternatives*, ed. T. Bever, pp. 133–152. Hillsdale, NJ: Erlbaum.

Miezin, F., Maccotta, L., Ollinger, J., Petersen, S. & Buckner, R. (2000): Characterizing the hemodynamic response: effects of presentation rate, sampling procedure, and the possibility of ordering brain activity based on relative timing. *Neuroimage* **11**, 735–759.

Miller, E.K. & Cohen, J.D. (2001): An integrative theory of prefrontal cortex function. *Annu. Rev. Neurosci.* **24**, 167–202.

Mills, D.L., Coffey-Corina, S. & Neville, H.J. (1997): Language comprehension and cerebral specialization from 13 to 20 months. *Dev. Neuropsychol.* **13**, 397–445.

Muzik, O., Chugani, D.C., Juhasz, C., Shen, C. & Chugani, H.T. (2000): Statistical parametric mapping: assessment of application in children. *Neuroimage* **12**, 538–549.

Nelles, J.L., Lugar, H.M., Coalson, R.S., Miezin, F.M., Petersen, S.E. & Schlaggar, B.L. (2003): An automated method for extracting response latencies of subject vocalizations in event-related fMRI experiments. *Neuroimage* **20**, 1865–1871.

Ojemann, J.G., Ojemann, G.A. & Lettich, E. (2002): Cortical stimulation mapping of language cortex by using a verb generation task: effects of learning and comparison to mapping based on object naming. *J. Neurosurg.* **97**, 33–38.

Passingham, R.E. (1996): Attention to action. *Philos. Trans. R. Soc. Lond. B. Biol. Sci.* **351**, 1473–1479.

Petersen, S.E., Fiez, J.A. (1993): The processing of single words studied with positron emission tomography. *Annu. Rev. Neurosci.* **16**, 509–530.

Petersen, S.E., Fox, P.T., Posner, M.I., Mintun, M. & Raichle, M.E. (1988): Positron emission tomographic studies of the cortical anatomy of single-word processing. *Nature* **331**, 585–589.

Petersen, S.E., Fox, P.T., Snyder, A.Z. & Raichle, M.E. (1990): Activation of extrastriate and frontal cortical areas by visual words and word-like stimuli. *Science* **249**, 1041–1044.

Petersen, S.E., van Mier, H., Fiez, J.A. & Raichle, M.E. (1998): The effects of practice on the functional anatomy of task performance. *Proc. Natl. Acad. Sci. USA* **95**, 853–860.

Pfefferbaum, A., Mathalon, D.H., Sullivan, E.V., Rawles, J.M., Zipursky, R.B. & Lim, K.O. (1994): A quantitative magnetic resonance imaging study of changes in brain morphology from infancy to late adulthood. *Arch. Neurol.* **51**, 874–887.

Posner, M.I. & Petersen, S.E. (1990): The attention system of the human brain. *Annu. Rev. Neurosci.* **13**, 25–42.

Posner, M.I., Petersen, S.E., Fox, P.T. & Raichle, M.E. (1988): Localization of cognitive operations in the human brain. *Science* **240**, 1627–1631.

Quartz, S.R. & Sejnowski, T.J. (1997): The neural basis of cognitive development: a constructivist manifesto. *Behav. Brain Sci.* **20**, 537–556 (discussion 556–596).

Raichle, M.E., Fiez, J.A., Videen, T.O., MacLoed, A.-M.K., Pardo, J.V., Fox, P.T. & Petersen, S.E. (1994): Practice-related changes in human brain functional anatomy during nonmotor learning. *Cereb. Cortex* **4**, 8–26.

Schlaggar, B.L., Brown, T.T., Lugar, H.M., Coalson, R.S., Petersen, S.E. (2002a): fMRI in performance-matched children and adults: modality dependent and independent age-related differences in lexical processing. *Paper presented at the Society for Neuroscience, Orlando, FL.*

Schlaggar, B.L., Brown, T.T., Lugar, H.M., Visscher, K.M., Miezin, F.M. & Petersen, S.E. (2002b): Functional neuroanatomical differences between adults and school-age children in the processing of single words. *Science* **296**, 1476–1479.

Seger, C.A., Rabin, L.A., Barella, M. & Gabrieli, J.D. (1997): Preserved verb generation priming in global amnesia. *Neuropsychologia* **35**, 1069–1074.

Shaywitz, B.A., Shaywitz, S.E., Pugh, K.R., Mencl, W.E., Fulbright, R.K., Skudlarski, P., Constable, R.T., Marchione, K.E., Fletcher, J.M., Lyon, G.R. & Gore, J.C. (2002): Disruption of posterior brain systems for reading in children with developmental dyslexia. *Biol. Psychiatry* **52**, 101–110.

Sowell, E.R., Peterson, B.S., Thompson, P.M., Welcome, S.E., Henkenius, A.L. & Toga, A.W. (2003): Mapping cortical change across the human life span. *Nat. Neurosci.* **6**, 309–315.

Stuss, D.T. & Benson, D.F. (1984): Neuropsychological studies of the frontal lobes. *Psychol. Bull.* **95**, 3–28.

Talairach, J. & Tournoux, P. (1988): *Co-planar stereotaxic atlas of the human brain.* New York: Thieme.

Tamm, L., Menon, V. & Reiss, A.L. (2002): Maturation of brain function associated with response inhibition. *J. Am. Acad. Child Adolesc. Psychiatry* **41**, 1231–1238.

Thelen, E. & Smith, L. (1994): *A dynamic systems approach to the development of cognition and action.* Cambridge, MA: MIT Press.

Thomas, K.M., King, S.W., Franzen, P.L., Welsh, T.F., Berkowitz, A.L., Noll, D.C., Birmaher, V. & Casey, B.J. (1999): A developmental functional MRI study of spatial working memory. *Neuroimage* **10**, 327–338.

Thompson-Schill, S.L., Swick, D., Farah, M.J., D'Esposito, M., Kan, I.P. & Knight, R.T. (1998): Verb generation in patients with focal frontal lesions: a neuropsychological test of neuroimaging findings. *Proc. Natl. Acad. Sci. USA* **22**, 15855–15860.

Turkeltaub, P.E., Gareau, L., Flowers, D.L., Zeffiro, T.A. & Eden, G.F. (2003): Development of neural mechanisms for reading. *Nat. Neurosci.* **6**, 767–773.

Van Essen, D.C. (2002): Windows on the brain: the emerging role of atlases and databases in neuroscience. *Curr. Opin. Neurobiol.* **12**, 574–579. See also http://pulvinar.wustl.edu:8081/sums/search.do?filename=ATLAS&filetype=tar.gz

Van Essen, D.C., Drury, H.A., Dickson, J., Harwell, J., Hanlon, D. & Anderson, C.H. (2001): An integrated software suite for surface-based analyses of cerebral cortex. *J. Am. Med. Inform. Assoc.* **8**, 443–459. See also http://brainmap.wustl.edu/caret

Wechsler, D. (1999): *Wechsler abbreviated scale of Intelligence.* San Antonio: The Psychological Corporation.

Weinberger, D.R. & Berman, K.F. (1998): Prefrontal function in schizophrenia: confounds and controversies. In: *The prefrontal cortex: executive and cognitive functions,* eds. A.C. Roberts, T.W. Robbins & L. Weiskrantz, pp. 165–180. New York: Oxford.

Wise, R., Chollet, F., Hadar, U., Friston, K., Hoffner, E. & Frackowiak, R. (1991): Distribution of cortical neural networks involved in word comprehension and word retrieval. *Brain* **114**, 1803–1817.

Yakovlev, P.I. & Lecours, A.R. (1967): The myelogenetic cycles of regional maturation of the brain. In: *Regional development of the brain in early life,* ed. A. Minkowski, pp. 3–70. Oxford: Blackwell Scientific.

Chapter 8

Functional magnetic resonance imaging in normal and pathological language development

William D. Gaillard[*,º], Erin N. Moore[*], Deborah A. Weber[*], Eva K. Ritzl[º] and Madison M. Berl[*]

[*] *Department of Neuroscience, Children's National Medical Center, George Washington University School of Medicine and Health Sciences, 111 Michigan Ave NW, Washington DC 20010, USA*
[º] *Clinical Epilepsy Section, NINDS, NIH, Bethesda, Maryland, USA*
wgaillar@cnmc.org

Summary

Functional magnetic resonance imaging (fMRI) studies of language allow non-invasive investigation of the normal and pathological organisation of neural networks that process language functions. Studies that stress both receptive and expressive aspects of language show that the networks that process language are well established by the age of 4 or 5 years, and that the patterns of activation – in location and in degree of left hemisphere laterality – are fundamentally the same by this age as in adults. Studies of stroke and epilepsy show reorganization of language to homologous regions in the typically non-dominant right hemisphere. Reorganization to the right hemisphere usually occurs in the setting of a brain injury or disorder before the age of 6 years. Reorganization may occur regionally, it may involve the widespread hemispheric language networks, or it may reflect implementation of an immature or less efficient strategy portrayed in weighted activation patterns within a larger distributed language network. Activation in regions outside traditional language processing areas, including right hemisphere homologues, is rare and therefore suggests that only evolutionarily defined brain areas maintain the capacity to process language. It cannot be discerned whether reorganization represents persistence of an immature network or a true shift of language function to the right hemisphere. Brain injury after age 6 years can be associated with right activation, but language function is not normal. Reorganization of language can occur in humans with diminishing degree into late childhood and early adolescence.

Introduction

In this chapter we will survey the use of functional magnetic resonance imaging (fMRI) to identify the neural networks implicated in language processing in normal children and in children with brain injury or neurological disease. fMRI studies in children with brain disorders provide insight into the developmental plasticity of language. In particular, information is gained on the timing, location, and extent of reorganized language processing. Other chapters in this volume discuss the behavioural assessment of children with brain lesions and the theories of language plasticity. Previous chapters on fMRI discuss the normal organization of auditory processing and lexical processing of language during normal development.

Brain networks processing language

The brain networks that process language in humans typically reside along the perisylvian areas in the left hemisphere. These networks derive evolutionarily from communication networks found in primates and other species. Evidence for left dominance may be seen in asymmetry in the planum temporale in macaques and in infants, and in the endocasts of hominid ancestors such as the australopithicines (Wada et al., 1975; Preis et al., 1999). This evidence suggests that the networks that process language are evolutionarily selected. However, the inability to master language without exposure to language in early life and the capacity to sustain language despite injury to the left hemisphere in early childhood suggest that a period of environmental exposure and consolidation is necessary for the mature language processing network. This observation supports the notion of a critical period for language development (Lenneberg, 1967; Krashen, 1973; Hécaen, 1983; Muter et al., 1997; Muller & Courchesne, 2000; Bates & Roe, 2001).

fMRI is a non-invasive method that allows the mapping of cognitive networks in children and adults. The principles of fMRI have been outlined in a previous chapter (p. 61). Group analysis methods are commonly employed to identify networks involved in various cognitive tasks. These studies typically employ small subject groups (8–15) and analyse datasets in a common anatomical atlas (for example, the atlas of Talairach and Tournoux, 1988). The statistical methods used seek to identify common areas of activation across the group. The most powerful of these methods, random effects analysis, allows extrapolation of findings to broad populations. A shortcoming of these studies and methods is that they assume a homogeneous population, and that only one valid network exists for any given task or cognitive process. Clinical experience in patient populations is confounded both by different developmental levels and by disease, and provides evidence that heterogeneity is to be expected. Furthermore, null activation maps or imaging results in patient populations analysed by group methods may provide misleading results and thus need to be interpreted with caution. These methods will not identify normal or pathological variants. For example, most humans are left-hemisphere dominant for language, but four to six per cent of the population are right-hemisphere dominant or bilateral for language (Pujol et al., 1999; Knecht et al., 2000). In another example, children who learn to read may employ a phonological strategy for reading (as do a minority of adults) which gives rise to a different pattern and weighting of activation from that seen in a mature, efficient semantic reading strategy (Gaillard et al., 2001a). In the following discussion, group maps in healthy populations are used to convey a sense of the expected typical activation. Individual subject analyses are used to examine the effect of disease states and developmental conditions on language networks.

Studies in healthy children

fMRI language studies in healthy paediatric populations show a distributed network of language processing fundamentally similar in location and hemisphere dominance to that found in adults *(Fig. 1)*. These studies show that 'receptive' language processing occurs along the left superior temporal sulcus, as can be seen in paradigms that stress whole language processing such as reading or text (sentences and stories) (Gaillard et al., 2001b; Gaillard et al., 2003b) or listening to sentences or descriptions of objects (Booth et al., 2000; Balsamo et al., 2002; Ahmad et al.,

Chapter 8 Functional magnetic resonance imaging in normal and pathological language development

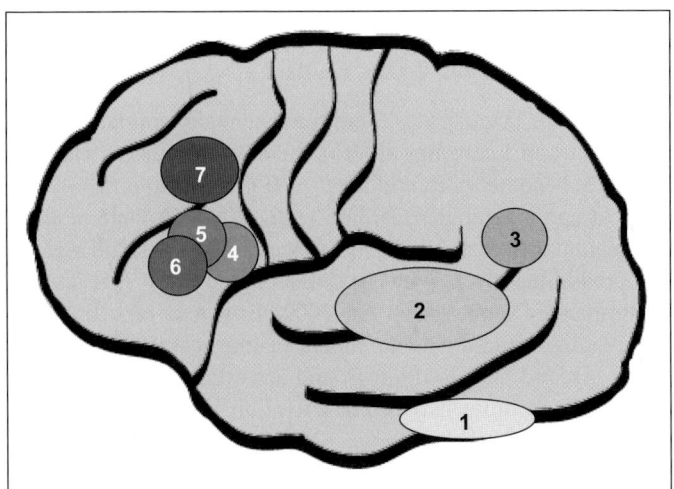

Fig. 1. Schema of areas activated by type of language task. Basal temporal/fusiform activation is seen with feature identification required for reading and object naming or recall (1). Activation along superior temporal gyrus (2) is enhanced with whole text language either auditory or reading. Single-word reading tends to activate BA 37, listening to stories more supramarginal areas (3). Inferior frontal activation (4, 5, 6) is seen in verbal fluency tasks that require either generation or decision. Tasks with phonological weighting yield more posterior IFG activation (4); semantic tasks give more anterior and superior activation (5). Decision tasks generate more anterior activation (BA 47) (6). Mid-frontal gyrus (7) is activated in recall, fluency, and reading tasks, probably because of working memory requirements.

2003). Tasks that require feature detection or identification, such as in naming objects or deciphering letters during reading, activate the basal temporal language area (left fusiform and lingual gyrus) (Gaillard et al., 2001b; Shaywitz et al., 2002; Balsamo et al., 2003; Gaillard et al., 2003a; Gaillard, 2004). Tasks that require some form of single word lexical processing (word generation or decision) activate the left inferior frontal gyrus (IFG) (Gaillard et al., 2000; Holland et al., 2001; Liegeois et al., 2002; Schlaggar et al., 2002; Shaywitz et al., 2002; Gaillard et al., 2003a; Brown et al., 2004; Wood et al., 2004). Semantic and grammatical decisions activate areas somewhat anterior the left IFG, BA 47 (Poldrack et al., 1999), whereas phonological processing tasks activate areas in more inferior and posterior left IFG (Bookheimer, 2002; McDermott et al., 2003). The left middle frontal gyrus (MFG) is activated when verbal working memory is required for task processing, as occurs in fluency tasks, decision based (lexical or grammatical) tasks, and reading tasks (Gaillard, 2004). The frontal activation is typically associated with 'expressive' language processing, such as fluency and recall and planning speech. The separation of anterior 'expressive' and posterior 'receptive' language processing is a simplification for the complex interplay necessary for language processing – for example frontal networks are required for accessing and implementing grammatical rules – but reflects a convenient way of interpreting the principal components of tasks.

A study of listening to speech in infants demonstrated left temporal activation, suggesting that the networks for early communication that will eventually sustain language are left-hemisphere dominant near birth (Dehaene-Lambertz et al., 2002). Studies of auditory comprehension (Ahmad et al., 2003), reading (Gaillard et al., 2003a), and verbal fluency (Byars et al., 2002) show that left hemisphere language activation and laterality is established in children aged 5 years. However, fMRI is unable to image awake children younger than 4 years in a systematic fashion. fMRI studies in younger children are increasingly susceptible to selection bias for cognitive capability, and hence they may not be representative of typically developing peers (Balsamo et al., 2003; Gaillard et al., 2003a; Gaillard et al., 2003b).

While the activation maps for language tasks are fundamentally similar to those found in adults, there are some important and interesting developmental differences. There is some evidence that verbal fluency tasks become more unilateral in IFG with time (5 to 7 year olds *vs.* older children) in both extent and magnitude (Gaillard et al., 2000; Holland et al., 2001; Gaillard et al., 2003a). Developmental differences in lexical processing show some regional developmental changes with time, predominantly in MFG and association areas that are age-dependent and independent of performance (Schlaggar et al., 2002; Brown et al., 2004). A study of covert implicit single word reading – based on a monitored feature search embedded within true words and a false font script – found increased left frontal activation that correlated with a combined language measure score, and more lateralized activation in temporal regions also correlated with phonological awareness (Turkeltaub et al., 2003).

Studies in children with neurological disorders

Behavioural studies show that children recover from brain injury (Hacaen, 1983; Muter et al., 1997; Muller & Courchesne, 2000; Bates & Roe, 2001) in diminishing capacity to late childhood and early adolescence. Behavioural evidence is available from brain injury from stroke, trauma, and brain tumours (especially following resection). Functional imaging data are available in epilepsy and congenital stroke populations. The greatest experience is in patients with epilepsy which informs our notions of language plasticity and reorganization. Historically, it has been important to identify hemisphere dominance for language and to localize language cortex in planning epilepsy surgery in order to minimize untoward postoperative aphasia and language deficits.

Studies using the intracarotid amobarbital test (IAT) show that there is a higher incidence of atypical language in patients with epilepsy: atypical language is present in four per cent of right-handed patients, in 30 per cent of left-handed patients, and in over 70 per cent of patients with acquired left handedness and evidence of left-hemisphere brain injury early in life (Rasmussen & Milner, 1977). These studies are not able to determine how language functions are differentially represented or where they reside anatomically. Cortical stimulation studies show some degree of intrahemispheric language organization in the left hemisphere (Ojemann et al., 1989; Devinsky et al., 1993; Duchowny et al., 1996). It is important to recall that there are no normative data for either IAT or cortical stimulation to help interpret these observations. Non-invasive studies using either fMRI of verbal fluency or optical imaging confirm observations of atypical language dominance in normal right- and left-handed individuals (Pujol et al., 1999; Knecht et al., 2000). fMRI has excellent agreement with IAT – 90 per cent concordance, 10 per cent partial disparity (one unilateral, the other bilateral), and rare overt disagreement (Binder et al., 1996; Bahn et al., 1997; Hertz-Pannier et al., 1997; Yetkin et al., 1998; Benson et al., 1999; Lehericy et al., 2000; Carpentier et al., 2001; Fernandez et al., 2001; Gaillard et al., 2002; Rutten et al., 2002a; Woermann et al., 2003; Gaillard, 2004). The language disruption methods of IAT and electrical cortical stimulation undertaken in epilepsy populations have validated the language activation methods of fMRI and ^{15}O-water PET. Comparison of electrical cortical stimulation with fMRI finds a sensitivity 90 per cent and specificity of 67 per cent (Bookheimer et al., 1997; Pouratian et al., 2002; Rutten, 2002b).

Epilepsy

In adults with childhood onset localization-related epilepsy, fMRI studies find 20–24 per cent atypical language representation (Springer *et al.*, 1999; Gaillard, 2004). Atypical language is associated with younger age of seizure onset (Springer *et al.*, 1999; Gaillard, 2004). In our series nearly all patients (here, predominantly with temporal lobe epilepsy) have a history of seizure onset before 6 years, left handedness, or MRI findings that suggest a developmental or acquired brain insult before 6 years (for example, mesial temporal sclerosis, dysplasia, tumours, stroke) (Gaillard, 2004). The overrepresentation of left handedness suggests the possibility of remote brain injury before the age of 3 years. As a result, it is difficult to discern from the current literature whether it is the intrinsic interictal/ictal process or epilepsy's remote cause that is forcing developmental reorganization of language – though it is likely that both contribute. Postoperative evaluation of patients with right temporal seizures is characterized by an increase in verbal IQ, suggesting a remote and deleterious effect of seizures on language function (Novelly *et al.*, 1984). MRI and FDG-PET studies also demonstrate remote effects of epilepsy on brain structure and cerebral metabolism (DeCarli *et al.*, 1995; Marsh *et al.*, 1997; DeCarli *et al.*, 1998; Lawson *et al.*, 2000; Spanaki *et al.*, 2000; Liu *et al.*, 2003; Theodore *et al.*, 2003).

fMRI allows the identification of brain areas that process language in patients with atypical language. In our epilepsy patient series (n=120; children and adults, 95 per cent with epilepsy onset before the age of 16 years) we identified five activation patterns in the atypical language patients (n=24) based upon performing a panel of language tasks targeted at probing different aspects of language processing (Fig. 2). These tasks are both auditory and reading based, place an emphasis on whole language comprehension, and also include tasks that require semantic decision and recall. Of patients with atypical language, one third are right-dominant with activation in right hemispheric regions homologous to those typically activated in left-dominant healthy volunteers (Berl *et al.*, 2004; Gaillard, 2004) (Fig. 3). The remainder show various forms of bilateral language: equal activation in right and left regions (12 per cent); a diaschisis of activation between temporal and frontal regions (12 per cent), or bifrontal but unilateral temporal (either right or left) activation (46 per cent). Rarely, patients will have laterality that is task-dependent (two per cent). Nearly all activation occurs in homologous right hemisphere regions. It is unusual to see activation outside these regions, suggesting neurophysiological constraints on brain regions that can sustain language functions. Occasionally a different weighting of activation within the distributed language is seen (for example, angular gyrus rather than mid-temporal gyrus for reading). Interhemispheric reorganization of language is common in epilepsy patients, and occurs in homologous regions in the right hemisphere.

Further evidence of the effect of epilepsy on distributed language networks is to be found in a study probing naming-to-description in 50 patients with childhood onset localization-related epilepsy compared with 33 healthy controls (Berl, 2005) (Fig. 4). In this visual task, participants covertly named an object described by a five or six letter sentence ('what is a long yellow fruit?', answer 'banana'). This paradigm elicits activation in left fusiform gyrus, left mid-temporal gyrus, left IFG, and left MFG (Gaillard *et al.*, 2002). Twenty per cent of left-hemisphere focus patients had atypical language dominance (bilateral or right dominant), no right-hemisphere focus patients had atypical language representation. Patients with a left-hemisphere (predominantly temporal) seizure focus who were left-hemisphere dominant for language – excluding patients with atypical language – had a lower degree of laterality in all language processing areas (temporal, IFG, MFG) than healthy controls. Right-hemisphere focus

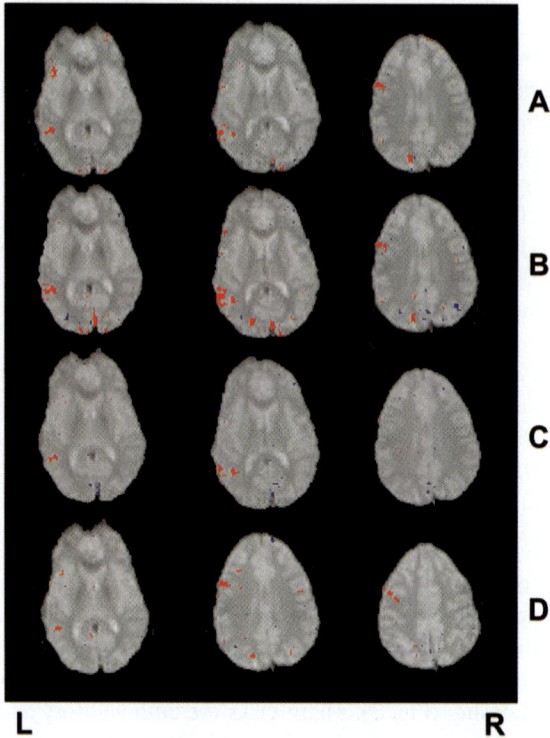

Fig. 2. Normal activation patterns for left-hemisphere dominant 10-year-old child. Different paradigms, using visual and auditory presentation, target frontal and temporal language processing regions. (A) Read-response naming ('What is a large grey animal'). (B) Reading a story. (C) Listening to a story. (D) Verbal fluency to categories. These images demonstrate activation in left inferior frontal gyrus, left mid-frontal gyrus, and left temporal lobe (mid- and superior temporal gyrus). Differences in activation patterns reflect task-dependent utilization of regions in the more widely distributed language processing network. For images, left image is left brain.

patients also had reduced laterality except for IFG. The reduced laterality is attributed to relatively greater activation in the right hemisphere regions. One explanation for these findings is greater recruitment of a distributed network required to perform tasks which require greater cognitive effort for patient populations, such as occurs with increasing task difficulty in sentence-reading paradigms in normal populations (Just *et al.*, 1996). The findings also suggest local and remote effects of the seizure focus on language-processing functions and networks – left-temporal focus patients have a lower laterality of activation in IFG than right-temporal focus patients. Intrahemispheric reorganization is harder to establish with fMRI. Preliminary evidence from the same reading response naming paradigm described above suggests that the location, extent, and magnitude of activation in temporal regions, IFG, and MFG are not different between patient populations and normal populations. Activation in the right hemisphere occurred within homologous right hemispheric areas based on healthy volunteer activation in the left hemisphere.

Remote effects of epilepsy on cognitive processes can be demonstrated in several other studies. A study of 10 patients with a variety of developmental and acquired frontal and temporal lesions showed that temporal lesions, paradoxically, were more likely to be associated with reorganization of activation to the right hemisphere than frontal lesions. This study used a verbal fluency task and thus was primarily targeted at frontal language networks; a probe of receptive temporal processing was not used. Frontal lesions were often adjacent to frontal language networks. As all patients had epilepsy, the findings probably reflect a remote effect of temporal lobe epilepsy on frontal language networks, as described above (Liegeois et al., 2004). Billingsley et al. also showed greater recruitment of frontal areas for single word semantic and phonological processing in adult patients with childhood onset temporal lobe epilepsy, seen in patients with a left, rather than right, temporal seizure focus (Billingsley et al., 2001). Jokeit and colleagues showed greater frontal activation and less hippocampal activation than normal controls with a memory task in adult patients with left-temporal lobe epilepsy (Jokeit et al., 2001). These studies suggest the use of alternative strategies, revealed by different activation maps, to perform cognitive tasks.

Reorganization of language in patients with seizure onset after the age of 6 is difficult to demonstrate, and in these rare instances it is hard to separate epilepsy from the co-morbid disease processes. There are a few case reports of recovery of language in children with late onset Rasmussen's encephalitis who had left (dominant) hemispherectomy after the age of 6 years. Such children have some recovery of speech – significantly more that an adult could achieve – but remain impaired in language function, with significantly diminished language capacity and verbal IQ (Vargha-Khadem et al., 1991; Vargha-Khadem et al., 1997; Boatman et al., 1999; Hertz-Pannier et al., 2002). One such patient, who was left-hemisphere dominant for a verbal fluency task (LIFG) before hemispherectomy, subsequently showed activation in broad right frontal dorsolateral prefrontal cortex following surgery (Hertz-Pannier et al., 2002). Language recovery was not normal in this child (verbal IQ 48) but right-sided areas were recruited to process whatever language recovery occurred.

Stroke

There are few systematic studies in children with stroke. Our data in four children with congenital stroke (and epilepsy) showed that activation occurred in homologous right frontal and temporal areas. Booth et al. demonstrated activation in homologous right areas for auditory processing of sentences of increasing grammatical complexity (Booth et al., 1999; Booth et al., 2000). Staudt and colleagues conducted an elegant study in adults with congenital ischaemic lesions affecting periventricular frontal white matter (Staudt et al., 2001; Staudt et al., 2002). They demonstrated that the likelihood of shift of activation to regions in right IFG/MFG for a verbal fluency task was proportional to the extent of white matter injury. They also showed that reorganization occurred in mirror image homologous right frontal cortex. In contrast, temporal activation with a listening task showed little interhemispheric reorganization of language. These investigators provided evidence for a region-specific effect on language processing with early focal injury.

Other disorders

In contrast to stroke, developmental tumours, without surgery, do not appear to transfer language as readily to the right hemisphere (Labate et al., 2004). Other developmental lesions such as dysplasia are more problematic. Dysplasia can sustain motor, sensory, and language function (personal observations; Duchowny et al., 1996; Janszky et al., 2003), but some dysplasia is associated with 'transfer' of language function intrahemispherically to dysplasia margins or interhemispherically to homologous right hemisphere regions. These studies are often complicated by epilepsy which may also be an important factor influencing the reorganization of language, as discussed above (Smith et al., 2004).

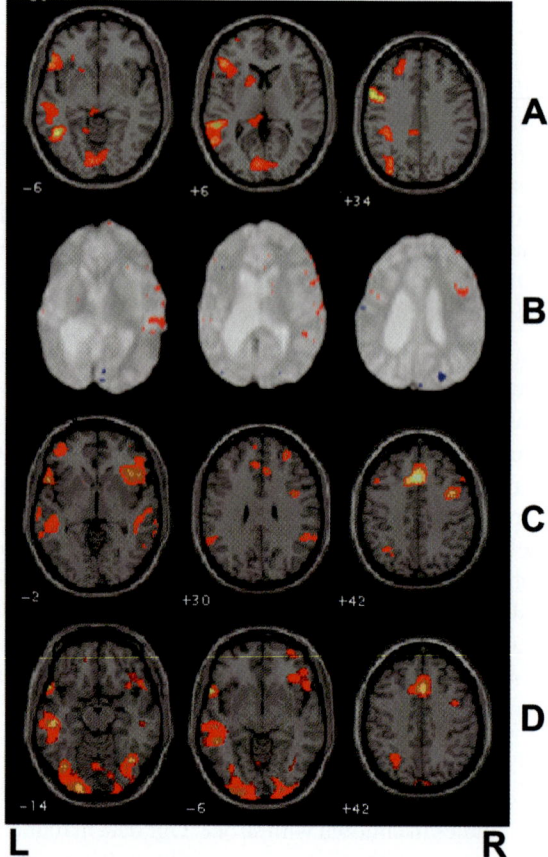

Fig. 3. Patient studies showing atypical language dominance. (A) Left dominant activation for an auditory responsive naming task (What is a large grey animal?). (B) Right hemisphere activation in patient with left temporal lobe epilepsy, perinatal ischaemia, periventricular nodular heterotopia, and left mesial temporal sclerosis. Task is auditory responsive naming. (C) and (D) are the same patient with a left frontal seizure focus showing diaschisis of activation. (C) is auditory responsive naming task and (D) is reading responsive naming. There is greater right frontal than left frontal activation, and greater left temporal than right temporal activation (seen better with reading version of the task). All patients had childhood onset epilepsy. For images, left image is left brain.

Studies of adults with childhood dyslexia suggest greater right and frontal activation for visually based semantic and phonological single word decision tasks, effectively recruiting immature networks to perform the task (Shaywitz et al., 2002). In this circumstance regions with sub-threshold activation in normal populations are recruited more strongly for task performance. Similar results are seen during a passive single-word processing task where premature children, who lag behind their typically developing peers, activate brain regions employed by typically developing peers in phonologic processing. The premature child uses a less mature phonological processing strategy to perform a lexical task that stresses semantic processing in typically developing children (Peterson et al., 2002). Together with studies in epilepsy patients, these group studies support a regional weighting of activation relying on recruiting right homologous regions, or on less mature strategies and their networks.

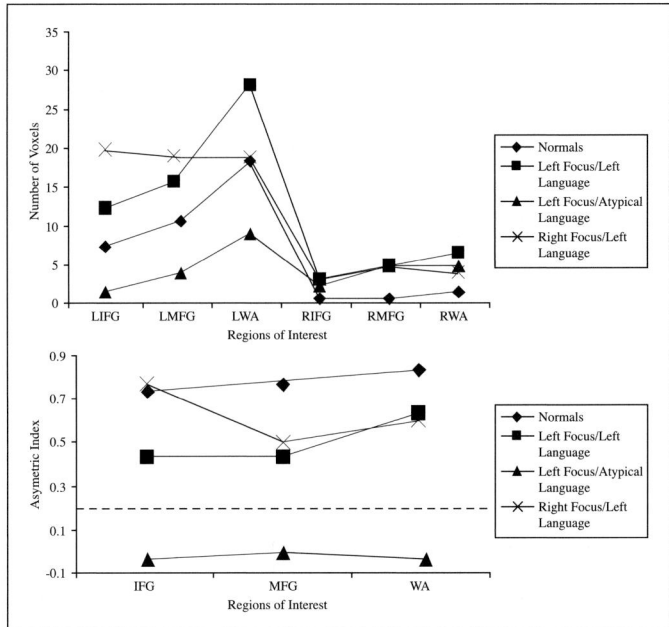

Fig. 4. Regional asymmetry indices (AI) and voxel counts in normal controls (diamonds), right-hemisphere focus/left language epilepsy patients (cross), left-hemisphere focus/left language epilepsy patients (square), and left-hemisphere focus/atypical language epilepsy patients (triangle). Regions include right (R) and left (L) inferior frontal gyrus (IFG), mid-frontal gyrus (MFG), and Wernicke's area (WA) (left mid/superior temporal gyrus/inferior parietal lobe). Dashed line for AI is 0.2 which represents threshold for typical (>0.2) and atypical (<0.2) language dominance, based on 2 SD normal volunteer regional data for several language tasks.

Conclusions

All studies of language processing that have examined individual data sets using a region of interest approach find some degree of bilateral activation for language tasks. The degree and extent of right activation varies from 10 to 40 per cent. Furthermore, the appearance and extent of right activation is apparent at lower 'less rigorous' thresholds (Gaillard et al., 2001a). Activation in right regions may be elicited by using more complex grammatical task items or by stressing pragmatic non-linguistic aspect of language (Just et al., 1996, Gaillard et al., 2001a). These observations suggest that the extent and degree of language recovery does not depend on the critical period of left language networks, but rather on the critical period for right-sided regions. Activation in regions outside traditional language processing areas – including right hemisphere homologues – is rare, which suggests that only evolutionarily defined brain areas maintain the capacity to process language. Current studies cannot distinguish between recovery of function in an effectively persistent immature pattern *versus* a true shift of language function from left to right. The history of early injury or disease onset may favour the later explanation. Early focal acute injury is more likely to be associated with a full recovery of language function, and when this occurs language processing networks are in a distributed network in the right hemisphere which mirrors the typical pattern seen in the left hemisphere language dominant population. Reorganization of language functions is possible, with diminishing degree and capacity, into later childhood and early adolescence.

Acknowledgments: Supported by NINDS R01 NS44280, NICHD P30HD40677, the Clinical Epilepsy Section, NINDS, NIH.

References

Ahmad, Z., Balsamo, L.M., Sachs, B.C., Xu, B. & Gaillard, W.D. (2003): Auditory comprehension of language in young children: neural networks identified with fMRI. *Neurology* **60**, 1598–1605.

Bahn, M.M., Lin, W., Silbergeld, D.L., Miller, J.W., Kuppusamy, K., Cook, R.J., Hammer, G., Wetzel, R., & Cross, D. (1997): Localization of language cortices by functional imaging compared with intracarotid amobarbital hemispheric sedation. *Am. J. Radiol.* **169**, 575–579.

Balsamo, L., Grandin, C.B., Xu, B., Elliott, T.K., Petrella, J.R., Basso, G., Braniecki, S., Theodore, W. & Gaillard, W. (2002): An fMRI study of auditory responsive naming in children. *Arch. Neurol.* **59**, 1168–1174.

Balsamo, L.M., Xu, B., Sachs, B. & Gaillard, W.D. (2003): Language networks underlying auditory based category decision in children identified with fMRI. *Ann. Neurol.* **54**, S105.

Bates, E. & Roe, K. (2001): Language development in children with unilateral brain injury. In: *Handbook of developmental cognitive neuroscience*, eds. C.A Nelson & M. Luciano. Cambridge, MA: MIT Press.

Benson, R.R., FitzGerald, D.B., LeSeuer, L.L., Kennedy, D.N., Kwong, K.K., Buchbinder, B.R., Davis, T.L., Weisskoff, R.M., Talavage, T.M., Logan, W.J., Cosgrove, G.R., Belliveau, J.W. & Rosen, B.R. (1999): Language dominance determined by whole brain functional MRI in patients with brain lesions. *Neurology* **52**, 798–809.

Berl, M.M., Moore, E.N., Xu, B., Pearl, P.L., Conry, J.A., Weinstein, S.L., Ritter, F.J., Theodore, W.H. & Gaillard, W.D. (2004): Atypical language dominance and patterns of reorganization in epilepsy as assessed by a panel of fMRI tasks. *Epilepsia* **45** (Suppl. 7), 366 (abstract G.02).

Berl, M.M., Balsamo, L.M. Xu, B., Moore, E.N., Weinstein, S.L., Conry, J.A., Pearl, P.L., Sachs, B.C., Grandin, C.B., Frattali, C., Ritter, F.J., Sato, S., Theodore, W.H. & Gaillard, W.D. (2005): Seizure focus affects regional language networks assessed by fMRI. *Neurology* **65**, 1604–1611.

Billingsley, R., McAndrews, M.P., Crawley, A.P. & Mikulis, D.J. (2001): Functional MRI of phonological and semantic processing in temporal lobe epilepsy. *Brain* **124**, 1218–1227.

Binder, J.R., Swanson, S.J., Hammeke, T.A., Morris, G.L., Mueller, W.M., Fischer, M., Benbadis, S., Frost, J.A., Rao, S.M. & Haughton, V.M. (1996): Determination of language dominance using functional MRI: a comparison with the Wada test. *Neurology* **46**, 978–984.

Boatman, D., Freeman, J., Vining, E., Pulsifer, M., Miglioretti, D., Minahan, R., Carson, B., Brandt, J. & McKhann, G. (1999): Language recovery after left hemispherectomy in children with late-onset seizures. *Ann. Neurol.* **46**, 579–586.

Bookheimer, S.Y., Dapretto, M., Black, K. & Cohen, M.S. (1997): FMRI of language in patients with aggressive brain tumors. *Soc. Neurosci. Abs.* 23.

Bookheimer, S. (2002): Functional MRI of language: new approaches to understanding the cortical organization of semantic processing. *Annu. Rev. Neurosci.* **25**, 151–188.

Booth, J.R., Macwhinney, B., Thulborn, K.R., Sacco, K., Voyvodic, J. & Feldman, H.M. (1999): Functional organization of activation patterns in children: whole brain fMRI imaging during three different cognitive tasks. *Prog. Neuropsychopharmacol. Biol. Psychiatry* **23**, 669–682.

Booth, J.R., MacWhinney, B., Thulborn, K.R., Sacco, K., Voyvodic, J.T. & Feldman, H.M. (2000): Developmental and lesion effects in brain activation during sentence comprehension and mental rotation. *Dev. Neuropsychol.* **18**, 139–169.

Brown, T.T., Lugar, H.M., Coalson, R.S., Miezin, F.M., Petersen, S. & Schlaggar, B.L. (2005): Developmental changes in human cerebral functional organization for word generation. *Cereb. Cortex.* **15** (Suppl. 3), 275–290.

Byars, A.W., Holland, S.K., Strawsburg, R.H., Bommer, W., Dunn, R.S., Schmithorst, V.J. & Plante, E. (2002): Practical aspects of conducting large-scale functional magnetic resonance imaging studies in children. *J. Child Neurol.* **17**, 885–890.

Carpentier, A., Pugh, K.R., Westerveld, M., Studholme, C., Skrinjar, O., Thompson, J.L., Spencer, D.D. & Constable, R.T. (2001): Functional MRI of language processing: dependence on input modality and temporal lobe epilepsy. *Epilepsia* **42**, 1241–1254.

DeCarli, C., McIntosh, A.R. & Blaxton, T.A. (1995): Use of positron emission tomography for the evaluation of epilepsy. *Neuroimaging Clin. North Am.* **5**, 623–645.

DeCarli, C., Hatta, J., Fazilat, S., Gaillard, W.D. & Theodore, W.H. (1998): Extratemporal atrophy in patients with complex partial seizures of left temporal origin. *Ann. Neurol.* **43**, 41–45.

Dehaene-Lambertz, G., Dehaene, S. & Hertz-Pannier, L. (2002): Functional neuroimaging of speech perception in infants. *Science* **298**, 2013–2015.

Devinsky, O., Perrine, K., Llinas, R., Luciano, D.J. & Dogali, M. (1993): Anterior temporal language areas in patients with early onset of temporal lobe epilepsy. *Ann. Neurol.* **34**, 727–732.

Duchowny, M., Jayakar, P., Harvey, A.S., Resnick, T., Alvarez, L., Dean, P. & Levin, B. (1996): Language cortex representation: effects of developmental versus acquired pathology. *Ann. Neurol.* **40**, 31–38.

Fernandez, G., de Greiff, A., von Oertzen, J., Reuber, M., Lun, S., Klaver, P., Ruhlmann, J., Reul, J. & Elger, C.E. (2001): Language mapping in less than 15 minutes: real-time functional MRI during routine clinical investigation. *Neuroimage* **14**, 585–594.

Gaillard, W.D. (2004): Functional MR imaging of language, memory, and sensorimotor cortex. *Neuroimaging Clin. North Am.* **14**, 471–485.

Gaillard, W.D., Hertz-Pannier, L., Mott, S.H., Barnett, A.S., LeBihan, D. & Theodore, W.H. (2000): Functional anatomy of cognitive development: fMRI of verbal fluency in children and adults. *Neurology* **54**, 180–185.

Gaillard, W.D., Grandin, C.B. & Xu, B. (2001a): Developmental aspects of pediatric fMRI: considerations for image acquisition, analysis, and interpretation. *Neuroimage* **13**, 239–249.

Gaillard, W.D., Pugliese, M., Grandin, C.B., Braniecki, S.H., Kondapaneni, P., Hunter, K., Xu, B., Petrella, J.R., Balsamo, L. & Basso, G. (2001b): Cortical localization of reading in normal children: an fMRI language study. *Neurology* **57**, 47–54.

Gaillard, W.D., Balsamo, L., Xu, B., Grandin, C.B., Braniecki, S.H., Papero, P.H., Weinstein, S., Conry, J., Pearl, P.L., Sachs, B., Sato, S., Jabbari, B., Vezina, L.G., Frattali, C. & Theodore, W.H. (2002): Language dominance in partial epilepsy patients identified with an fMRI reading task. *Neurology* **59**, 256–265.

Gaillard, W.D., Balsamo, L.M., Ibrahim, Z., Sachs, B.C. & Xu, B. (2003a): fMRI identifies regional specialization of neural networks for reading in young children. *Neurology* **60**, 94–100.

Gaillard, W.D., Sachs, B.C., Whitnah, J.R., Ahmad, Z., Balsamo, L.M., Petrella, J.R., Braniecki, S.H., McKinney, C.M., Hunter, K., Xu, B. & Grandin, C.B. (2003b): Developmental aspects of language processing: fMRI of verbal fluency in children and adults. *Hum. Brain Mapp.* **18**, 176–185.

Hécaen, H. (1983): Acquired asphasia in children: revisited. *Neuropsychologia* **21**, 581–587.

Hertz-Pannier, L., Gaillard, W.D., Mott, S.H., Cuenod, C.A., Bookheimer, S.Y., Weinstein, S., Conry, J., Papero, P.H., Schiff, S.J., Le Bihan, D. & Theodore, W.H. (1997): Noninvasive assessment of language dominance in children and adolescents with functional MRI: a preliminary study. *Neurology* **48**, 1003–1012.

Hertz-Pannier, L., Chiron, C., Jambaque, I., Renaux-Kieffer, V., Van de Moortele, P.F., Delalande, O., Fohlen, M., Brunelle, F. & Le Bihan, D. (2002): Late plasticity for language in a child's non-dominant hemisphere: a pre- and post-surgery fMRI study. *Brain* **125**, 361–372.

Holland, S.K., Plante, E., Weber Byars, A., Strawsburg, R.H., Schmithorst, V.J. & Ball, W.S. (2001): Normal fMRI brain activation patterns in children performing a verb generation task. *Neuroimage* **14**, 837–843.

Janszky, J., Ebner, A., Kruse, B., Mertens, M., Jokeit, H., Seitz, R.J., Witte, O.W., Tuxhorn, I. & Woermann, F.G. (2003): Functional organization of the brain with malformations of cortical development. *Ann. Neurol.* **53**, 759–767.

Jokeit, H., Okujava, M. & Woermann, F.G. (2001): Memory fMRI lateralizes temporal lobe epilepsy. *Neurology* **57**, 1786–1793.

Just, M.A., Carpenter, P.A., Keller, T.A., Eddy, W.F. & Thulborn, K.R. (1996): Brain activity modulated by sentence comprehension. *Science* **274**, 114–116.

Knecht, S., Deppe, M., Drager, B., Bobe, L., Lohmann, H., Ringelstein, E.B. & Henningsen, H. (2000): Language lateralization in healthy right-handers. *Brain* **123**, 74–81.

Krashen, S.D. (1973): Lateralization, language learning, and the critical period: some new evidence. *Lang. Learn.* **23**, 63–74.

Labate, A., Briellmann, R., Waites, A.B., Harvey, A.S., & Jackson, G. (2004): Temporal lobe developmental tumors: an fMRI study for language lateralization. *Epilepsia* **45** (Suppl. 7), 301–302.

Lawson, J.A., Vogrin, S., Bleasel, A.F., Cook, M.J. & Bye, A.M. (2000): Cerebral and cerebellar volume reduction in children with intractable epilepsy. *Epilepsia* **41**, 1456–1462.

Lehericy, S., Cohen, L., Bazin, B., Samson, S., Giacomini, E., Routgetet, R., Hertz-Pannier, L., LeBihan, D., Marsault, C. & Baulac, M. (2000): Functional MR evaluation of temporal and frontal language dominance compared with the Wada test. *Neurology* **54**, 1625–1633.

Lenneberg, E.H. (1967): *Biological foundations of language*. New York: John Wiley.

Liégeois, F., Connelly, A., Salmond, C.H., Gadian, D.G., Vargha-Khadem, F. & Baldeweg, T. (2002): A direct test for lateralization of language activation using fMRI: comparison with invasive assessments in children with epilepsy. *Neuroimage* **17**, 1861–1867.

Liegeois, F., Connelly, A., Cross, J.H., Boyd, S.G., Gadian, Vargha-Khadem, F. & Baldeweg, T. (2004): Language reorganization in children with early-onset lesions of the left hemisphere: an fMRI study. *Brain* **127**, 1229–1236.

Liu, R.S., Lemieux, L., Bell, G.S., Hammers, A., Sisodiya, S.M., Bartlett, P.A., Shorvon, S.D., Sander, J.W. & Duncan, J.S. (2003): Progressive neocortical damage in epilepsy. *Ann. Neurol.* **53**, 312–324.

Marsh, L., Morrell, M.J., Shear, P.K., Sullivan, E.V., Freeman, H., Marie, A., Lim, K. O. & Pfefferbaum, A. (1997): Cortical and hippocampal volume deficits in temporal lobe epilepsy. *Epilepsia* **38**, 576–587.

McDermott, K.B., Petersen, S.E., Watson, J.M. & Ojemann, J.G. (2003): A procedure for identifying regions preferentially activated by attention to semantic and phonological relations using functional magnetic resonance imaging. *Neuropsychologia* **41**, 293–303.

Muller, R.A. & Courchesne, E. (2000): *The duplicity of plasticity: a conceptual approach to the study of early lesion and developmental disorders*. New York: Cambridge University Press.

Muter, V., Taylor, S. & Vargha-Khadem, F. (1997): A longitudinal study of early intellectual development in hemiplegic children. *Neuropsychologia* **35**, 289–298.

Novelly, R.A., Augustine, E.A., Mattson, R.H., Glasser, G.H., Williamson, P.D., Spencer, D.D. & Spencer, S.S. (1984): Selective memory improvement and impairment in temporal lobectomy for epilepsy. *Ann. Neurol.* **15**, 64–67.

Ojemann, G., Ojemann, J., Lettich, E. & Berger, M. (1989): Cortical language localization in left, dominant hemisphere. An electrical stimulation mapping investigation in 117 patients. *J. Neurosurg.* **71**, 316–326.

Peterson, B.S., Vohr, B., Kane, M.J., Whalen, D.H., Schneider, K.C., Katz, K.H., Zhang, H., Duncan, C.C., Makuch, R., Gore, J.C. & Ment, L.R. (2002): A functional magnetic resonance imaging study of language processing and its cognitive correlates in prematurely born children. *Pediatrics* **110**, 1153–1162.

Poldrack, R.A., Wagner, A.D., Prull, M.W., Desmond, J.E., Glover, G.H. & Gabrieli, J.D. (1999): Functional specialization for semantic and phonological processing in the left inferior prefrontal cortex. *Neuroimage* **10**, 15–35.

Pouratian, N., Bookheimer, S.Y., Rex, D.E., Martin, N.A. & Toga, A.W. (2002): Utility of preoperative functional magnetic resonance imaging for identifying language cortices in patients with vascular malformations. *J. Neurosurg.* **97**, 21–32.

Preis, S., Jancke, L., Schmitz-Hillebrecht, J. & Steinmetz, H. (1999): Child age and planum temporale asymmetry. *Brain Cogn.* **40**, 441–452.

Pujol, J., Deus, J., Losilla, J.M. & Capdevila, A. (1999): Cerebral lateralization of language in normal left-handed people studies by functional fMRI. *Neurology* **52**, 1038–1043.

Rasmussen, T. & Milner, B. (1977): The role of early left-brain injury in determining lateralization of cerebral speech functions. *Ann. N.Y. Acad. Sci.* **299**, 355–369.

Rutten, G.J., Ramsey, N.F., van Rijen, P.C., Alpherts, W.C. & van Veelen, C.W. (2002a): fMRI-determined language lateralization in patients with unilateral or mixed language dominance according to the Wada test. *Neuroimage* **17**, 447–460.

Rutten, G.J., Ramsey, N.F., van Rijen, P.C. & van Veelen, C.W. (2002b): Reproducibility of fMRI-determined language lateralization in individual subjects. *Brain Lang.* **80**, 421–437.

Schlaggar, B.L., Brown, T.T., Lugar, H.M., Visscher, K.M., Miezin, F.M. & Petersen, S.E. (2002): Functional neuroanatomical differences between adults and school-age children in the processing of single words. *Science* **296**, 1476–1479.

Shaywitz, B.A., Shaywitz, S.E., Pugh, K.R., Mencl, W.E., Fulbright, R.K., Skudlarski, P., Constable, R.T., Marchione, K.E., Fletcher, J.M., Lyon, G.R. & Gore, J.C. (2002): Disruption of posterior brain systems for reading in children with developmental dyslexia. *Biol. Psychiatry* **52**, 101–110.

Smith, M.L., Bernal, B., Duchowny, M., Dunoyer, C., Jayakar, P. & Altman, N.R. (2004): Severity of focal cortical dysplasia and functional organization of the brain. *Epilepsia* **45**, 357.

Spanaki, M.V., Kopylev, L., Liow, K., DeCarli, C., Fazilat, S., Gaillard, W.D. & Theodore, W.H. (2000): Relationship of seizure frequency to hippocampus volume and metabolism in temporal lobe epilepsy. *Epilepsia* **41**, 1227–1229.

Springer, J., Binder, J., Hammeke, T., Swanson, S., Frost, J., Bellgowan, P., Brewer, C., Perry, H., Morris, G. & Mueller, W. (1999): Language dominance in neurologically normal and epilepsy subjects: a functional MRI study. *Brain* **122**, 2033–2045.

Staudt, M., Grodd, W., Niemann, G., Wildgruber, D., Erb, M. & Krageloh-Mann, I. (2001): Early left periventricular brain lesions induce right hemispheric organization of speech. *Neurology* **57**, 122–125.

Staudt, M., Lidzba, K., Grodd, W., Wildgruber, D., Erb, M.& Krageloh-Mann, I. (2002): Right-hemispheric organization of language following early left-sided brain lesions: functional MRI topography. *Neuroimage* **16**, 954–967.

Talairach, J. & Tournoux, P. (1988): *Co-planar stereotaxic atlas of the human brain*. New York: Thieme Medical Publishers.

Theodore, W.H., DeCarli, C. & Gaillard, W.D. (2003): Total cerebral volume is reduced in patients with localization-related epilepsy and a history of complex febrile seizures. *Arch. Neurol.* **60**, 250–252.

Turkeltaub, P.E., Gareau, L., Flowers, D.L., Zeffiro, T.A. & Eden, G.F. (2003): Development of neural mechanisms for reading. *Nat. Neurosci.* **6**, 767–773.

Vargha-Khadem, F., Isaacs, E., Papaleloudi, Polkey, C.E. & Wilson, J. (1991): Development of language in six hemispherectomized patients. *Brain* **114**, 473–495.

Vargha-Khadem, F., Carr, L.J., Isaacs, E., Brent, E., Adams, C. & Miskhkin, M. (1997): Onset of speech after left hemispherectomy in a 9-year-old boy. *Brain* **120**, 159–182.

Wada, J.A., Clark, R. & Hamm, A. (1975): Cerebral hemispheric asymmetry in humans. *Arch. Neurol.* **32**, 329.

Woermann, F.G., Jokeit, H., Luerding, R., Freitag, H., Schulz, R., Guertler, S., Okujava, M., Wolf, P., Tuxhorn, I. & Ebner, A. (2003): Language lateralization by Wada test and fMRI in 100 patients with epilepsy. *Neurology* **61**, 699–701.

Wood, A.G., Harvey, A.S., Wellard, R.M., Abbott, D.F., Anderson, V., Kean, M., Saling, M.M. & Jackson, G.D. (2004): Language cortex activation in normal children. *Neurology* **63**, 1035–1044.

Yetkin, F.Z., Swanson, S., Fischer, M., Akansel, G., Morris, G., Mueller, W. & Haughton, V. (1998): Functional MR of frontal lobe activation: comparison with Wada language results. *Am. J. Neuroradiol.* **19**, 1095–1098.

Language in congenital and acquired brain lesions/maldevelopment

Chapter 9

Language and its development in the autism spectrum disorders

Isabelle Rapin

In: J.M. Pérez, P.M. González, M.L. Comí and C. Nieto (eds.), New Developments in Autism. The future is Today.
London: Jessica Kingsley Publishers. Copyright © Asociación de Padres de Personas con Autismo (APNA) 2007.
Reproduced with permission from Jessica Kingsley Publishers
rapin@aecom.yu.edu

Introduction

The autism spectrum disorders (pervasive developmental disorders in DSM-IV and ICD-10 (American Psychiatric Association, 2000; World Health Organization, 1992), referred to as autism for short in this chapter) are developmental disorders of the immature brain characterized by: (1) impaired social skills, empathy and insight into others' thinking, (2) inadequate development of non-verbal and verbal communication, especially conversational skills, and impoverished imagination, and (3) cognitive and behavioral rigidity and repetitive behaviors. Neither the level of cognitive competence, nor the presence of any other handicap, nor the biologic cause (aetiology) of the brain dysfunction responsible for the disorder is a defining feature or rules it out. It is well established that the complex phenotype of autism can result, in a minority of cases, from a purely environmental relatively non selective insult to the immature brain, for example an early infection like intrauterine rubella (Chess *et al.*, 1971), or from a single Mendelian gene defect like fragile-X or tuberous sclerosis with a widespread impact on brain development. In the majority of affected individuals autism reflects the cumulative consequences of a number of mutations or polymorphisms affecting some of the many genes that orchestrate the sequential unfolding of brain development (Muhle *et al.*, 2004). This multigenic aetiology, in concert with the unique environmental impacts which each individual experiences, accounts for the wide variation in severity and symptomatology of the autistic phenotype (autism spectrum), and for a recurrence risk of less than 10 per cent within sibships.

Language is a rule-governed set of arbitrary signals every society develops as a means for communicating with others; it is also an important modality for thought. The auditory-vocal channel (speech) dominates communication, but there are many others, for example the visual-manual (sign languages, reading/writing) and tactile-vocal (Braille). All languages are arbitrarily multicoded systems created and shared by any communicating group. Some non-vocal coded language systems, like alphabets, map more or less directly onto the speech code; others such as music and mathematical notations or blue prints do not.

Language acquisition and levels of language encoding

A schematic view of the multiple levels of language encoding is shown in Box 9.1. All normal children learn the oral language(s) of their speaking community rapidly and effortlessly as infants and preschoolers, although the age at which mastery of the various levels of language is achieved differs. The ear is mature at the end of the second trimester of pregnancy so that the infant hears *in utero*, mostly the sounds emanating from the mother, including her voice. Acquisition of the *phonologic (speech sound) code of speech* starts at birth. Infant hone their ability to perceive and segment phonologic contrasts relevant to the language(s) they hear and within months start practicing producing them, whereas contrasts they do not hear wither (Kuhl et al., 1997). Phonology encompasses not only the several dozen distinct phonemes (phonetics or individual speech sounds of languages) but also suprasegmental sound codes (prosody) that signal boundaries between longer utterances and the type of communication intended, for example a question, a declarative sentence, an angry outburst, or an endearment.

Box 9.1. Levels of language encoding

Phonology (speech sounds)
Phonetics segmental
Prosody suprasegmental
Grammar (connected utterances)
Syntax word order, use of closed or small class words (articles, prepositions, etc.)
Morphology word endings, etc.
Semantics (meaning of language)
Lexicon dictionary of words in the brain
Meaning of connected utterances
Pragmatics (intent of communication – conversational use of language)
Verbal word choices, referencing, etc.
Non-verbal direction of gaze, facial expression, turn-taking, gestures, body posture, prosody, etc.

Also starting at birth is the acquisition of *pragmatics* which convey the intent of the communication. *Non-verbal pragmatics* includes direction of gaze, gestures, facial expression, and body posture, nods and other indicators of comprehension or reaction to the content of the received message; *verbal pragmatics* encompasses turn-taking, choice of intonation, topic and words appropriate to the particular communicative interchange. Acquisition of non-verbal pragmatics comes first: it takes only a few weeks for infants to become aware that communication involves turning toward and fixating on the face of the person speaking to them, especially the eyes, and turn-taking with alternating periods of silence and vocal production. Infants' first expressive communication ('word') is generally pointing toward a desired target or to draw attention to it. Pointing usually emerges by about one year and is the clear indication that the infant understands that communication is power over another person's behaviour.

Semantics encompasses the acquisition of a 'dictionary' of words (of signs in the deaf infant with signing parents) or lexicon stored in the brain and of the meaning of longer utterances. The lexicon also emerges around one year and grows throughout life. *Grammar*, the rules for creating multiword utterances that conform to the rules of the language of a speaking community, does not start to emerge until the child's lexicon has reached a critical size, usually between 50 and 100 words at around age two years. It takes a number of years for infants to master all the complicated rules for word order (syntax) or word inflections (morphology) that clarify the meaning of complex utterances by indicating the role of each word in multiword utterances and in longer strings like paragraphs.

Inadequate language acquisition – developmental language disorders (DLDs)

Given the complexities of the language code it is not surprising that the pace and ease of acquisition depend on and are influenced by many neuropsychologic abilities. Deficits like *inadequate hearing* and impaired conduction and processing of auditory signals in the brain will preclude the acquisition of language if severe, or jeopardize it to a greater or lesser degree if milder, because decoding phonology is the necessary first step toward language comprehension and acquisition. Memory and attention are also requisites for language learning. Infants must have an innate drive to communicate and seek social contact in order to orient toward other speakers and to work to make themselves intelligible to others. Although language generally develops in the face of less-than-severe cognitive disability, mental retardation does slow its emergence and decreases the richness of the lexicon and the ability to comprehend complex communications.

Because language is an input-processing-output function with parallel top-down loops to assist bottom-up operations, input disorders will preclude all subsequent operations at the language-learning age. Consequently *receptive deficits* in young children are necessarily mixed receptive-expressive disorders. In contrast *expressive disorders* may be 'pure', in the sense that reception and processing develop normally when impairment is at the level of output operations. Because the four levels of language (phonology, grammar, semantics and pragmatics), take place in part hierarchically or sequentially and in part in parallel, phonologic and syntactic disorders are requisite for semantic processing, whereas *higher-order processing (semantic) disorders* may exist in the absence of phonologic deficits and with deficits limited to complex grammatical and semantic comprehension, processing and formulation. Disordered *verbal pragmatics* may be associated with any type of language deficit that impairs the comprehension of language, be it at the level of phonology, grammar, or semantics. Pragmatics is almost always adequate in children with isolated expressive disorders that spare phonologic, syntactic and semantic comprehension and processing as the children are aware of the intent and power of communication. Inadequate *non-verbal pragmatics* sharply differentiates autism from DLD.

Thus one can simplify the DLDs by dividing them clinically into two broad groups with subtypes (Box 9.2). In the first group (A), production of well articulated, well formed sentences is impaired because phonology and basic grammatic rules are inadequate. This group encompasses two disorders, each with subtypes, differentiated on the basis of comprehension: mixed receptive/expressive disorders and expressive disorders. The second broad group (B) is characterized by adequate acquisition of the phonologic and grammatical codes and vocabulary, therefore the children produce intelligible well formed utterances, but with impaired semantics and acquisition of the more abstract grammatical rules of language. A salient deficit is often comprehension of such open-ended questions as 'who', 'what' and 'where' in the absence of a proximate referent, 'either/or', and especially 'why', 'when' and 'how' which normally-developing children learn to understand and use gradually, usually between ages three and five. Because children with language disorders at the level of semantics speak clearly and understand simple multiword utterances such as one or two level commands and 'what's that' and concrete 'what', 'who' and 'where' questions in context, their comprehension deficits often pass unnoticed early on. Their failure to respond to more complex questions or their propensity to respond to a word rather than the gist of questions is regularly misinterpreted as failure to cooperate or as a thought disorder.

Box 9.2. Clinically defined subtypes of developmental language disorders (DLDs) in young children

A LOWER LEVEL PROCESSING DISORDERS
phonology (and syntax) affected, therefore the production of well articulated speech is impaired
1 **Input disorders**
mixed receptive/expressive disorders affecting phonology, grammar and semantics
Verbal auditory agnosia (VAA) inability to decode phonology:
precludes all subsequent language operations. Language development extremely delayed or absent *via* the acoustic channel, though it may develop *via* the visual or tactile channel if pragmatics is spared:
– Comprehension: little or none
– Expression: child nonverbal or minimally verbal with very poor phonologic production, generally very few poorly articulated and labored single words May be associated with (not caused by!) oromotor deficit or *dysarthria* which is an oromotor deficit that affects swallowing and production of non-speech sounds and mouth movements as well as speech
Mixed phonologic-syntactic disorder language development delayed and impoverished at all levels
– Comprehension: limited, equal to or somewhat better than expression
– Expression: dysfluent, often labored. May be associated with (not caused by!) dysarthria
  o Phonology: impaired
  o Grammar: simplified, short utterances
  o Lexicon impoverished
2 **Expressive disorders**
speech development delayed, comprehension and higher level language processing not affected
Dysfluent (verbal dyspraxia) often associated with, but not caused by, dysarthria
– Comprehension: unimpaired
– Expression: extremely impaired, especially if associated with a severe dysarthria (which is not causative but contributory!). Verbal output may be limited to vowel sounds or to a few consonant sounds in the face of intact or relatively intact comprehension at all levels of language
Fluent (or more fluent) speech programing deficit
– Comprehension: unimpaired
– Expression
  o Phonology: may produce a more or less unintelligible jargon
  o Grammar: unimpaired or impaired by difficulty programming coherent discourse
  o Semantics: unimpaired or may have word retrieval difficulty

B HIGHER ORDER PROCESSING DISORDERS
phonology and syntax basically not impaired
Lexical-syntactic disorder language development delayed
– Comprehension: adequate at the word level, impaired for connected speech
– Expression: fluency variable
  o Phonology: early – frequent jargon, later OK
  o Grammar: early – immature, later OK
  o Semantics: early – severe word finding problems: pseudo-stuttering, lexicon impoverished. Impaired programing of discourse
Semantic-pragmatic disorder expressive language development usually not delayed
– Comprehension: unimpaired at the word or simple sentence level, impaired for discourse, especially open-ended questions forms. Typically comprehension is paradoxically worse than expression
– Expression: fluency unimpaired, chatty, may be verbose
  o Phonology: unimpaired
  o Grammar: unimpaired
  o Semantics: average or (extremely) large often atypical lexicon, perseverative or poorly constrained discourse
  o Pragmatics: impaired conversational skill

NOTE 1 PRAGMATICS:
– *Non-verbal pragmatics* universally impaired in the autism spectrum disorders (ASDs); preserved or at most mildly impaired in 'specific' (uncomplicated) developmental language disorders (DLDs, also known as specific language impairment or SLI)
– *Verbal pragmatics* depends largely on the severity of the language disorder, notably comprehension, in both DLDs and ASDs

NOTE 2 ABNORMAL FEATURES SUGGESTING AN ASD RATHER THAN A DLD
– *Striking pragmatic impairment non-verbal and verbal*, lack of awareness of the power of language and of a drive to communicate, speaking to speak rather than to communicate
– *Atypical prosody*
– *Echolalia* immediate or delayed (formulaic language, scripted speech), perseveration
– *Esoteric word choices*
– *Comprehension of discourse paradoxically more impaired than expression*
– *Purely expressive disorders* not characteristic of children with an ASD!

As stated earlier, the most salient language differences between children on the autism spectrum and those with isolated DLDs are that (1) pragmatics, especially non-verbal pragmatics, is universally deficient in autism, (2) the language of verbal children with autism has abnormal features that are infrequent in children with DLD, and (3) the relative frequency of various types of language disorders differs in autism compared to DLDs, with 'pure' expressive disorders rare in autism and frequent in DLD and the so-called semantic-pragmatic disorder considerably more frequent in autism than in DLD (Table 9.1).

Table 9.1. Most salient differences between the language disorders of children with autism and those with developmental language disorders

Differentiating deficits	Autism spectrum disorders (ASD)	Developmental language disorders (DLD)
Non-verbal pragmatics	⇓ ⇓ ⇓	OK
Verbal pragmatics	⇓ ⇓ ⇓	OK or ⇓ ⇓ ⇓
Prosody	⇓ ⇓ ⇓	OK
Abnormal features (e.g., echolalia, scripts and pronoun reversal)	+++	essentially 0
Verbal auditory agnosia	More common than in DLD	Uncommon (but frequent in acquired epileptic aphasia)
Mixed receptive/expressive disorders	Common	Common
Expressive disorders	essentially 0	Common
Semantic/pragmatic disorder	Common	Uncommon
Lexical/syntactic disorder	Common	Common

Early studies of language disorders in children with autism

There are a variety of plausible reasons for children on the autism spectrum to have inadequate and, in most cases, delayed development of language. Early formal studies focused on pragmatic deficits because lack of the drive to communicate non-verbally is so salient in these children. Even verbal children and adults on the spectrum have prominent pragmatic deficits such as inadequate conversational skills, sparse and unpredictable speech or inability to switch topics with their conversational partner, gaze avoidance, failure to respond when addressed and other obviously deviant characteristics. It was assumed for a long time that non-verbal or minimally verbal children with autism chose not to speak rather than were unable to speak. The fact that the rare utterances of some children were spoken clearly and were often sparse multiword exclamations was viewed as corroborating the interpretation that the children's problem was not language itself but a manifestation of their social deficit. Persistent failure for the emergence of any speech was attributed to their mental retardation; the possibility that lack of language might play a major contributing role to the retardation was not considered, perhaps because early investigators did not view autism as an organic brain disorder.

Many studies focused on the peculiarities of speech in children on the autism spectrum who did speak and spoke clearly (Tager-Flusberg, 2003). Their vocabularies are often remarkably large but atypical, and their speech is marked by such obviously deviant features as immediate echolalia, delayed echolalia or formulaic language (the reciting of overlearned scripts in more or less appropriate context), incessant repetitive questioning, and atypical prosody such as a singsong or uninflected (robotic) voice or a rising tone in utterances that make assertions sound like questions. Immediate and delayed echolalia and compulsive questioning may mask incomprehension as they obviate the need to formulate an apt response or initiate communication (Prizant & Rydell, 1984). Lack of insight into an other persons' agenda (theory of mind) (Leslie & Frith, 1988) and inattention to facial expression and body language (Schultz et al., 2003; Klin et al., 2002), which are contributory features to or consequences of autistic individuals' social inadequacies, may play a role in lack of sensitivity to prosody (suprasegmental phonologic code) and nonverbal pragmatics and, therefore, in their inadequate acquisition. Young verbal children's pragmatic deficits are salient in that they do not take the point of view of their conversational partner into account, often speak ad nauseam of their topic and have a great deal of difficulty switching topics or listening to what their partner has to say.

It was not until my late colleague, the developmental psycholinguist Dr Doris Allen, and I studied the language skills of children who were nonverbal or minimally verbal as well as those of verbal children that it became clear that language disorders involving phonology and grammar occur in children with autism as well as in those with DLD (Rapin, 1997; Rapin & Dunn, 2003). Recent genetic studies have provided a biologic basis for our behavioral observations (Bradford et al., 2001; Wassink et al., 2001) by disclosing linkage to chromosome 7q31–33 and the *WNT2* gene, but only in late-talking individuals with autism who had first-order relatives who were either late talkers or late readers. As it is clear that the most prevalent cause of both developmental language disorders and of dyslexia is phonologic processing deficiency (Shaywitz, 2003), the implication is that impairment of phonologic decoding akin to that in these families is largely responsible for severely compromised comprehension and impoverished poorly articulated expressive language in some non-verbal or poorly verbal children with autism. Dr Allen and I proposed that taking into consideration both the input-processing-output operations of language in the brain and the four encoded levels of language indicates that young children with autism have several subtypes of language disorders, and that these are similar in many ways to those we had identified clinically in young children with DLD (Table 9.2). What follows is a description of these subtypes as a function of age.

Age-defined clinical subtypes of language deficits in individuals on the autism spectrum

Infants

Autism is rarely diagnosed in infancy despite the fact that many parents are aware before the age of one year that there is something wrong with their infant, and despite the fact that recent research has shown that it is often possible to spot an affected child by analyzing home videos of infants on their first birthday parties (Osterling et al., 2002). What parents are sensitive to are early social/pragmatic deficits: infants who do not sustain gaze, infants who do not like the parent-child interaction of cuddling and who may arch their backs and scream at attempts to hug them, infants who do not put up their arms and greet a parent who comes to pick them up after a nap and are content to stay in their crib making no demands for attention for unusually long periods, and quiet infants who do not babble a great deal. Whether lack of babbling (repetitive consonant-vowel utterances which appear in the second half of the first year) is the first sign of a phonologic processing deficit has not been determined formally, but is plausible.

Toddlers/preschoolers

There are three main ways in which autism presents in this age group: (1) delayed or failure to develop expressive language; (2) language that develops at the expected age but that has aberrant features; and (3) regression of language skills.

1) Potential deficits in children with absent or delayed expressive language

Parents' first awareness that something is amiss with their child is likely to be *delay or failure of first words to emerge*. Parents will often bring this concern to their physician, only to be reassured that there is a great deal of variability among children in the unfolding of early language abilities (Thal & Bates, 1990). Many physicians cite the tendency for boys, who are of course those most likely to be on the autism spectrum (and to have DLDs), to speak later than girls as a reason for the delay. The parents may be told not to compare one of their children with the others and to come back in several months. Instead, the following possibilities need to be considered:

Hearing impairment

In toddlers/preschoolers who do not speak or in whom language develops very late, the first order of business is to determine whether hearing is normal. This mandates a competent pure tone audiogram, but as behavioral testing requires the infant to tolerate earphones and to respond reliably by orienting toward the stimulated ear in order to see a visual reinforcer that appears on that side of the booth, the child must be able to tolerate earphones and to be at least somewhat cooperative. Unless the test provides unequivocal results, physiologic tests, that is otoacoustic emissions and auditory brain-stem evoked responses to tonal stimuli, must be obtained without delay. It is never enough to accept the parents' report that the child hears as there are unfortunate children who are both hearing impaired and autistic (Jure *et al.*, 1991), and overlooking a hearing loss, in particular a high-tone loss that may pass unnoticed clinically, is an egregious error.

Inadequate comprehension of speech

Once hearing has been shown to be normal, the question is how well the child comprehends speech. This is often difficult to determine because of uncertainty about whether lack of response to a question or of compliance to a verbal command denotes failure to understand speech, inattention, lack of motivation, or negativism. Lack of comprehension is therefore necessarily inferential and is based on verbal and nonverbal responses to a verbal input. It is imperative not to base this inference on a single instance or a parents' report as they are likely to provide inadvertent visual cues. Evaluating comprehension is crucial because it is requisite to the emergence of speech.

Non-fluent phonologic decoding deficits

Children whose hearing is demonstrably normal yet are non-verbal or minimally verbal and who appear to comprehend very few or essentially no verbal commands without visual cues may be suffering from the most severe input disorder, *verbal auditory agnosia*, in which lack of ability to decode phonology precludes all further language operations (Table 9.2). Some of these children have epileptiform activity in their perisylvian cortex which is presumed to interfere with the function of the primary or secondary auditory cortex (Klein *et al.*, 2000). This language disorder is infrequent. If the decoding disorder for phonology is less severe and speech comprehension impaired rather than absent, children's utterances are likely to be sparse, imperfectly articulated, effortful, their vocabulary to be limited and their grammar simplified, in some cases to the point of speech consisting mostly of single words or uninflected two-word utterances. Verbal auditory agnosia and the less severe and considerably more prevalent *mixed receptive/expressive dysfluent language deficit* are likely to be variants on a continuum, as both are characterized by impaired receptive and expressive phonology, deficient grammar and a meager lexicon. What differentiates children with autism from those with the same developmental language disorder without autism is their profoundly impaired pragmatics.

Pragmatic deficits

These need to be looked for specifically. Caretakers must be asked whether the child attempts to communicate by gesture, whether the infant points to desired objects or to draw parents' attention to a salient event or object of interest. Does the infant have a means for expressing wants besides attempting to reach the desired object without help, pulling the parent by the hand toward it, or screaming? Does the infant shake the head to communicate 'no', or just push away an undesirable object, or sink to the floor to indicate refusal to comply? Does the infant look up when called by name? Deaf toddlers and those with specific language deficits without autism attempt to communicate by any mean available to them and in fact will invent their own gesture language to do so, in contrast to toddlers on the autism spectrum who appear to have little or no need to communicate and, when they do, it is in the very primitive ways just described.

Non-fluent higher-order language processing deficits

Rather than having difficulty with the phonologic code, with its resultant mixed receptive/expressive deficit and curtailed and inadequate phonologic and grammatic production, there are toddlers/preschoolers on the autism spectrum whose deficit is at the semantic and, of course, at the pragmatic level as well. If expressive language is delayed, it may start with a fluent jargon, often produced without clear communicative intent, namely speaking with the back turned and without expecting a response or the need for a communicative partner. When intelligible speech develops, the semantic deficit is characterized by an impoverished lexicon and, in some children, with such severe word retrieval deficits that the children sound like stutterers. When words appear, phonology improves rapidly to the point where speech is intelligible. Grammar may be simplified early on but also tends to catch up. Some of them have prominent echolalia, repeating what was just said rather than responding with a self-generated utterance. Prominent and persistent echolalia (echolalia is a normal but transient stage in learning to speak) should bring up the possibility of either inadequate comprehension or difficulty with sentence generation. These are the children who understand simple commands but whose deficit can be brought out by asking them questions, especially open ended wh- questions like 'why', 'when', and 'how'. Allen and Rapin's name for this quite frequent type of language deficit is the *lexical-syntactic deficit*, which is also quite prevalent in non-autistic children, but without the salient pragmatic deficits and characteristic features of autistic speech.

2) Higher-order language processing deficits in fluent children without delayed speech

Not all toddlers/preschoolers fail to speak at the expected age, but when early language develops it is likely to have aberrant features (e.g., Tager-Flusberg, 2003). They have another subtype of higher order language processing deficit, the fluent so-called *semantic-pragmatic subtype*. Because they speak at the expected age, this earns such children the label of Asperger syndrome provided they are not mentally retarded, that is, provided their IQ is at least 70. Although they share many of the features with the less fluent children just described, they differ from them in their chattiness and large, often esoteric vocabularies. Their speech is characterized less by immediate echoes than by the production of overlearned scripts and perseveration on favorite topics, and by incessant questioning. These children are the 'little professors' with prodigious rote memories who may endear themselves to admiring adults by the depth of their knowledge of some obscure topic but whose peers shun them because they would rather talk than play. Whether the semantic-pragmatic subtype exists in non-autistic children as well was disputed (Boucher, 1998). It is seen in some hydrocephalic children (Fletcher *et al.*, 2002) and children with Williams syndrome (Laws & Bishop, 2004), most of whom do not qualify for an autism spectrum deficit because social skill may be one of their strengths.

A great deal of linguistic research has been devoted to the study of the semantic-pragmatic language disorder and its associated deficits. Good resources are the series of papers devoted to this topic (Boucher, 1998), the studies by Bishop and colleagues reviewed in her book on receptive language disorders (Bishop, 1997), Tager-Flusberg's review of language in autism (Tager-Flusberg, 2003), and a study of electrophysiologic correlates of semantic deficits in intelligent children with autism (Dunn & Bates, 2004).

3) Language stagnation or regression, relation to acquired epileptic aphasia

The third way in which autism presents in toddlers/preschoolers is *loss of language skills, together with a regression in sociability and play*. At least one in three parents reports that, at a mean age of 18-24 months, but in some cases as early as one year, whatever communication skill the infant had developed fades insidiously or, occasionally, abruptly or, in some cases, fails to develop further for many months. Some of the toddlers seemed entirely normal prior to the regression although, in retrospect, other parents had overlooked evidence for delay in the use of gestures or the appearance of single words. In some very young toddlers what goes away is imitation of meaningful gestures such as waving goodbye or of the gestures called for in a nursery song. When regression occurs very early it is difficult to be certain of the antecedent normality of the child, although availability of home videos (Osterling *et al.*, 2002) has vindicated clinicians who elicited a history of language regression by direct questioning of parents (Kurita *et al.*, 1992; Kurita, 1996).

Our group has performed a number of studies of the relation of language regression and autism to epilepsy (defined in all of these studies as a history of at least two unprovoked seizures). In a cohort of 585 children on the autism spectrum evaluated by Tuchman (Tuchman & Rapin, 1997), parents reported that language had regressed at a mean age of 21 months in 30 per cent, and that 11 per cent had epilepsy as just defined. Among 392 children (two-thirds of the cohort) with an available sleep EEG, the EEG was epileptiform in 21 (19 per cent) of the 113 nonepileptic children who had undergone a regression and in 22 (10 per cent) of 222 with neither regression nor epilepsy [EEGs were of course much more likely (about 60 per cent) to be epileptiform in children who had epilepsy, whether or not they had regressed]. In another study of 176 preschoolers with autism, 27 per cent of parents reported regression of single words (Rapin, 1996). A brief questionnaire to 177 parents in a third cohort disclosed that age at language regression was an important variable: regression before age three years was associated with autistic features in 91 per cent of children and with epilepsy in 14 per cent, whereas the trend was reversed after age three years: epilepsy in 58 per cent and autism in 53 per cent of children (Shinnar *et al.*, 2001). This effect of age was duplicated in a fourth cohort of 196 children with histories of language regression, 98 per cent of whom had autistic features (Sy *et al.*, 2003). Asked whether there were antecedent events that might have triggered the regression, parents invoked a variety of non-specific intercurrent illnesses, reactions to immunizations and traumatic life events, although the relevance of these memories is unproven as some parents reported several potential triggers, but the time between alleged trigger and regression varied a great deal casting doubt on the reliability of their answers (Shinnar *et al.*, 2001). Extensive epidemiologic evidence has not persuaded parents, who understandably seek an explanation for untoward events, that vaccines and environmental intoxications are contemporary with, but not responsible for, the emergence of autism. As stated earlier, the principal aetiology of the autism spectrum disorders is complex multigenic effects on prenatal brain development that vary among affected individuals, even, occasionally, within the same family (Muhle *et al.*, 2004). This is not to deny that the vagaries of each individual's environmental circumstances influence the behavioral expression of these genetic traits.

There has been a great deal of speculation about the potential role of clinical or subclinical epilepsy in language/autistic regression of toddlers (Deonna, 1991; Lewine *et al.*, 1999; Holmes *et al.*, 1981). The reason is that the very much rarer unexplained loss of language in later childhood is invariably associated with epilepsy or an epileptiform EEG that is exacerbated by slow-wave sleep (acquired epileptic aphasia or Landau-Kleffner syndrome) (Klein *et al.*, 2000; Ballaban-Gil & Tuchman, 2000). A recent study of 149 children with histories of language regression who underwent all-night EEG monitoring (McVicar *et al.*, 2000) indicates that 69 per cent of them were on the autism spectrum. Once again regression occurred earlier, at 26 months on average, in those on the autism spectrum than in those who were not whose mean age at regression was 39 months. Eight per cent of children with autistic features had had at least two unprovoked seizures but only 2 per cent of them had an epileptiform overnight EEG; in contrast, 33 per cent of children who were not on the autism spectrum had epilepsy and 57 per cent had an epileptiform EEG and thus fulfilled criteria for acquired epileptiform aphasia.

In summary, this series of studies on the relation of epilepsy to language loss in autism shows unequivocally that a history of very early language regression must be taken very seriously because it is the harbinger of an autism spectrum disorder in the great majority of toddlers. It also shows that epilepsy or an epileptiform EEG is unlikely to be the major culprit in early language/autistic regression even though it may play a role in a minority of the children, and that the opposite is true of children whose language regresses at school-age, with a considerable overlap between the two ages.

If epilepsy plays a subsidiary role in language/autistic regression, other possibilities need to be considered. Some cases might plausibly arise because of enhanced genetic predisposition to the deleterious effects of unidentified environmental influences. Linkage to genes relevant to immunity (Torres *et al.*, 2002), together with an increased prevalence of autoimmune disorders in the families of children with autism (Comi *et al.*, 1999) suggested that immunology might increase susceptibility to autism or autistic regression upon exposure to generally benign non-specific infections or well tolerated immunizations (Korvatska *et al.*, 2002). Live measles vaccine (Miller, 2003) and toxic effects of the ethyl mercury (thimerosal) used as a preservative in many vaccines have recently received a great deal of publicity (Kimmel, 2002). Reports of an increase in the prevalence of the autism spectrum disorders (a so-called autistic epidemic) (Croen *et al.*, 2002), together with an escalating number of vaccines administered to infants and toddlers at the peak age of language regression and of the diagnosis of autism fueled the hypothesis of a causal relation. This remains a hypothesis to be investigated further, although extensive epidemiological studies have failed to corroborate these hypotheses (e.g., Madsen *et al.*, 2002; Pichichero *et al.*, 2002; Heron & Golding, 2004; Andrews *et al.*, 2004). The evidence for an autism epidemic seems to reflect mostly an increase in the identification of mild cases by both professionals and the public, fueled by awareness that a diagnosis of autism buys more intensive intervention for toddlers/preschoolers than a non-specific label like developmental delay (Fombonne, 2003).

School-age children

The good news is that in most children with autism, like in those with uncomplicated developmental language disorders, language generally improves with maturation, provided the child is not profoundly autistic or cognitively impaired. The most informative study of outcome as a function of the clinically-defined language deficits subtypes of toddlers and preschoolers would be a longitudinal study of children whose language was evaluated several times between its emergence and later ages. Most of the studies to date are cross-sectional studies, the majority of them of verbal children. As part of a larger study, a group of specifically trained neurologists had the opportunity to score 83 children on the autism spectrum at preschool, seven or nine years. Preliminary analysis indicates that the neurologists had scored the expressive language of two-thirds of lower-functioning children *versus* one-third of the higher-functioning group (whose expressive skills started out higher of course) as improved and as had the receptive skills of slightly more than half of both groups.

The classic descriptions of the language of children on the autism spectrum have focused on school-age and adolescence, with particular emphasis on bright individuals labeled Asperger syndrome even though some of them had delayed onset of language, and therefore rigorous application of the DSM-IV/ICD-10 criteria would classify them as having either high-functioning autism (autistic disorder without mental retardation and with adequate verbal ability) or pervasive developmental disorders not otherwise specified (PDD-NOS). Whether there is a biologic difference between Asperger syndrome, high-functioning autism, and PDD-NOS is questionable (Myhr, 1998). It is well established that emergence by age five years of functional speech (that is, speech used for communication, not just echolalia, scripts, or elicited utterances) is a more reliable predictor of a favorable outcome than the severity of the dysfunction at preschool (Eisenmajer *et al.*, 1998; Lord & Paul, 1997), this despite the infrequent later emergence of speech in a heretofore nonverbal or minimally verbal older child. Provision of a visual mode of communication such as pictures (Bondy & Frost, 1998) or sign language (Bonvillian *et al.*, 1981) for those who remain non-verbal greatly enhances their quality of life. An occasional non-verbal child with an ASD will learn to read prior to the emergence of speech since reading may serve as scaffolding for speech.

I know of no study which used the clinical classification described in this chapter to determine whether the language subtypes in children on the spectrum were stable or predictive of school-age language. Clinical experience suggests that as children receive language training and mature, those who were classified in the lexical subtype at preschool, and probably some of the less severely affected children in the mixed phonologic-syntactic subtype, develop the characteristics of those with the classic semantic-pragmatic subtype, but longitudinal research based on the analysis of spontaneous language samples is needed.

Many of the children who underwent a language regression as toddlers regain speech and it seems to me (but again without formal data to support this supposition) that they do not fall exclusively into any one of the clinically defined language subtypes. The majority recover language, some completely or virtually completely except for residual pragmatic, prosodic and semantic deficits. The vast majority of those who 'recover' retain enough autistic features to remain at the mild end of the autism spectrum. A few remain non-verbal or minimally verbal with impaired phonologic production and limited comprehension; as expected, such children are generally moderately to severely mentally retarded and more severely autistic than those able to speak.

It is important to mention here that there are children who undergo a catastrophic autistic regression *(disintegrative disorder)* as preschoolers or at school-age (Fombonne, 2002). Almost all become and remain mute life-long, severely autistic and retarded. Although disintegrative disorder is generally stated to have a worse outcome than autism (Volkmar & Cohen, 1989), a recent study (Kurita *et al.*, 2004) disputes this, albeit in a small number of children because the disorder is mercifully rare. Whether disintegrative disorder and the infinitely more prevalent autistic regression are distinct or related disorders is not known, but both appear to have heterogeneous aetiologies.

Adolescents and adults

Despite many descriptions of language in adolescence and adulthood, long-term longitudinal studies are sparse. Ballaban-Gil and colleagues (Ballaban-Gil *et al.*, 1996), on the basis of structured phone interviews to a parent, re-evaluated 48 individuals without severe mental retardation, 26 with documented or estimated normal or near-normal intelligence and 22 with mild to moderate cognitive impairment; one neurologist had diagnosed all of them in childhood as being on the autism spectrum. Expressive language had improved in 54 per cent and was stable in 19 per cent of the 26 with normal or near-normal intelligence, compared to improvement in 36 per cent and stability in 59 per cent of the 22 with mild or moderate cognitive impairment. Parents reported that expressive ability had worsened in 15 per cent and 5 per cent of the children in these two groups, but numbers are so small as to make this difference unreliable. The language of children seen for the first time below age six years was twice as likely to have improved as that of children seen between ages 6 and 12 years. Mawhood and colleagues (Mawhood *et al.*, 2000) reassessed at age 23–24 18 men who had been given a diagnosis of autism in childhood and whose mean non-verbal IQ (performance IQ or PIQ) at the time was 70 or better [mean PIQ 94, verbal IQ(VIQ) 66]. They found that VIQ had increased substantially to 82 in the nine individuals retested but that their PIQ had dropped by ten points. Only 8 of the 18 were speaking in full sentences and four were still essentially nonverbal. Language comprehension in childhood was the strongest predictor not only of language in adulthood but also of social skills and overall function. As was true in their early twenties, all the men's social skills remained deficient in mid-adult life and only one had obtained independent employment (Howlin *et al.*, 2000).

Neurologic correlates of language impairment in the autism spectrum disorders

Imaging

There is now a growing literature on morphometric imaging in autism, but very few of them address language specifically. In a series of studies, Herbert and colleagues compared 16 school-age boys identified at preschool as having autistic disorder and a non-verbal IQ of at least 80 to two groups of age and handedness-matched controls: normally-developing boys and boys with DLD. The many similarities between the brains of boys with DLD and autism brains were salient and included increased white matter volume in both, due to selective enlargement of superficial white matter which contains late myelinating intrahemispheric corticocortical fibers (Herbert *et al.*, 2004b). Even though, at the whole brain level, there was no asymmetry between the hemispheres in any of the three groups, there were cortical differences between regions, a notable one being that language-related frontal cortex was larger on the right in autism, larger on the left in normal controls (Herbert *et al.*, 2002). Parcellation into smaller cortical areas revealed that this rightward shift was more marked in autism than DLD, that more parcellation units in other association cortices were asymmetrical in autism than DLD, and that the asymmetry reflected enlargement on the right rather than loss of volume on the left, consonant with brain enlargement in both disorders (Herbert et al., 2004a). A single functional MRI study disclosed failure of voice-selective activation of the left superior temporal sulcus despite normal activation to non-vocal sounds in autism (Gervais et al., 2004).

Electrophysiology

In hearing children with autism, refined behavioral and physiologic studies have failed to demonstrate any impairment of peripheral or subcortical auditory function (Gravel et al., 2004). There are a small number of children with both peripheral hearing losses and an autism spectrum disorder (Jure et al., 1991), many of them with either syndromic deafness or a hearing loss due to a definable condition like an infection that damaged both the ear and the brain. No doubt these presumably unrelated deficits interact, but I know of no convincing evidence for an increase in the prevalence of autism in early non-syndromic deafness unassociated with brain dysfunction, in contrast with blindness which does seem to be a risk factor for autism (Hobson et al., 1999), although both are still controversial statements in need of further research based on modern diagnostic criteria.

Severely impaired four- to eight-year-old children with autism, compared to children with mental deficiency and normal controls, were found to have a significant delay and lower amplitude in the early obligatory cortical event-related response (ERP) component N1c to tones, (Bruneau et al., 1999), pointing to deficient processing of auditory stimuli in very young severely impaired children with autism. This component, which has a latency of 130-170 msec, appears to be generated in lateral temporal auditory association cortex, as opposed to the earlier N1b component with a latency of 100-110 msec generated in primary auditory cortex in the supratemporal plane which is not delayed following either tones or speech sounds in autism. In eight- to ten-year-old children with autism, N1c latency to tones was similar to normally developing controls but delayed over the left hemisphere in response to words. This N1c finding was replicated in another sample of eight- to nine-year-old but not found in 11- to 12-year-old children with autism (Dunn & Bates, 2004b). Another study of high-functioning children provided physiologic evidence for a deficit in language presented to the auditory modality: there was no deviance in the early automatic response (mismatch negativity) to occasional deviance in simple or complex tones or vowels, whereas the P3a component, an index of attentional orienting, was absent but only for vowel changes, which points to the 'speechiness' of the auditory stimulus as determinant of deviance (Ceponiene et al., 2003).

Differences in semantic processing at both the word (lexical) and sentence levels have been identified comparing normal children to those with autism. Children with autism have difficulty automatically organizing words presented to the visual or auditory modality into superordinate categories for efficient storage. For example, when asked to generate categorical words, such as 'animals', young children with autism offered atypical exemplars (Dunn et al., 1996); this suggested that they had stored each exemplar individually so that rare exemplars were just as likely to be retrieved from the lexicon as prototypic exemplars of the abstract superordinate category 'animal' which summarizes features shared by many familiar members of the group. Even high-functioning adults have deficits integrating new meaning into a context, which jeopardizes the creating of networks in memory to categorize words and ideas efficiently (Frith & Happe, 1994). A physiologic abnormality of the N4 wave which occurs some 400 msec post stimulus presentation and indexes processing of the semantic relatedness between a word and its context was found only in eight- to nine-year-old but not 11- to 12-year-old children with autism; it consisted of failure of the infrequent presentation of an out-of-category word to produce the expected increase in the amplitude of the N4 wave (Dunn & Bates, 2004a). That the abnormality was limited to the younger children confirms improvement of lexical semantic function with longer exposure to language.

Implications for language intervention in autism

As detailed in this chapter, research to date indicates that children with autism suffer from a variety of language deficits. As effective intervention requires that remediation addresses each child's particular deficits, this mandates a searching evaluation of the child's receptive and expressive deficits at each level of language. The first step is always to make sure that there is no peripheral hearing loss. In hearing children with severe comprehension deficits for speech it is mandatory to supplement the auditory modality by the visual. The most immediate measure is to limit the complexity and length of utterances and to speak mostly of the here-and-now, that is, to speak of what is happening as it is happening, for example of shoes as they are going onto the feet and of cookies as they are being offered. What this strategy does is provide a visual referent to the words being spoken. Presenting communications using sign language (Bonvillian, 1991), pictures (Frost & Bondy, 1994), a communication book, written language, a computer or other augmentative communication devices (National Research Council, 2001), far from retarding the emergence of speech may help it and, in any case, may reduce frustration significantly by enhancing comprehension and providing the child with an alternate channel for expression. In fluent children, it is important to keep in mind that comprehension of discourse and of question forms may be deficient in the face of an extensive vocabulary so that strategies to improve comprehension and conversational skills need to be provided (Minshew *et al.*, 2003).

As all children on the autism spectrum have pragmatic deficits, these must be addressed in all of them. Children must be taught and given the opportunity to practice pragmatic skills such as glancing up when addressed, looking a conversational partner in the eye, responding verbally or non-verbally when spoken to, and curtailing perseveration on favorite topics and repeated questioning. The techniques to assist non-fluent children to develop better articulation and grammatical skills are similar to those used with nonautistic children who have a mixed receptive/expressive DLD, but they can only be introduced effectively to children on the spectrum who have improved their joint attentional and pragmatic skills sufficiently to be reasonably motivated to interact and comply with demands (Allen *et al.*, 1989; Allen & Mendelson, 2000; Koegel, 2000). This is where systematic conditioning approaches like Applied Behavior Analysis (ABA) come into play because they are often rather rapidly effective for eliciting imitative speech in young nonverbal preschoolers, provided, that is, that their cognitive deficits are not severe or profound (Lovaas, 1981). But children with autism need to progress beyond echolalia and speech on demand. This is the focus of the many other language interventions in current use which share the common goal of fostering in more naturalistic functional contexts the communicative use of speech, or a visual language in nonverbal or poorly intelligible children (Ozonoff *et al.*, 2003).

References

Allen, D.A. & Mendelson, L. (2000): Parent, child, and professional: meeting the needs of young autistic children and their families in a multidisciplinary therapeutic nursery model. In: *Autistic spectrum disorders and psychoanalytic ideas: reassessing the fit*, ed. S. Epstein, pp. 704–731. Hillsdale, NJ: The Analytic Press.

Allen, D.A., Mendelson, L. & Rapin, I. (1989): Syndrome specific remediation in preschool developmental dysphasia. In: *Child neurology and developmental disabilities*, eds. J. H. French, S. Harel, P. Casaer, M. I. Gottlieb, I. Rapin & D. C. De Vivo, pp. 233–243. Baltimore: Paul Brookes.

American Psychiatric Association (2000): *Diagnostic and statistical manual of mental disorders*. 4th ed., text revision: DSMIV-TR 4th ed. Washington DC: American Psychiatric Association.

Andrews, N., Miller, E., Grant, A., Stowe, J., Osborne, V. & Taylor, B. (2004): Thimerosal exposure in infants and developmental disorders: a retrospective cohort study in the United Kingdom does not support a causal association. *Pediatrics* **114**, 584–591.

Ballaban-Gil, K. & Tuchman, R. (2000): Epilepsy and epileptiform EEG: association with autism and language disorders. Mental retardation and developmental disabilities research. *Reviews* **6**, 300–308.

Ballaban-Gil, K., Rapin, I., Tuchman, R.F. & Shinnar, S. (1996): Longitudinal examination of the behavioural, language, and social changes in a population of adolescents and young adults with autistic disorder. *Pediatric Neurology* **15**, 217–223.

Bishop, D.V.M. (1997): *Uncommon understanding: development and disorders of comprehension in children*. Hove, East Sussex, UK: Psychology Press.

Bondy, A.S. & Frost, L.A. (1998): The picture exchange communication system. *Semin. Speech Lang.* **19**, 373–388.

Bonvillian, J.D. (1991): Manual communication and autism: factors relating to sign language acquisition. In: *Theoretical issues in sign language and research*, eds. P. Siple & S.D. Fisher, Vol. 2 Psychology. Chicago, IL: University of Chicago Press.

Bonvillian, J.D., Nelson, K.E. & Rhyne, J.M. (1981): Sign language and autism. *J. Autism Dev. Disord.* **11**, 125–137.

Boucher, J. (1998): Clinical forum. SPD as a distinct diagnostic entity: logical considerations and directions for future research. *Int. J. Lang. Commun. Disord.* **33**, 71–81.

Bradford, Y., Haines, J., Hutcheson, H., Gardiner, M., Braun, T. & Sheffield, V. (2001): Incorporating language phenotypes strengthens evidence of linkage to autism. *Am. J. Med. Genet.* **105**, 539–547.

Bruneau, N., Roux, S., Adrien, J.L. & Barthelemy, C. (1999): Auditory associative cortex dysfunction in children with autism: evidence from late auditory evoked potentials (N1 wave-T complex). *Clin. Neurophysiol.* **110**, 1927–1934.

Ceponiene, R., Lepisto, T., Shestakova, A., Vanhala, R., Alku, P. & Naatanen, R. (2003): Speech-sound-selective auditory impairment in children with autism: they can perceive but do not attend. *Proc. Natl. Acad. Sci. USA* **100**, 5567–5572.

Chess, S., Korn, S.J. & Fernandez, P.B. (1971): *Psychiatric disorders of children with congenital rubella*. New York: Brunner/Mazel.

Comi, A.M., Zimmerman, A.W., Frye, V.H., Law, P.A. & Peeden, J.N. (1999): Familial clustering of autoimmune disorders and evaluation of medical risk factors in autism. *J. Child Neurol.* **14**, 388–394.

Croen, L.A., Grether, J.K., Hoogstrate, J. & Selvin, S. (2002): The changing prevalence of autism in California. *J. Autism Dev. Disord.* **32**, 207–215.

Deonna, T.W. (1991): Acquired epileptiform aphasia in children (Landau-Kleffner syndrome). *J. Clin. Neurophysiol.* **3**, 288–298.

Dunn, M. & Bates J. (in press): A cross-sectional study of change in electrophysiologic correlates of semantic classification in autism. *J. Autism Dev. Disord.*

Dunn, M.A. & Bates, J.C. (2005): Developmental change in neutral processing of words by children with autism. *J. Autism Dev. Disord.* **35** (3), 361–376.

Eisenmajer, R., Prior, M., Leekam, S., Wing, L., Ong, B. & Gould, J. (1998): Delayed language onset as a predictor of clinical symptoms in pervasive developmental disorders. *J. Autism Dev. Disord.* **28**, 527–533.

Fletcher, J.M., Barnes, M. & Dennis, M. (2002): Language development in children with spina bifida. *Semin. Pediatr. Neurol.* **9**, 201–208.

Fombonne, E. (2002): Prevalence of childhood disintegrative disorder. *Autism* **6**, 149–157.

Fombonne, E. (2003): Epidemiological surveys of autism and other pervasive developmental disorders: an update. *J. Autism Dev. Disord.* **33**, 365–382.

Frith, U. & Happe, F. (1994): Autism: beyond 'theory of mind'. *Cognition* **50**, 115–132.

Frost, L. & Bondy, A. (1994): *PECS: the Picture Exchange Communication System training Manual*. Cherry Hill, NJ: Pyramid Educational Consultants.

Gervais, H., Belin, P., Boddaert, N., Leboyer, M., Coez, A. & Sfaello, I. (2004): Abnormal cortical voice processing in autism. *Nat. Neurosci.* **7**, 801–802.

Gravel, J.S., Dunn, M., Lee, W. & Ellis, M.A. (2004): Peripheral audition of children on the autistic spectrum. *J. Speech Lang. Hear. Res.*

Herbert, M.R., Harris, G.J., Adrien, K.T., Ziegler, D.A., Makris, N. & Kennedy, D.N. (2002): Abnormal asymmetry in language association cortex in autism. *Ann. Neurol.* **52**, 588–596.

Herbert, M.R., Ziegler, D.A., Deutsch, C.K., O'Brien, L.M., Kennedy, D.N. & Filipek, P.A. (2004a): Brain asymmetries in autism and developmental language disorders: a nested whole-brain analysis. *Brain*, on-line publishing (doi:10.1093/brain/awh330).

Herbert, M.R., Ziegler, D.A., Makris, N., Filipek, P.A., Kemper, T.L. & Normandin, J.J. (2004b): Localization of white matter volume increase in autism and developmental language disorder. *Ann. Neurol.* **55**, 530–540.

Heron, J. & Golding, J. (2004): Thimerosal exposure in infants and developmental disorders: a prospective cohort study in the United kingdom does not support a causal association. *Pediatrics* **114**, 577–583.

Hobson, R.P., Lee, A. & Brown, R. (1999): Autism and congenital blindness. *J. Autism Dev. Disord.* **29**, 45–56.

Holmes, G.L., McKeever, M. & Saunders, Z. (1981): Epileptiform activity in aphasia of childhood: an epiphenomenon? *Epilepsia* **22**, 631–639.

Howlin, P., Mawhood, L. & Rutter, M. (2000): Autism and developmental receptive language disorder – a follow-up comparison in early adult life. II: Social, behavioural, and psychiatric outcomes. *J. Child Psychol. Psychiatry* **41**, 561–578.

Jure, R., Rapin, I. & Tuchman, R.F. (1991): Hearing-impaired autistic children. *Dev. Med. Child Neurol.* **33**, 1062–1072.

Kimmel, S.R. (2002): Vaccine adverse events: separating myth from reality. *Am. Fam. Physician* **66**, 2113–2120.

Klein, S.K., Tuchman, R.F. & Rapin, I. (2000): The influence of premorbid language skills and behavior on language recovery in children with verbal auditory agnosia. *J. Child Neurol.* **15**, 36–43.

Klin, A., Jones, W., Schultz, R., Volkmar, F. & Cohen, D. (2002): Visual fixation patterns during viewing of naturalistic social situations as predictors of social competence in individuals with autism. *AMA Arch. Gen. Psychiatry* **59**, 809–816.

Koegel, L.K. (2000): Interventions to facilitate communication in autism. *J. Autism Dev. Disord.* **30**, 383–391.

Korvatska, E., Van de, W.J., Anders, T.F. & Gershwin, M.E. (2002): Genetic and immunologic considerations in autism. *Neurobiol. Dis.* **9**, 107–125.

Kuhl, P.K., Andruski, J.E., Chistovich, I.A., Chistovich, L.A., Kozhevnikova, E.V. & Ryskina, V.L. (1997): Cross-language analysis of phonetic units in language addressed to infants. *Science* **277**, 684–686.

Kurita, H. (1996): Specificity and developmental consequences of speech loss in children with pervasive developmental disorders. *Psychiatry Clin. Neurosci.* **50**, 181–184.

Kurita, H., Kita, M. & Miyake, Y. (1992): A comparative study of development and symptoms among disintegrative psychosis and infantile autism with and without speech loss. *J. Autism Dev. Disord.* **22**, 175–188.

Kurita, H., Osada, H. & Miyake, Y. (2004): External validity of childhood disintegrative disorder in comparison with autistic disorder. *J. Autism Dev. Disord.* **34**, 355–362.

Laws, G. & Bishop, D. (2004): Pragmatic language impairment and social deficits in Williams syndrome: a comparison with Down syndrome and specific language impairment. *Int. J. Lang. Commun. Disord.* **39**, 45–64.

Leslie, A.M. & Frith, U. (1988): Autistic children's understanding of seeing, knowing and believing. *Br. J. Clin. Psychol.* **6**, 315–324.

Lewine, J.D., Andrews, R., Chez, M., Patil, A.A., Devinsky, O. & Smith, M. (1999): Magnetoencephalographic patterns of epileptiform activity in children with regressive autism spectrum disorders. *Pediatrics* **104**, 405–418.

Lord, C. & Paul, R. (1997): Language and communication in autism. In: *Handbook of autism and pervasive developmental disorders*, eds. D.J. Cohen & F.R. Volkmar (2n edn.), pp. 195–225. New York: John Wiley and Sons.

Madsen, K.M., Hviid, A., Vestergaard, M., Schendel, D., Wohlfahrt, J. & Thorsen, P. (2002): A population-based study of measles, mumps, and rubella vaccination and autism. *N. Engl. J. Med.* **347**, 1477–1482.

Mawhood, L., Howlin, P. & Rutter, M. (2000): Autism and developmental receptive language disorder – a comparative follow-up in early adult life. I: Cognitive and language outcomes. *J. Child Psychol. Psychiatry* **41**, 547–559.

McVicar, K.A., Ballaban-Gil, K., Rapin, I., Moshé, S.L. & Shinnar, S. (2005): Epileptiform EEG abnormalities in children with language regression. *Neurology* **65**, 129–131.

Miller, E. (2003): Measles-mumps-rubella vaccine and the development of autism. *Semin. Pediatr. Infect. Dis.* **14**, 199–206.

Minshew, N.J., Meyer, J.A. & Dunn, M. (2003): Autism spectrum disorders. In: *Child Neuropsychology*, eds. S. Segalowitz & I. Rapin (2nd edn.), pp. 863–896. Amsterdam: Elsevier Science.

Muhle, R., Trentacoste, S.V. & Rapin, I. (2004): The genetics of autism. *Pediatrics* **113**, e472–e486.

Myhr, G. (1998): Autism and other pervasive developmental disorders: exploring the dimensional view. *Can. J. Psychiatry* **43**, 589–595.

National Research Council (2001): *Educating children with autism*. Washington, DC: National Academy Press.

Osterling, J.A., Dawson, G. & Munson, J.A. (2002): Early recognition of 1-year-old infants with autism spectrum disorder *versus* mental retardation. *Dev. Psychopathol.* **14**, 239–251.

Ozonoff, S., Rogers, S.J. & Hendren, R.L. (2003): *Autism spectrum disorders: a research review for practitioners.* Washington, DC: American Psychiatric Publishing.

Pichichero, M.E., Cernichiari, E., Lopreiato, J. & Treanor, J. (2002): Mercury concentrations and metabolism in infants receiving vaccines containing thimerosal: a descriptive study. *Lancet* **360**, 1737–1741.

Prizant, B.M. & Rydell, P. (1984): An analysis of the functions of immediate echolalia in autistic children. *J. Speech Hear. Res.* **27**, 183–192.

Rapin, I. (1996): *Preschool children with inadequate communication: developmental language disorders, autism, low IQ.* London: Mac Keith Press.

Rapin, I. (1997): Trastornos de la communicación en el autismo infantil. In: *El languaje del niño*, eds. J. Narbona & C. Chevrie-Muller. Barcelona: Masson.

Rapin, I. & Dunn, M. (2003): Update on the language disorders of individuals on the autistic spectrum. *Brain Dev.* **25**, 166–172.

Schultz, R.T., Grelotti, D.J., Klin, A., Kleinman, J., Van der, G.C. & Marois, R. (2003): The role of the fusiform face area in social cognition: implications for the pathobiology of autism. *Philos. Trans. R. Soc. Lond., B, Biol. Sci.* **358**, 415–427.

Shaywitz, S.E. (2003): *Overcoming dyslexia: a new and complete science-based program for overcoming reading problems at any level.* New York: Alfred A. Knopf.

Shinnar, S., Rapin, I., Arnold, S., Tuchman, R.F., Shulman, L. & Ballaban-Gil, K. (2001): Language regression in childhood. *Pediatr. Neurol.* **24**, 185–191.

Sy, W., Djukic, A., Shinnar, S., Dharmani, C. & Rapin, I. (2003): Clinical characteristics of language regression in children. *Dev. Med. Child Neurol.* **45**, 508–514.

Tager-Flusberg, H. (2003): Language impairments in children with complex neurodevelopmental disorders: the case of autism. In: *Language competence across populations: toward a definition of specific language impairment*, eds. Y. Levy & J. Schaeffer, pp. 297–321. Mahwah, NJ: Lawrence Erlbaum Associates.

Thal, D. & Bates, E. (1990): Continuity and variation in early language development. In: *Individual differences in infancy: reliability, stability, and prediction*, eds. J. Colombo & J. Sagan. Hillsdale, NJ: Erlbaum.

Torres, A.R., Maciulis, A., Stubbs, E.G., Cutler, A. & Odell, D. (2002): The transmission disequilibrium test suggests that HLA-DR4 and DR13 are linked to autism spectrum disorder. *Hum. Immunol.* **63**, 311–316.

Tuchman, R.F. & Rapin, I. (1997): Regression in pervasive developmental disorders: seizures and epileptiform EEG correlates. *Pediatrics* **99**, 560–566.

Volkmar, F.R. & Cohen, D.J. (1989): Disintegrative disorder or 'late onset' autism. *J. Child Psychol. Psychiatry* **5**, 717–724.

World Health Organization (1992): *The ICD-10 classification of mental and behavioural disorders: clinical descriptions and diagnostic guidelines* (10th edn.). Geneva, CH: World Health Organization.

Chapter 10

Language regression in autism: pathogenesis and differential diagnosis

Barış Korkmaz

*Istanbul University, CERRAHPASA Medical Faculty, Department of Neurology, Division of Child Neurology,
P.K. 18 Cerrahpasa, 34301 Istanbul, Turkey
bkorkmaz@istanbul.edu.tr*

Summary

Language regression in childhood is most likely to occur within the context of autism or of a more generalized cognitive regression in many different disorders, with or without epilepsy and/or epileptiform EEG discharges – including Landau-Kleffner syndrome (LKS), epilepsy with continuous spike and wave during slow sleep (ECSWS), autistic regression, and disintegrative disorder. Regression typically occurs before the age of 5, mostly between 8 months and 2 years. Clinical onset of language regression is usually gradual and takes place over weeks or months. Boys and children less than 3 years of age who regress have a higher probability of developing autistic behaviors. EEG abnormalities are reported in about a third of the children with language regression and are more common in those with seizures. However, the causal connection between language regression and epilepsy or epileptiform electroencephalographic (EEG) abnormalities remains unclear. Prognosis in cognitive/language regression is variable. In many children some improvement occurs in their adaptive skills, while problems with language and learning tend to persist. A sleep EEG may be appropriate in some patients presenting with language/cognitive/behavioral regression. Although there is no conclusive evidence that anticonvulsant drugs will have a therapeutic effect on the behavioral or language abnormalities, antiepileptic agents such as sodium valproate or ACTH may be considered as a treatment in some cases.

Introduction

Language regression is the loss of previously acquired language abilities affecting comprehension, expression, or both, and is usually accompanied by cognitive deterioration after normal or near normal neurological and mental development. Isolated language regression, except in Landau-Kleffner syndrome (LKS or acquired epileptic aphasia), is rare.

Language regression occurs commonly within the context of autism or of a more generalized cognitive regression in many different disorders of childhood, with or without epilepsy or epileptiform discharges on electroencephalography (EEG) (Table 1). LKS and some other epileptic disorders characterized by electroclinical status epilepticus during slow sleep (ESES), autistic regression and disintegrative disorder of childhood, and developmental language disorders should specifically be included in the differential diagnosis of language or cognitive regression.

Table 1. Neurological disorders characterized by language/cognitive deterioration*

1. Critical epileptiform discharges with or without epilepsy
    i. Transient cognitive impairment
    ii. Non-convulsive status epilepticus
    iii. Epileptic syndromes with cognitive/language/autistic regression and EEG abnormalities
       – Landau-Kleffner syndrome (LKS),
       – Continuous spike and wave during slow sleep (CSWS)
       – Other epileptic syndromes (*e.g.*, Lennox-Gastaut syndrome, infantile spasms, rolandic epilepsy, acquired epileptiform opercular syndrome etc.)

2. Pervasive developmental disorder of childhood
    – Autistic regression
    – Rett syndrome
    – Disintegrative disorder of childhood

3. Developmental language disorders
4. Other neurological causes including dementia of childhood (SSPE, Wilson's disease, leukodystrophies etc.)
5. Psychiatric and psychological causes

* Binnie *et al.*, 1987; Shafrir & Prensky, 1995; Rogers, 2004.

Although most of these disorders have distinctive features, they have many overlapping clinical and laboratory findings, and one disorder may evolve into another over time (Hirsch *et al.*, 1995; McVicar & Shinnar, 2004). Some investigators (Deonna *et al.*, 1997; Metz-Lutz & Massa, 1999; Stefanatos *et al.*, 2002; Deonna & Roulet-Perez, 2005) suggest that any kind of developmental regression with paroxysmal EEG abnormalities (with or without clinical epilepsy) should be classified under the spectrum of acquired cognitive/behavioral disturbances. Indeed, different syndromes and clinical disorders result from the involvement of different brain regions (Roulet-Perez *et al.*, 1993) with diverse aetiologies, although they share a common pathogenic mechanism.

Epileptic disorders with cognitive/autistic/language regression and EEG abnormalities

Epilepsy can cause problems in the acquisition, development, and maintenance of new skills and, ultimately, can be responsible for selective deficits such as a specific regression of graphomotor skills (Dubois *et al.*, 2003). Prolonged focal and generalized non-convulsive epileptic activity (lasting for several hours or days) may present with psychiatric symptoms and acquired cognitive dysfunction, including altered or blunted consciousness (Trimble *et al.*, 2000). On the other hand, epileptiform bioelectric discharges were shown to have a direct and transient effect on some aspects of cognitive function which can accumulate and result in detrimental effects on intelligence (Binnie *et al.*, 1987; Tromp *et al.*, 2003). In fact, there are specific epileptic syndromes characterized by language and cognitive regression with epileptic seizures and epileptiform EEG abnormalities (Bureau, 1995). They are included in the group of epileptic syndromes whose focal or generalized origin remains undetermined in the International Classification of Epilepsies (Commission of the International League Against Epilepsy, ILAE, 1989).

Landau-Kleffner syndrome (acquired epileptic aphasia)

Landau-Kleffner syndrome is defined by gradual or sudden loss of speech and language, together with unilateral or, more often, bilateral epileptiform EEG abnormalities with or without clinical seizures (Landau & Kleffner, 1957). It is most commonly seen in the 3- to 9-year age range, with a 2:1 predominance in boys. The youngest age reported is 18 months (Uldall *et al.*,

2000). Occasionally it starts as late as 10 to 12 years (Dugas *et al.*, 1995). Epileptic seizures may be present, but in one third of cases there is no history of seizures. These may precede or follow the onset of the language disorder. The most common types of seizures are partial motor seizures with secondary generalization (usually nocturnal), generalized tonic-clonic seizures, atypical absences, atonic seizures with head drops, minor automatisms, eyelid myoclonias, and eye blinking (Deonna *et al.*, 1977; Rossi *et al.*, 1999). Complex partial seizures of temporal lobe origin are rare and tonic seizures are probably incompatible with the diagnosis (Panayiotopoulos, 1999). Patients usually have a normal history of psychomotor and language development, although some may have preexisting language problems (Soprano *et al.*, 1994). The cardinal feature of clinically typical Landau-Kleffner syndrome (acquired aphasia with convulsive disorder) is the language regression, although hyperactivity, temper tantrums, aggressiveness, or impaired social communication may be accompanying features. In classic Landau-Kleffner syndrome, cognitive deficits are language-domain-specific. Psychotic or autistic features may be present in cases with an early onset of language disturbance (Klein *et al.*, 2000), but it is currently controversial whether to consider those cases as part of an extended Landau-Kleffner spectrum (McVicar & Shinnar, 2004).

The aetiology of LKS is unclear. Although most cases are idiopathic, LKS may represent a final common pathway with multiple potential etiologies (Pearl *et al.*, 2001), as it has been reported in the context of a variety of disorders ranging from arachnoidal cyst (De Volder *et al.*, 1994) to perisylvian polymicrogyria (Huppke *et al.*, 2005). The awake EEG usually shows brief bursts of temporal or temporo-occipital spike-and-wave discharges, either symmetrical or asymmetrical, while in many cases continuous 1.5 Hz to 5 Hz spike-and-wave discharges typically appear during slow sleep (Beaumanoir, 1992; Deonna & Roulet-Perez, 1995; De Negri, 1997).

Epilepsy with continuous spike and wave during slow sleep (ECSWS)

ECSWS is a clinical epileptic syndrome characterized by a general regression in neuropsychological abilities, often associated with behavioral disorders such as hyperactivity, learning disabilities, and in some instances psychotic regression (Bureau, 1995) and with the typical EEG pattern of ESES (electroclinical status epilepticus during slow sleep) which consists of sleep-induced continuous or discontinuous paroxysmal EEG activity, lasting several months or years. Premorbid cognitive development is normal. As with Landau-Kleffner syndrome, there are many symptomatic forms of ECSWS (Guerrini *et al.*, 1998; Ben-Zeev *et al.*, 2004).

It is not a settled issue whether LKS and ECSWS should be considered two separate entities or subtypes of a single syndrome, as they display many common features (De Negri, 1997; Maquet *et al.*, 1999; Tassinari *et al.*, 2002; Deonna & Roulet-Perez, 1995). However, the common origin of the two syndromes is suggested by recent functional brain imaging and by neurophysiological and neurosurgical techniques (Rossi *et al.*, 1999; Hirsch *et al.*, 1995; Morrell, 1995; Neville *et al.*, 1997). While some researchers think that LKS and ECSWS may blend into one another as the clinical picture evolves into ECSWS which is characterized by a later more severe and global cognitive regression (Rossi *et al.*, 1999), others clearly support the differentiation into two syndromes on the basis of several clinical and EEG features (Genton & Guerrini, 1993). Furthermore, as many of the neuropsychological and neuropsychiatric symptoms seen in these children may resemble those found in disintegrative disorder of childhood or autistic regression (Roulet-Perez *et al.*, 1993), some investigators apply the term disintegrative disorder to the severe global regression and use ESES or ECSWS synonymously for the EEG. Hence, nosological boundaries of ECSWS in relation to other clinical entities presenting either with the same EEG and/or similar clinical features, remains to be established (Tassinari et al., 1995).

The major feature differentiating ECSWS from the other clinical disorders with language regression is the typical ESES pattern, as well as the more generalized involvement of cognitive functions. ESES usually disappears during the waking state and during REM sleep. It is usually bilaterally diffuse, although it sometimes appears unilaterally or with predominance in a certain area. However, there are patients who demonstrate continuous activation of spikes, or spike-and-wave potentials (without clinical seizures) during eye closure. Although the strict definition implies the presence of epileptiform discharges during at least 85 per cent of non-REM sleep, some investigators include children with less than that if other clinical features are present (Ballaban-Gil & Tuchman, 2000). ESES, as an electroclinical pattern, may be relatively independent of the underlying aetiology but may affect the brain areas differentially with respect to their age-specific development (Tassinari et al., 1992; Galanopoulou et al., 2000). While localization of the spike-and-wave discharges is predominantly temporal or parietotemporal in LKS and tends to remain focal and to be activated during all sleep stages, it is predominantly frontal in ECSWS and it tends to spread bilaterally to become diffuse during slow sleep (Genton & Guerrini, 1993).

ESES, although typically seen in ECSWS, can develop in a broad spectrum of childhood epileptic conditions, including some with a favorable neuropsychological prognosis. No single feature seems to be common to all conditions within this spectrum, except the evolution of the bioelectric abnormalities in the EEG and, to a certain extent, the apparent relation of the clinical features to the localization and the diffusion of those abnormalities (Tassinari et al., 1995; Saltik et al., 2005). The continuum of ESES includes LKS and epilepsy with continuous spike-and-wave during slow sleep (ECSWS) at one end, and benign epilepsy of childhood with Rolandic spikes at the other, with some intermediate forms (Pearl et al., 2001).

Other epileptic syndromes

Several authors previously reported a relationship between LKS and the benign epilepsies of childhood (Deonna & Roulet-Perez, 1995). Indeed, some children with benign epileptic syndromes such as Rolandic epilepsy have neuropsychological deficits, including language impairment, which may persist even though the children were in remission; these children may never have had any demonstrable ESES feature on EEG (Monjauze et al., 2005). An early form of Rolandic epilepsy was reported to interfere with prelinguistic skills in a very young child, associated with an early regression of babbling and delay in the emergence of language; this deficit recovered completely with anti-epileptic treatment (Dubois et al., 2004). There are reported cases of benign childhood epilepsy with centro-temporal spikes evolving into Landau-Kleffner syndrome (Fejerman et al., 2000) or ECSWS (Saltik et al., 2005). An increase in seizure frequency or development of new seizure types, the appearance of behavioral problems, decrease in cognitive performance, or a tendency for previously focal abnormalities to spread in follow-up EEGs may be alerting features to a developing ESES in children with idiopathic partial epilepsies (Saltik et al., 2005). Intermediate forms between benign childhood epilepsy with centro-temporal spikes and Landau-Kleffner syndrome, which occasionally display typical ESES pattern, include Panayiotopoulos syndrome, Foix-Chavany-Marie syndrome, and atypical benign partial epilepsy (Shafrir & Prensky, 1995; Pearl et al., 2001).

Panayiotopoulos syndrome is one of the benign, age-related, idiopathic focal epilepsies of childhood. It is characterized by autonomic seizures (predominantly nocturnal) such as vomiting, behavioral disturbances, deviation of the eyes, and often impairment of consciousness that can progress to convulsions (Ferrie et al., 2006). The interictal EEG frequently shows occipital paroxysms or occipital spikes, although one-fifth of the cases have only extraoccipital spikes in a normal EEG background. A few patients with initially typical early-onset benign childhood occipital epilepsy (Panayiotopoulos type) syndrome were reported to have language impairment secondary to continuous spike-and-wave discharges during slow sleep (Caraballo et al., 2001; Ferrie et al., 2002).

Foix-Chavany-Marie syndrome (FCMS) is characterized by linguo-bucco-facial apraxia with facial weakness, drooling, palatal and lingual speech disorders, masticatory problems, and increased jaw reflex (Weller, 1993). Functional cases of FCMS on an epileptic and ictal basis are reported in relation to benign Rolandic epilepsy presenting with status epilepticus in which the interictal EEG displayed ESES (Colamaria et al., 1991).

'Atypical benign partial epilepsy of childhood', described by Aicardi and Chevrie in 1982, is also known as 'pseudo-Lennox syndrome' or 'Doose syndrome' (Doose & Baier, 1989). It is characterized by several types of seizures, notably partial motor seizures, atypical absences, and myoclonic-atonic seizures, with an onset between 2 and 6 years of age. Its hallmark is that the neurological and mental functions remain essentially normal throughout its course, although there may be some degree of temporary mental slowing or behavioral disturbance during the active seizure periods. Sleep EEGs display the ESES pattern particularly during the active period of atonic seizures (Aicardi & Chevrie, 1982; Aicardi, 2000).

The Lennox-Gastaut syndrome may occasionally begin in a normal child and eventually causes cognitive regression (Besag, 1988). Generalized bursts of 2–2.5 Hz spike-wave complexes may be continuous, but the EEG does not show dramatic changes between awake and sleep EEG recordings. In addition to atypical absences, atonic seizures and head drops, typical tonic seizures occur mostly during non-REM sleep and are sometimes associated with runs of generalized rhythmical 10 Hz spikes (Ferrie et al., 1998). Cases with hypsarrhythmia without clinical signs may also be classified within the group of electrical or bioelectrical status. In some cases, a continuous hypsarrhythmia is observed only during sleep. The correlations between sleep and prolonged epileptic activity are reviewed in relation to several forms of status epilepticus and epileptic encephalopathies (Froscher, 1991)

Pervasive Developmental Disorder (PDD) spectrum

Several clinical entities are listed under the eponym of pervasive developmental disorders (American Psychiatric Association, 1994). Most of these are related to cognitive-language regression. Autistic disorder appears to be the most frequent condition in which regression occurs (Rogers, 2004), whereas it is less likely to occur in Asperger syndrome when compared with other PDD subgroups (Whiteley, 2004).

Autistic regression (setback-type autism, acquired autistic syndrome)

Autism is a dynamic disorder, as its manifestations change with age and in many cases it improves with early intervention. However, approximately one third of autistic children (usually between the ages of 18 and 24 months) show regressive changes affecting overall development, including language, sociability, and play, after normal or near-normal development before the onset of the regression (Tuchman & Rapin, 1997). This mode of progression is not indicative of a typical degenerative disease of the brain, as it leads to a prolonged plateau after which development resumes (Luyster et al., 2005).

Disintegrative disorder of childhood

This disorder, sometimes called Heller's syndrome or Heller's dementia (progressive disintegrative psychosis, pervasive disintegrative disorder), refers to a subgroup of children on the PDD spectrum who were developing entirely normally, including speaking in sentences, but in whom regression occurs after 2 years of age and occasionally as late as mid-childhood (2 to 10 years). The severity of the cognitive and behavioral manifestations and the later age of the regression, and the presence of problems during earlier development help to differentiate disintegrative disorder from others such as Landau-Kleffner syndrome and autistic regression. In comparison to children with autistic regression, those with disintegrative disorder of childhood more often show fearfulness during the period of speech loss, are more likely to have epilepsy, and more commonly show stereotypies at their first visit after speech loss (on average about 6 years of age), and a significantly less uneven intellectual profile (Kurita *et al.*, 2004). The risk of epilepsy is as high as 70 per cent (Mouridsen *et al.*, 1999). In disintegrative disorder of childhood, regression is more profound, with a general cognitive regression. These children may become permanently demented. There is no detectable cause in most cases. The aetiology is heterogeneous in others and includes some known causes such as tuberous sclerosis (Mouridsen *et al.*, 1998). Although prognosis is widely accepted to be much worse than for autistic regression, a recent study showed that there was no significant difference in the retardation level between these two groups with regard to short-term outcome (Kurita *et al.*, 2004).

Rett syndrome

Rett syndrome is a disorder characteristically seen in girls which is associated with several different mutations in the gene encoding methyl-CpG-binding protein 2 (MeCP2). Regression is a defining feature of the disorder. After a period of normal development, at around 6 months of age, the growth of the head circumference decelerates and autistic features appear. These include loss of communication and social skills, poor eye contact, and lack of interest, psychomotor retardation, and spasticity (Kerr & Engerström, 2001). Seizures, especially generalized seizures, occur at various stages of the illness and may be intractable. Mutations have been discovered in Rett syndrome variants, mentally retarded males, and occasional autistic children. As there are several atypical cases within a broad spectrum of clinical manifestations – because of variable clinical severity, perhaps reflecting the type and site of the MeCP2 gene mutation coupled with possible variation in X-chromosome inactivation – Rett syndrome should always be considered in the differential diagnosis of any cognitive regression, particularly in autistic girls (Chae *et al.*, 2004; Neul & Zoghbi, 2004; Schanen *et al.*, 2004).

Other causes of language regression

Developmental language disorders

Although regression is not typical of most cases of developmental language disorders, language regression may occur as the worsening of already abnormally developing language in some cases (Ballaban-Gill & Tuchman, 2000; Klein *et al.*, 2000), without any evidence of bioelectric abnormality suggestive of a known disorder or any other apparent cause. In early-onset cases of Landau-Kleffner syndrome, the differential diagnosis with developmental dysphasia associated with EEG discharges can be difficult. The same applies to children with autistic features, regression, and epileptiform EEGs (Tuchman & Rapin, 1997). Epileptiform activities in the

EEG are also seen in some children with developmental dysphasia (Maccario *et al.*, 1982; Echenne *et al.*, 1992; Picard *et al.*, 1998), adding difficulties to the differential diagnosis of Landau-Kleffner syndrome and related disorders.

Other neurological conditions

Cognitive/language deterioration of children may be a feature of many progressive degenerative neurologic disorders of childhood such as the leucodystrophies, subacute sclerosing panencephalitis, Wilson's disease, and Huntington's chorea (Fenichel, 1997). Rarely some sleep disorders (Archbold *et al.*, 2004) and some drugs (Gross-Tsur & Shalev, 2004) may cause acquired cognitive dysfunction. Neuropsychological dysfunction, and especially language problems in children less than 5 years of age, may be clinically subtle due to the plasticity of the brain, and therefore may pass unnoticed. Finally, a progressive hearing loss acquired during the critical stages of language acquisition, may give rise to language regression so that an extensive workup for acquired deafness may need to be considered.

Psychiatric and psychological causes

Schizophrenia, depression (Pollard & Prendergast, 2004), and severe emotional disturbance due to difficult life events or disasters (for example, earthquakes) may cause transient, episodic, or permanent cognitive/language regression, or fluctuation in the mental functions. Selective mutism is a disorder in which children consistently fail to speak in specific social situations where they are expected to speak (*e.g.*, in school), while they demonstrate language competence in other situations. It typically starts at preschool or during the early school years. Onset is usually slow, and for a definitive diagnosis it should last longer than 4 weeks. Biologically mediated temperament and anxiety components seem to play a major role. It is more common among girls than boys (Kumpulainen, 2002; APA, 1994). Selective mutism can be easily differentiated from other disorders that cause language regression on the basis of typical clinical features and the absence of EEG and other laboratory findings, but it needs to be documented by a recording of the child's speech in an environment where she is comfortable and able to converse.

Clinical features of language regression

Isolated language regression is much rarer than general cognitive regression, and in the great majority of cases it is associated with autistic regression (Sy *et al.*, 2003). In a recent study it was shown that boys and children less than 3 years of age who regressed were at highest risk for developing autistic behaviors (Shinnar *et al.*, 2001).

Indeed, one-third of all autistic children show cognitive regression, almost always with some speech/language loss (Tuchman & Rapin, 1997). Parents usually report gradual regression of language, most commonly the loss of their child's first few words, typically occurring over weeks or months before the age of 5, mostly spanning between 8 months and 2 years. Changes in language may be subtle and insidious although, rarely, a sudden overnight loss of vocabulary may occur. Loss of acquired language may involve only the loss of communicative gestures (Shinnar *et al.*, 2001).

There may be developmental language disorder, language delay, or some cognitive deficits before regression begins. Epilepsy may or may not be an associated feature. During adolescence, a further cognitive/behavioral regression may be seen (Goldberg *et al.*, 2003).

In some cases (38 per cent) – especially in the children who had a rapid clinical regression – a triggering factor is identified (Sy et al., 2003). The parents tend to attribute the regression to environmental causes such as accidents, birth of a new sibling, or rarely, to medical interventions (Kobayashi & Murata, 1998). The detection of language regression depends largely on parental report and clinical recognition and reporting of skills (Goldberg et al., 2003).

Some linguistic features of language regression

The spectrum of linguistic problems is broad in cases with language regression. The typical language profile of Landau-Kleffner syndrome is verbal auditory agnosia (Rapin et al., 1992) but different types of aphasia (Soprano et al., 1994) and, in the most severe cases, auditory agnosia and cortical deafness are reported (Kaga, 1999). In one-tenth of the cases there is no receptive language disorder and expressive language problems predominate (Marien et al., 1993). There may be articulation problems, telegraphic speech, or total mutism. During the evolution of the disorder, the type of speech/language difficulty may change.

Verbal auditory agnosia (VAA) is at the core of various overlapping clinical disorders with language/cognitive regression (Tuchman & Rapin, 2002). VAA is the inability to decode speech presented to the auditory channel, with preserved ability to decode language presented to the visual channel (Rapin et al., 1992; Metz-Lutz & Massa, 1999). In VAA, speech sounds lose their significance; a child no longer responds to commands even when voices are raised. Word deafness may deteriorate into total unresponsiveness and impaired expressive communication over a variable time interval. Expression is marked by a gradual increase in misarticulations and telegraphic speech. A fluent jargon or total mutism may occur. Hence these children have a severe receptive and expressive language disorder (Rapin et al., 1992) which is believed to arise from inadequate auditory or phonologic processing that engages activity in primary or secondary auditory cortices (Hecaen & Albert, 1978). There are acquired (Landau-Kleffner syndrome) and developmental forms of VAA (Klein et al., 1995). VAA is the most likely subtype of language disorder to be associated with epilepsy – a disorder not infrequently caused by temporal lobe dysfunction (Tuchman et al., 1991a; Tuchmann & Rapin, 2002).

Non-linguistic auditory agnosia is the severest form of language regression. The child does not react to even familiar noises such as bells, whistles, or a ringing phone (Kaga, 1999). The affected child is incapable of attributing a semantic value to acoustic signals. These children are usually mistakenly thought to be deaf or autistic, as they do not respond to sounds. It is because of this that the diagnosis is often delayed, and mistaken for acquired deafness or mutism (Panayiotopoulos, 1999).

Although verbal auditory agnosia is one of the major types of language deficit, particularly in severe autism, children with VAA are not always autistic; not infrequently, the rare pure case VAA is misidentified as autistic. These non-autistic children may develop a crude sign system of their own or some communicative gestures. Children with acquired VAA, especially those with subclinical epileptiform EEG discharges, are more likely to experience fluctuations in language skills than those in other groups (Sy et al., 2003).

Language regression and (subclinical) epilepsy

The complex relationship between language regression and epilepsy is not well understood. Even in cases of LKS with clinical epilepsy there is not necessarily a tight temporal correlation between loss of language and seizure onset or the occurrence of fluctuations.

Epilepsy is common in autism, as it develops in about one third of autistic adolescents (Rapin & Katzman, 1998). However, the causal connection between autism and epilepsy in general, and autistic regression and epilepsy in particular, is also unclear.

A temporal relationship between the onset of seizures and regression of language occurred in 36 per cent of children with verbal auditory agnosia and epilepsy (Tuchman et al., 1991b). In another large cohort of autistic patients, regression had occurred equally among children without seizures and in those with epilepsy (Tuchman & Rapin, 1997). On the other hand, still another study revealed a high incidence of epilepsy in the cases with regression (31 per cent in those with regression vs. 15 per cent in those without) (Kobayashi & Murata, 1998). However, in a more recent study, there was a history of seizures in 15 per cent of 196 children with language regression (Sy et al., 2003). Seizures were more common in children who regressed after they reached 3 years of age, and children with seizures were less likely to have associated autistic regression.

Bioelectric features and pathophysiology

The relation between the epileptiform EEG abnormalities and autistic or cognitive (including language) regression remains controversial, even in relation to LKS. EEG abnormalities are reported in 37–61 per cent of patients with language regression They were found to be more common in children with seizures (Shinnar et al., 2001; Nasr et al., 2001; McVicar et al., 2005) and in children with isolated language regression. Autistic regression was associated with an epileptiform EEG in 14 per cent of non-epileptic children who had undergone regression, as opposed to 6 per cent of children with neither regression nor epilepsy (Tuchman & Rapin, 1997). A recent study indicated autism with regression was not influenced by either the paroxysmal abnormalities or epilepsy (Canitano et al., 2005).

Magnetoencephalography (MEG), more sensitive to deeper sulcal foci of bioelectric discharges than EEG, identified epileptiform activity in 41 of 50 children with autistic regression (82 per cent), while the simultaneous EEG detected only 68 per cent (Lewine et al., 1999). However, there may have been a selection bias in this study because children with epilepsy or epileptiform EEGs were overrepresented as they were referred to an epilepsy center for the consideration of epilepsy surgery; the likely consequence was an atypically high proportion of children with uncontrolled seizures.

Many clinical and electrophysiological studies suggest that epileptiform discharges in the EEG without clinical seizures can be responsible for behavioral and cognitive impairment (Binnie et al., 1987; Maquet et al., 1995, Deonna & Roulet-Perez, 2005). A recent study suggests a correlation between the location of spikes and selective cognitive deficits in children with benign partial epilepsies, suggesting that focal interictal spikes may interfere with complex cognitive functions (Wolff et al., 2005)

MEG studies, alone or with EEG, indicated that the source of spike-and-wave discharges was mainly in the intrasylvian and perisylvian regions (Paetau, 2002) well known to be associated with language development and functions. The major site of the epileptic zone in LKS seems to be the dorsolateral surface of the superior temporal gyrus, especially in the auditory cortex, with the spike dipole being oriented tangentially to the scalp surface (Morrell et al., 1995). Discharges from this site may result in widespread epileptiform activity causing significant language and cognitive dysfunction (Deonna & Roulet-Perez, 2005). In LKS the earliest spike activity originates in the intrasylvian cortex, and secondary spikes in ipsilateral perisylvian, temporooccipital, and parietooccipital areas (Paetau et al., 1999), in contrast to Rolandic spikes which have a precentral origin (Ishitobi *et al.*, 2005). In cases with autistic regression, MEG reveals additional non-sylvian zones of independent epileptiform activity (Lewine *et al.*, 1999).

The neurobiological findings suggest three possible interacting levels of involvement with regard to the pathophysiology of language regression

First, focal epileptic discharges might have changed the cortical organization of language (Maquet *et al.*, 1999; Metz-Lutz & Massa, 1999), presumably causing aberrant development of synaptic connections. As the neuropathology of Rett syndrome shares certain features with other neurodevelopmental disorders, including autism, it may be a prototype for the genetic, molecular, and neurobiological analysis of regressive neurodevelopmental disorders likely to share a similar mechanism involving MeCP2 regulation and expression (Neul & Zoghbi, 2004). Neuropathological findings in Rett syndrome include mainly the selective reduction of dendritric spines in the pyramidal cells and abnormalities in synapse maintenance and modulation, features which have also been reported in autism (Glaze, 2004).

It was proposed that persistence of residual inappropriate synaptic contacts in the developing temporo-parietal cortex because of a persistent paroxysmal activity opposing normal apoptotic loss of synapses by falsely strengthening them, produces a permanent language dysfunction (Morrell *et al.*, 1995; Smith, 1998). This would also explain why eventual normalization of the EEG is not necessarily paralleled with improvement of aphasia. Recently, volumetric MR analysis (done at ages 5 to 6.5 years) in children with typical Landau-Kleffner syndrome (age of onset: 3–4.5), showed volume reduction in bilateral superior temporal areas, specifically in the planum temporale and superior temporal gyrus, where receptive language is localized (Takeoka *et al.*, 2004). Although volume reduction might have existed before language regression (due either to dysgenesis or as a consequence of steroid use), it is likely that early temporal lobe epileptiform activity caused focal cortical atrophy which prevented language recovery despite disappearance of the epileptiform activity (Bourgeois & Landau, 2004).

Second, thalamocortical dysfunction shown in these children – such as altered patterns in the decay of auditory memory traces and dysfunction of auditory sensory gating mechanism (Paetau, 1994; Isnard *et al.*, 1995; Seri *et al.*, 1998; Maquet *et al.*, 1999; Hurley *et al.*, 2000) – may well be responsible for inefficient analysis of sounds, which could eventually give rise to problems in language learning mechanisms.

Third, bilateral spread of discharges is likely to interfere with the hemispheric organization of language and other related cognitive functions. In fact, the mechanism of bilateral secondary synchronies after an initial functional spike focus is hypothesized to be the basis of the language impairment (Beaumanoir, 1985).

Despite the accumulation of data on the harmful and permanent effects of the bioelectric discharges, it is still possible that the EEG discharges and seizures are manifestations of underlying primary abnormalities of the cortex in the speech areas, rather than the cause of the language problems (Holmes *et al.*, 1981).

Laboratory investigations

Except in symptomatic cases, neurologic examination in many cases of language/autistic regression is normal. Neuropsychological evaluation, including a full language assessment, is important to define the nature of the language disorder, especially the detection of verbal auditory agnosia and level of intelligence.

The EEG is invaluable for the differentiation of the several disorders with language/cognitive regression. Except in occasional cases associated with cerebral structural pathologies, structural brain imaging is usually normal (Gordon, 1990). Functional imaging with PET and SPECT may well reveal unilateral or bilateral metabolic disturbances involving the temporal lobes (Maquet *et al.*, 1990; Mouridsen *et al.*, 1993; Guerreiro *et al.*, 1996; Da Silva *et al.*, 1997), but the value of these techniques is limited to the consideration of surgery in cases with intractable seizures or to research.

Prognosis, management, and treatment

Prognosis in cognitive/language regression is variable. Both improvement and aggravation of the aphasia have been reported (Deonna, 1991; Deonna *et al.*, 1997). While the seizures are usually controlled with antiepileptic drugs, the EEG abnormalities disappear after a few years. Prognosis in LKS may be inversely related to age at onset (Bishop, 1985). Many children reach the peak of the regression and remain at that state for many months or even years before showing later improvement; however, complete recovery is rare (Tuchman & Rapin, 2002; Shinnar *et al.*, 2001). The language disorder may persist in almost half of the patients (Mantovani & Landau, 1980; Paquier *et al.*, 1992). Despite language regression, these children may have a normal performance IQ (Tuchman & Rapin, 1997). Improvement is more likely in the patients who were entirely developmentally normal before the regression (Sy *et al.*, 2003). Some children recover good language function as adolescents or adults. Long-term deterioration of intellectual functions is uncommon in LKS (Dugas *et al.*, 1995). However a residual impairment in verbal short-term memory is frequent (Majerus *et al.*, 2003).

The location of the interictal EEG focus during the active phase may also influence prognosis in LKS and ECSWS. The best long-term prognoses were seen in those without a clear-cut focus on the wake EEG. However, a slow-wave focus and/or focal spikes during the acute phase were associated with focal and/or multifocal neuropsychological problems (Praline *et al.*, 2003; Deonna *et al.*, 1982). In clinical disorders with ESES, seizures and other EEG features usually disappear and, although some neuropsychological improvement often occurs, most patients are left with persistent cognitive problems and, sometimes, with a discrepancy between performance and verbal IQs (Roulet-Perez *et al.*, 1993).

In patients presenting with language/cognitive/behavioral regression, it is necessary to seek consultation with an experienced child neurologist who will evaluate treatment options on the basis of one or more sleep EEG examinations. However, there is no conclusive evidence that the use of anticonvulsant drugs or surgery in children with language or autistic regression without seizures but with epileptiform activity in their EEGs will have a therapeutic effect on the behavioral abnormalities of PDD and autism (Tharp, 2004). While the seizures associated with LKS can be easily treated, improvement in language function often does not follow their successful control (Trevathan, 2004).

Despite these controversial reports, when prolonged epileptiform activity is present on the EEG in children with severe language or cognitive regression, consideration of therapeutic intervention such as antiepileptic drugs, steroids, and, rarely, neurosurgery to control the possible harmful effects of prolonged subclinical discharges seems justified, particularly in children with the encephalopathic course seen in a small percentage of those with benign focal epilepsies in childhood (Fejerman *et al.*, 2000). In well selected cases there is the possibility of significant improvement in language and autistic features (Morrell *et al.*, 1995; Tuchman & Rapin, 2002).

Phenytoin, phenobarbital, and carbamazepine may worsen the EEG discharges and neuropsychological deficit even though they may be effective against the seizures (Marescaux *et al.*, 1990). Other antiepileptic agents such as sodium valproate, ethosuximide, and the benzodiazepines tend to be partially or transiently effective (Plioplys, 1994; Holmes & Riviello, 2001). Sulthiame may be another drug to consider (Lerman & Lerman-Sagie, 1995; Fejerman *et al.*, 2000; Huppke *et al.*, 2005). However, antiepileptic drugs, even valproate, may induce continuous spike-wave discharges and worsen clinical features (Prats *et al.*, 1998; Fejerman *et al.*, 2000) or not affect the language impairment (Scholtes *et al.*, 2005). Prolonged chronic or intermittent therapy with corticosteroids (hydrocortisone, ACTH, prednisolone) (Marescaux *et al.*, 1990; Lerman *et al.*, 1991; Tsuru *et al.*, 2000) or immunoglobulins in isolated cases may also be tried (Fayad *et al.*, 1997). This recommendation is based on the fact that early treatment of cryptogenic infantile spasms with high-dose ACTH is often associated with a favorable long-term cognitive outcome, whereas once major developmental regression has lasted for a month or more, the prognosis for normal cognitive outcome is poor (Kivity *et al.*, 2004). Large multisite trials are needed to determine treatment efficacy among children with language or cognitive regression, including LKS, and to establish whether there is a cause-effect relationship between electrographic status epilepticus in sleep or continuous spike-wave in slow-wave sleep and autistic language regression (Trevathan, 2004). Surgical intervention (multiple subpial transection of the cortex), though successful in abolishing epileptic discharges and behavioral problems in selected cases, was less effective in ameliorating language problems (Morrell *et al.*, 1995).

Speech/language therapy, educational interventions, and psychological counseling are also very important in the management of these patients. Some children with longstanding VAA may even be integrated into schools for the deaf. An effective communication system including sign language should always be considered.

Acknowledgments: I am grateful to Dr. I. Rapin who made several important suggestions and comments on the earlier drafts of the manuscript.

References

Aicardi, J. (2000): Atypical semiology of Rolandic epilepsy in some related syndromes. *Epileptic Disord.* **2** (Suppl. 1), S5–9.

Aicardi, J., & Chevrie J.J. (1982): Atypical benign partial epilepsy of childhood. *Dev. Med. Child. Neurol.* **24**, 281–292.

American Psychiatric Association (1994): Diagnostic and statistical manual of mental disorders, 4th edition, pp. 65–78. Washington, DC: American Psychiatric Association.

Archbold, K.H., Giordani, B., Ruzicka, D.L. & Chervin, R.D. (2004): Cognitive executive dysfunction in children with mild sleep-disordered breathing. *Biol. Res. Nurs.* **5**, 168–176.

Ballaban-Gil, K. & Tuchman, R. (2000): Epilepsy and epileptiform EEG: association with autism and language disorders. *Ment. Retard. Dev. Disabil. Res. Rev.* **6**, 300–308.

Beaumanoir, A (1985): The Landau-Kleffner syndrome. In: *Epileptic syndromes in infancy, childhood and adolescence*, eds. J. Roger, Ch. Dravet, M. Bureau, F.E. Dreifuss & P. Wolf, pp. 181–191. London: John Libbey Eurotext.

Beaumanoir, A. (1992): The Landau-Kleffner syndrome. In: *Epileptic syndromes in infancy, childhood and adolescence*, eds. J. Roger, Ch. Dravet, M. Bureau, F.E. Dreifuss & P. Wolf, 2nd edition. pp. 231–244. London: John Libbey Eurotext.

Ben-Zeev, B., Kivity, S., Pshitizki, Y., Watemberg, N., Brand, N. & Kramer, U. (2004): Congenital hydrocephalus and continuous spike wave in slow-wave sleep – a common association? *J. Child. Neurol.* **19**, 129–134.

Besag, F.M.C. (1988): Cognitive deterioration in children with epilepsy. In: *Epilepsy, behavior and cognitive function*, eds. M.R. Trimble & E.H. Reynolds, pp. 113–129. Reynolds, Chichester; John Wiley and Sons.

Binnie, C.D., Kasteleijn, N.T., Smit, A.M. & Wilkins, A.J. (1987): Interactions of epileptiform EEG discharges and cognition. *Epilepsy Res.* **1**, 239–245.

Bishop, D.V.M. (1985): Age of onset and outcome in acquired aphasia with convulsive disorder (Landau-Kleffner syndrome). *Dev. Med. Child. Neurol.* **27**, 705–712.

Bourgeois, B.F. & Landau, W.M. (2004): Landau-Kleffner syndrome and temporal cortical volume reduction: cause or effect? *Neurology* **63** (7), 1152–1153.

Bureau, M. (1995): Continuous spikes and waves during slow sleep: definition of the syndrome. In: *Continuous spikes and waves during slow sleep-Electrical status epilepticus during slow sleep*, Mariani Foundation Paediatric Neurology Series, vol. 3, eds. A. Beaumanoir, M. Bureau, T. Deonna, L. Mira & C.A. Tassinari, pp. 17–27. London: John Libbey.

Canitano, R., Luchetti, A. & Zappella, M. (2005): Epilepsy, electroencephalographic abnormalities, and regression in children with autism. *J. Child. Neurol.* **20** (1), 27–31.

Caraballo, R.H., Astorino, F., Cersosimo, R., Soprano, A.M. & Fejerman, N. (2001): Atypical evolution in childhood epilepsy with occipital paroxysms (Panayiotopoulos type). *Epileptic Disord.* **3** (3), 157–162.

Chae, J.H., Hwang, H., Hwang, Y.S., Cheong, H.J. & Kim, K.J. (2004): Influence of MECP2 gene mutation and X-chromosome inactivation on the Rett syndrome phenotype. *J. Child. Neurol.* **19**, 503–508.

Colamaria, V., Sgro, V., Caraballo, R., Simeone, M., Zullini, E., Fontana, E., Zanetti, R., Grimau-Merino, R. & Dalla Bernardina, B. (1991): Status epilepticus in benign Rolandic epilepsy manifesting as anterior operculum syndrome. *Epilepsia* **32** (3), 329–334.

Commission on Classification and Terminology of the International League Against Epilepsy. (1989): Proposal for revised classification of epilepsies and epileptic syndromes. *Epilepsia* **30**, 389–399.

Da Silva, E.A., Chugani, D.C., Muzik, O.& Chugani, H.T. (1997): Landau-Kleffner syndrome: metabolic abnormalities in temporal lobe are a common feature. *J. Child. Neurol.* **12**, 489–495.

De Negri, M. (1997): Electrical status epilepticus during sleep (ESES). Different clinical syndromes: towards a unifying view. *Brain Dev.* **19**, 447–451.

De Volder, A.G., Michel, C., Thauvoy, C., Willems, G.& Ferriere, G. (1994): Brain glucose utilization in acquired childhood aphasia associated with a Sylvian arachnoid cyst: recovery after shunting as demonstrated by PET. *J Neurol. Neurosurg. Psychiatry* **57**, 296–300.

Deonna, T. (1991): Acquired epileptiform aphasia in children (Landau-Kleffner syndrome). *J. Clin. Neurophysiol.* **8**, 288–298.

Deonna, T., Beaumanoir, A., Gaillard, F., Assal, G. (1977): Acquired aphasia in childhood with seizure disorder: a heterogeneous syndrome. *Neuropediatrie* **8**, 263–273.

Deonna, T., Davidoff, V., Maeder-Ingvar, M., Zesiger, P. & Marcoz, J.P. (1997): The spectrum of acquired cognitive disturbances in children with partial epilepsy and continuous spike-waves during sleep. *Eur. J. Paediatr. Neurol.* **1**, 19–29.

Deonna, T., Fletcher, P., Voumard, C. (1982): Temporary regression during language acquisition: a linguistic analysis of a $2^1/_2$-year-old child with epileptic aphasia. *Dev. Med. Child. Neurol.* **24**, 156–163.

Deonna, T. & Roulet-Perez, E. (1995): Acquired epileptic aphasia (AEA): definition of the syndrome and current problems. In: *Continuous spikes and waves during slow sleep-Electrical status epilepticus during slow sleep*, Mariani Foundation Paediatric Neurology Series, vol. 3, eds. A. Beaumanoir, M. Bureau, T. Deonna, L. Mira & C.A. Tassinari, pp. 37–45. London: John Libbey.

Deonna, T. & Roulet-Perez, E. (2005): *Cognitive and behavioral disorders of epileptic origin in children*. London UK: MacKeith Press.

Doose, H., & Baier, W.K. (1989): Benign partial epilepsy and related condition: multifactorial pathogenesis with hereditary impairment of brain mutation. *Eur. J. Pediatr.* **149**, 152–158.

Dubois, C.M., Zesiger, P., Perez, E.R., Ingvar, M.M. & Deonna, T. (2003): Acquired epileptic dysgraphia: a longitudinal study. *Dev. Med. Child. Neurol.* **45**, 807–812.

Dubois, C.M., Gianella, D., Chaves-Vischer, V., Haenggeli, C.A., Deonna, T. & Roulet Perez, E. (2004): Speech delay due to a prelinguistic regression of epileptic origin. *Neuropediatrics* **35**, 50–53.

Dugas, M., Franc, S., Loic, G.C. & Lecendreux, M. Evolution of acquired epileptic aphasia with or without continuous spikes and waves during slow sleep. In: *Continuous spikes and waves during slow sleep-Electrical status epilepticus during slow sleep*, Mariani Foundation Paediatric Neurology Series, vol. 3, eds. A. Beaumanoir, M. Bureau, T. Deonna, L. Mira & C.A. Tassinari, pp. 47–55. London: John Libbey.

Dugas, M., Gerard C.L., Franc, S. & Lecendreux, M. (1995): Late onset acquired epileptic aphasia. In: *Continuous spikes and waves during slow sleep-Electrical status epilepticus during slow sleep*, Mariani Foundation Paediatric Neurology Series, vol. 3, eds. A. Beaumanoir, M. Bureau, T. Deonna, L. Mira & C.A. Tassinari, pp. 143–149. London: John Libbey.

Echenne, B., Cheminal, R., Rivier, F., Negre, C., Touchon, J. & Billiard, M. (1992): Epileptic encephalopathic abnormalities and developmental dysphasias: study of 32 patients. *Brain Dev.* **14**, 216–225.

Fayad, M.N., Choueiri, R. & Mikati, M. (1997): Landau-Kleffner syndrome: consistent response to repeated intravenous gamma-globulin doses: a case report. *Epilepsia* **38**, 489–494.

Fejerman, N., Caraballo, R. & Tenembaum, S. (2000): Atypical evolutions of benign localization-related epilepsies in children: Are they predictable? *Epilepsia* **41** (4), 380–390.

Fenichel, G.M. (1997): *Clinical Pediatric Neurology*, 3rd edition, pp. 118–153. Philadelphia: WB Saunder Company.

Ferrie, C., Caraballo, R., Covanis, A., Demirbilek, V., Dervent, A., Kivity, S., Koutroumanidis, M., Martinovic, Z., Oguni, H., Verrotti, A., Vigevano, F., Watanabe, K., Yalçin, D. & Yoshinaga, H. (2006): Panayiotopoulos syndrome: a consensus view. *Dev. Med. Child. Neurol.* **48**, 236–240.

Ferrie, C.D., Agathonikou, A. & Panayiotopoulos, C.P. (1998): Electroencephalography and video-electroencephalography in the classification of childhood epilepsy syndromes. *Journal of the Royal Society of Medicine* **91** (5), 251–259.

Ferrie, C.D., Koutroumanidis, M., Rowlinson, S., Sanders S. & Panayiotopoulos, C.P. (2002): Atypical evolution of Panayiotopoulos syndrome: a case report. *Epileptic Disord.* **4** (1), 35–42.

Froscher, W. (1991): Sleep and prolonged epileptic activity (status epilepticus). *Epilepsy Res.* (Suppl. 2): 165–176.

Galanopoulou, A.S., Bojko, A., Lado, F. & Moshe, S.L. (2000): The spectrum of neuropsychiatric abnormalities associated with electrical status epilepticus in sleep. *Brain Dev.* **22**, 279–295.

Genton, P. & Guerrini, R. (1993): What differentiates Landau-Kleffner syndrome from the syndrome of continuous spikes and waves during slow sleep? *Arch. Neurol.* **50**, 1008–1009.

Glaze, D.G. (2004): Rett syndrome: of girls and mice – lessons for regression in autism. *Ment. Retard Dev. Disabil. Res. Rev.* **10**, 154–158.

Goldberg, W.A., Osann, K., Filipek, P.A., Laulhere, T., Jarvis, K., Modahl, C., Flodman, P. & Spence M.A. (2003): Language and other regression: assessment and timing. *J. Autism Dev. Disord.* **33**, 607–616.

Gordon, N. (1990): Acquired aphasia in childhood: the Landau-Kleffner syndrome. *Dev. Med. Child. Neurol.* **32**, 267–274.

Gross-Tsur, V. & Shalev, R.S. (2004): Reversible language regression as an adverse effect of topiramate treatment in children. *Neurology* **62**, 299–300.

Guerreiro, M.M., Camargo, E.E., Kato, M., Menezes Netto, J.R., Silva, E.A., Scotoni A.E., Silveira, D.C. & Guerreiro, C.A. (1996): Brain single photon emission computed tomography imaging in Landau-Kleffner syndrome. *Epilepsia* **37**, 60–67.

Guerrini, R., Genton, P., Bureau, M., Parmeggiani, A., Salas-Puig, X., Santucci, M., Bonanni, P., Ambrosetto, G. & Dravet, C. (1998): Multilobar polymicrogyria, intractable drop attack seizures, and sleep-related electrical status epilepticus. *Neurology* **51**, 504–512.

Hécaen, H. & Albert, M.L. (1978): *Human neuropsychology*, pp. 270–276. New York: John Wiley.

Hirsch, E., Maquet, P., Metz-Lutz, M., Motte, J., Finck, S. & Marescaux, C. (1995): The eponym 'Landau-Kleffner syndrome' should not be restricted to childhood-acquired aphasia with epilepsy. In: *Continuous spikes and waves during slow sleep-Electrical status epilepticus during slow sleep*, Mariani Foundation Paediatric Neurology Series, vol. 3, eds. A. Beaumanoir, M. Bureau, T. Deonna, L. Mira & C.A. Tassinari, pp. 57–62. London: John Libbey.

Holmes, G.L., McKeever, M. & Saunders, Z. (1981): Epileptiform activity in aphasia of childhood: an epiphenomenon? *Epilepsia* **22**, 631–639.

Holmes, G.L. & Riviello, J.J. (2001): Treatment of childhood idiopathic language deterioration with valproate. *Epilepsy Behav.* **2**, 272–276.

Huppke, P., Kallenberg, K. & Gartner, J. (2005): Perisylvian polymicrogyria in Landau-Kleffner syndrome. *Neurology* **64** (9), 1660.

Hurley, R.A., Lewine, J.D., Jones, G.M., Orrison, W.W. & Taber, K.H. (2000): Application of magnetoencephalography to the study of autism. *J. Neuropsychiatry Clin. Neurosci.* **12**, 1–3.

Ishitobi, M., Nakasato, N., Yamamoto, K. & Iinuma, K. (2005): Opercular to interhemispheric source distribution of benign rolandic spikes of childhood. *Neuroimage* 1; **25** (2), 417–423.

Isnard, J., Fischer, C., Bastuji, H., Badinand, N. & de Villard, R. (1995): Auditory early (BAEP) and middle-latency (MLAEP) evoked potentials in patients with CSWS and Landau-Kleffner syndrome. In: *Continuous spikes and waves during slow sleep-Electrical status epilepticus during slow sleep*, Mariani Foundation Paediatric Neurology Series, vol. 3, eds. A. Beaumanoir, M. Bureau, T. Deonna, L. Mira & C.A. Tassinari, pp. 99–103. London: John Libbey.

Kaga, M. (1999): Language disorders in Landau-Kleffner Syndrome. *J. Child. Neurol.* **14**, 118–122.

Kerr, A. & Engerström, I.W. (2001): The clinical background to the Rett syndrome. In: *Rett disorder and the developing brain*, eds. A. Kerr & I.W. Engerström, pp. 1–27. New York: Oxford University Press.

Kivity, S., Lerman, P., Ariel, R., Danziger, Y., Mimouni, M. & Shinnar, S. (2004): Long-term cognitive outcomes of a cohort of children with cryptogenic infantile spasms treated with high-dose adrenocorticotropic hormone. *Epilepsia* **45**, 255–262.

Klein, S.K., Kurtzberg, D., Brattson, A., Kreutzer, J.A., Stapells, D.R., Dunn, M.A., Rapin, I. & Vaughan, H.G. Jr. (1995): Electrophysiologic manifestations of impaired temporal lobe auditory processing in verbal auditory agnosia. *Brain Lang.* **51**, 383–405.

Klein, S.K., Tuchman, R.F. & Rapin, I. (2000): The influence of premorbid language skills and behavior on language recovery in children with verbal auditory agnosia. *J. Child. Neurol.* **15**, 36–43.

Kobayashi, R. & Murata, T. (1998): Setback phenomenon in autism and long-term prognosis. *Acta Psychiatr. Scand.* **98**, 296–303.

Kurita, H., Koyama, T., Setoya, Y., Shimizu, K. & Osada, H. (2004): Validity of childhood disintegrative disorder apart from autistic disorder with speech loss. *Eur. Child. Adolesc. Psychiatry* **13**, 221–226.

Kumpulainen, K. (2002): Phenomenology and treatment of selective mutism. *CNS Drugs* **16** (3), 175–180.

Lagae, L.G., Silberstein, J., Gillis, P.L. & Casaer, P.J. (1998): Successful use of intravenous immunoglobulins in Landau-Kleffner syndrome. *Pediatr. Neurol.* **18**, 165–168.

Landau, W.M. & Kleffner, F.R. (1957): Syndrome of acquired aphasia with convulsive disorder in children. *Neurology* **17**, 523–530.

Lerman, P. & Lerman-Sagie, T. (1995): Sulthiame revisited. *J. Child. Neurol.* **10** (3), 241–242.

Lerman, P., Lerman-Sagie T, & Kivity, S. (1991): Effect of early corticosteroid therapy for Landau-Kleffner syndrome. *Dev. Med. Child Neurol.* **33**, 257–260.

Lewine, J.D., Michael, A., Patil, A.A., Devinsky, O., Smith, M.C., Kanner, A., Davis, J.T., Funke, M., Jones, G., Chong, B., Provencal, S., Weisend, M., Lee, R.R. & Orrison, W.W.J. (1999): Magnetoencephalographic patterns of epileptiform activity in children with regressive autism spectrum disorder. *Pediatrics* **104**, 405–418.

Luyster, R., Richler, J., Risi, S., Hsu, W.L., Dawson, G., Bernier, R., Dunn, M., Hepburn, S., Hyman, S.L., McMahon, W.M., Goudie-Nice, J., Minshew, N., Rogers, S., Sigman, M., Spence, M.A., Goldberg, W.A., Tager-Flusberg, H., Volkmar, F.R.& Lord, C. (2005): Early regression in social communication in autism spectrum disorders: a CPEA study. *Dev. Neuropsychol.* **27**, 311–336.

Maccario, M., Hefferen, S.J., Keblusek, S.J.& Lipinski, K.A. (1982): Developmental dysphasia and electroencephalographic abnormalities. *Dev. Med. Child. Neurol.* **24**, 141–155.

Majerus, S., Laureys, S., Collette, F., Del Fiore, G., Degueldre, C., Luxen, A., Van der Linden, M., Maquet, P. & Metz-Lutz, M.N. (2003): Phonological short-term memory networks following recovery from Landau and Kleffner syndrome. *Hum. Brain Mapp.* **19** (3), 133–144.

Maquet, P., Hirsch, E., Dive, D., Salmon, E., Marescaux, C., & Franck, G. (1990): Cerebral glucose utilization during sleep in Landau-Kleffner syndrome: a PET study. *Epilepsia* **31**, 778–783.

Maquet, P., Hirsch, E., Metz-Lutz, M.N., Marescaux, C. & Franck, G. (1999): PET studies of Landau-Kleffner syndrome and related disorders. In: *Childhood epilepsies and brain development*, eds. A. Nehlig, J. Motte, S.L. Moshe & P. Plouin, pp. 135–145. London: John Libbey.

Maquet, P., Hirsch, E., Metz-Lutz, M.N., Motte, J., Dive, D., Marescaux, C. & Franck, G. (1995): Regional cerebral glucose metabolism in children with deterioration of one or more cognitive functions and continuous spike-and-wave discharges during sleep. *Brain* **118**, 1497–1520.

Marescaux, C., Hirsch, E., Finck, S., Maquet, P., Schlumberger, E., Sellal, F., Metz-Lutz, M.N., Alembik, Y., Salmon, E. & Franck, G. (1990): Landau-Kleffner syndrome: a pharmacologic study of five cases. *Epilepsia* **31**, 768–777.

Marien, P., Saerens, J., Verslegers, W., Borggreve, F. & De Deyn, P.P. (1993): Some controversies about type and nature of aphasic symptomatology in Landau-Kleffner's syndrome: a case study. *Acta Neurol. Belg.* **93**, 183–203.

McVicar, K.A. & Shinnar, S. (2004): Landau-Kleffner syndrome, electrical status epilepticus in slow wave sleep, and language regression in children. *Ment. Retard Dev. Disabil. Res. Rev.* **10**, 144–149.

McVicar, K.A., Ballaban-Gil, K., Rapin, I., Moshe, S.L. & Shinnar, S. (2005): Epileptiform EEG abnormalities in children with language regression. *Neurology.* 12; **65** (1), 129–131.

Metz-Lutz, M. & Massa, R. (1999) : Cognitive and behavioral consequences of epilepsies in childhood. In: *Childhood epilepsies and brain development*, eds. A. Nehlig, J. Motte, S.L. Moshe & P. Plouin, pp. 123–135. London: John Libbey.

Mikati, M.A., Saab, R., Fayad, M.N., Choueiri, R.N. (2002): Efficacy of intravenous immunoglobulin in Landau-Kleffner syndrome. *Pediatr. Neurol.* **26** (4), 298–300.

Monjauze, C., Tuller, L., Hommet, C., Barthez, M.A. & Khomsi, A. (2005): Language in benign childhood epilepsy with centro-temporal spikes abbreviated form: Rolandic epilepsy and language. *Brain and Language* **92**, 300–308.

Morrell, F., Whisler, W.W., Smith, M.C., Hoeppneer, T.J., de Toledo-Morrell, L., Pierre-Louis, S.J.C., Kanneer, A.M., Buelow, J.M., Ristanovic, R., Bergen, D., Chez, M. & Hasegawa, H. (1995): Landau-Kleffner syndrome: treatment with subpial intracortical transection. *Brain* **118**, 1529–1546.

Morrell, F. (1995): Electrophysiology of CSWS in Landau-Kleffner syndrome. In: *Continuous spikes and waves during slow sleep-Electrical status epilepticus during slow sleep*, Mariani Foundation Paediatric Neurology Series, vol. 3, eds. A. Beaumanoir, M. Bureau, T. Deonna, L. Mira & C.A. Tassinari, pp. 77–91. London: John Libbey.

Mouridsen, S.E., Rich, B. & Isoger, T. (1998): Validity of childhood disintegrative psychosis. General findings of a long term follow-up study. *Br. J. Psychiatry* **172**, 263–267.

Mouridsen, S.E., Rich, B. & Isoger, T. (1999): Epilepsy in disintegrative psychosis and infantile autism: a long-term validation study. *Dev. Med. Child. Neurol.* **41** (2), 110–114.

Mouridsen, S.E., Videbaek, C., Sogaard, H. & Andersen, A.R. (1993): Regional blood-flow measured by HMPAO nd SPECT ion a 5-year-old boy with Landau-Kleffner syndrome. *Neuropediatrics* **24**, 47–50.

Nasr, J.T., Gabis, L., Savatic, M. & Andriola, M.R. (2001): The electroencephalogram in children with developmental dysphasia. *Epilepsy Behav.* **2**, 115–118.

Neul, J.L. & Zoghbi, H.Y. (2004): Rett syndrome: a prototypical neurodevelopmental disorder. *Neuroscientist* **10**, 118–128.

Neville, B.G., Harkness, W.F., Cross, J.H., Cass, H.C., Burch, V.C., Lees, J.A., Taylor, D.C. (1997): Surgical treatment of severe autistic regression in childhood epilepsy. *Pediatr. Neurol.* **16** (2), 137–140.

Paetau, R. (1994): Sounds trigger spikes in the Landau-Kleffner syndrome. *J. Clin. Neurophysiol.* **11**, 231–241.

Paetau, R. (2002): Magnetoencephalography in pediatric neuroimaging. *Dev. Sci.* **5**, 361–370.

Panayiotopoulos, C.P. (1999): Other benign childhood partial seizures with the exceptional severe syndromes of mainly linguistic and neuropsychological deficits, seizures or both. In: *Benign childhood partial seizures and related epileptic syndromes*, ed. C.P. Panayiotopoulos, pp. 337–361. London: John Libbey.

Paquier, P.F., Van Dongen, H.R. & Loonen, C.B. (1992): The Landau-Kleffner syndrome or 'acquired aphasia with convulsive disorder'. Long-term follow-up of six children and a review of the recent literature. *Arch. Neurol.* **49**, 354–359.

Paetau, R., Granstrom, M.L., Blomstedt, G., Jousmaki, V., Korkman, M. & Liukkonen, E. (1999): Magnetoencephalography in presurgical evaluation of children with the Landau-Kleffner syndrome. *Epilepsia* **40** (3), 326–335.

Pearl, P.L., Carrazana, E.J. & Holmes, G.L. (2001): The Landau-Kleffner syndrome. *Epilepsy Currents* **1**, 39–45.

Picard, A., Cheliout Heraut, F., Bouskraoui, M., Lemoine, M., Lacert, P. & Delattre, J. (1998): Sleep EEG and developmental dysphasia. *Dev. Med. Child. Neurol.* **40**, 595–599.

Plioplys, A.V. (1994): Autism: electroencephalogram abnormalities and clinical improvement with valproic acid. *Arch. Pediatr. Adolesc. Med.* **148**, 220–222.

Pollard, A.J. & Prendergast, M. (2004): Depressive pseudodementia in a child with autism. *Dev. Med. Child. Neurol.* **46**, 485–489.

Praline, J., Hommet, C., Barthez, M.A., Brault, F., Perrier, D., Passage, G.D., Lucas, B., Bonnard, J., Billard, C., Toffol, B.D. & Autret, A. (2003): Outcome at adulthood of the continuous spike-waves during show sleep and Landau-Kleffner syndromes. *Epilepsia* **44** (11), 1434–1440.

Prats, J.M., Garaizar, C., García-Nieto, M.L, & Madoz, P. (1998): Antiepileptic drugs and atypical evolution of idiopathic partial epilepsy. *Pediatr. Neurol.* **18**, 402–406.

Rapin, I. & Katzman, R. (1998): Neurobiology of autism. *Ann. Neurol.* **43**, 7–14.

Rapin, I., Allen, D.A. & Dunn, M.A. (1992): Developmental language disorders. In: *Handbook of neuropsychology*, eds. S.J. Segalowitz & I. Rapin, vol. 7, pp. 111–139. Amsterdam: Elsevier.

Rogers, S.J. (2004): Developmental regression in autism spectrum disorders. *Ment. Retard Dev. Disabil. Res. Rev.* **10**, 139–143.

Rossi, P.G., Parmeggiani, A., Posar, A., Scaduto, M.C., Chioda, S. & Vatti, G. (1999): Landau-Kleffner syndrome (LKS): long term follow-up and links with electrical status epilepticus during sleep (ESES). *Brain Dev.* **21**, 90–98.

Roulet Perez, E., Davidoff, V., Despland, P.A. & Deonna, T. (1993): Mental and behavioural deterioration of children with epilepsy and CSWS: acquired epileptic frontal syndrome. *Dev. Med. Child Neurol.* **35**, 661–674.

Saltik, S., Uluduz, D., Cokar, O., Demirbilek, V. & Dervent, A. (2005): Idiopathic partial epilepsies with evolution into ESES spectrum disorders. *Epilepsia* **46** (4), 524–533.

Schanen, C., Houwink, E.J., Dorrani, N., Lane, J., Everett, R., Feng, A., Cantor, R.M. & Percy, A. (2004): Phenotypic manifestations of MECP2 mutations in classical and atypical Rett syndrome. *Am. J. Med. Genet.* **126**, 129–140.

Scholtes, F.B., Hendriks, M.P. & Renier, W.O. (2005): Cognitive deterioration and electrical status epilepticus during slow sleep. *Epilepsy Behav.* **6** (2), 167–173.

Seri, S., Cerquiglini, A. & Pisani, F. (1998): Spike-induced interference in auditory sensory processing in Landau-Kleffner syndrome. *Electroencephalogr. Clin. Neurophysiol.* **108**, 506–510.

Shafrir, Y. & Prensky, A.L. (1995): Acquired epileptiform opercular syndrome: a second case report, review of the literature, and comparison to the Landau-Kleffner syndrome. *Epilepsia* **36**, 1050–1057.

Shinnar, S., Rapin, I., Arnold, S., Tuchman, R., Shulman, L., Ballaban-Gill, K., Maw, M., Deuel, R.K. & Volkmar, F.R. (2001): Language regression in childhood. *Pediatr. Neurol.* **24**, 185–191.

Smith, M.C. (1998): Landau-Kleffner syndrome and continuous spikes and waves during slow sleep. In: *Epilepsy: a comprehensive textbook*, eds. J. Engel & T.A. Pedley, pp. 2367–2377. Philadelphia, New York: Lippincott-Raven.

Soprano, A.M., Garcia, E.F., Caraballo, R. & Fejerman, N. (1994): Acquired epileptic aphasia: neuropsychologic follow-up of 12 patients. *Pediatr. Neurol.* **11** (3), 230–235.

Stefanatos, G.A., Kinsbourne, M. & Wasserstein, J. (2002): Acquired epileptiform aphasia: a dimensional view of Landau-Kleffner syndrome and the relation to regressive autistic spectrum disorders. *Neuropsychol. Dev. Cogn. C. Child. Neuropsychol.* **8**, 195–228.

Sy, W., Djukij, A., Shinnar, S., Dharmani, C. & Rapin, I. (2003): Clinical characteristics of language regression in children. *Dev. Med. Child. Neurol.* **45**, 508–514.

Takeoka, M., Riviello, J.J., Duffy, F.H., Kim, F., Kennedy, D.N., Makris, N., Caviness, V.S. & Holmes, G.L. (2004): Bilateral volume reduction of the superior temporal areas in Landau-Kleffner syndrome. *Neurology* **63**, 1289–1292.

Tassinari, CA., Bureau, M., Dravet, C., Dalla Bernardina, B. & Roger, J. (1992): Epilepsy with continuous spikes and waves during slow sleep – otherwise described as ESES (epilepsy with electrical status epilepticus during slow sleep). In: *Epileptic syndromes in infancy, childhood and adolescence*, 2nd edition, eds. J. Roger, M. Bureau, C. Dravet, F. Dreifus, A. Perret & P. Wolf, pp. 245–256. London: John Libbey.

Tassinari, C.A., Daniele, O. & Dalla Bernardina, B. (1995): The problems of 'continuous spikes and waves during slow sleep' or 'electrical status epilepticus during slow sleep' today. In: *Continuous spikes and waves during slow sleep-Electrical status epilepticus during slow sleep*, Mariani Foundation Paediatric Neurology Series, vol. 3, eds. A. Beaumanoir, M. Bureau, T. Deonna, L. Mira & C.A. Tassinari, pp. 251–255. London: John Libbey.

Tassinari, C.A., Rubboli, G., Volpi, L., Billard, C. & Bureau, M. (2002): Electrical status epilepticus during slow sleep (ESES or CSWS) including acquired epileptic aphasia (Landau-Kleffner syndrome). In: *Epileptic syndromes in infancy, childhood and adolescence*, 3rd ed., eds. J. Roger, M. Bureau, C.H. Dravet, P. Genton, C.A. Tassinari & P. Wolf, pp. 265–283. Eastleigh: John Libbey.

Tharp, B.R. (2004): Epileptic encephalopathies and their relationship to developmental disorders: do spikes cause autism? *Ment. Retard. Dev. Disabil. Res. Rev.* **10**, 132–134.

Trevathan, E. (2004): Seizures and epilepsy among children with language regression and autistic spectrum disorders. *J. Child. Neurol.* **19** (Suppl. 1), 49–57.

Trimble, M.R., Ring, H.A. & Schmitz, B. (2000): Epilepsy. In: *Synopsis of neuropsychiatry*, eds. B.S. Fogel, R.B. Schiffer & S.M. Rao, pp. 469–491. Philadelphia: Lippincott Williams & Wilkins.

Tromp, S.C., Weber, J.W., Aldenkamp, A.P., Arends, J., van der Linden, I. & Diepman, L. (2003): Relative influence of epileptic seizures and of epilepsy syndrome on cognitive function. *J. Child. Neurol.* **18**, 407–412.

Tsuru, T., Mori, M. & Mizuguchi, M. (2000): Effects of high-dose intravenous corticosteroid therapy in Landau-Kleffner syndrome. *Pediatr. Neurol.* **22** (2), 145–147.

Tuchman, R.F. & Rapin, I. (1997): Regression in pervasive developmental disorders: seizures and epileptiform electroencephalogram correlates. *Pediatrics* **99**, 560–566.

Tuchman, R.F. & Rapin, I. (2002). Epilepsy in autism. *Lancet Neurol.* **1**, 353–358.

Tuchman, R.F., Rapin, I. & Shinnar, S. (1991a): Autistic and dysphasic children. I: Clinical characteristics. *Pediatrics* **88**, 1211–1218.

Tuchman, R.F., Rapin, I. & Shinnar, S. (1991b): Autistic and dysphasic children. II: Epilepsy. *Pediatrics* **88**, 1219–1225.

Uldall, P., Sahlholdt, L. & Alving, J. (2000): Landau-Kleffner syndrome with onset at 18 months and an initial diagnosis of pervasive developmental disorder. *Eur. J. Paediatr. Neurol.* **4**, 81–86.

Weller, M. (1993): Anterior opercular cortex lesions cause dissociated lower cranial nerve palsies and anarthria but no aphasia: Foix-Chavany-Marie syndrome and 'automatic voluntary dissociation' revisited. *J. Neurol.* **240**, 199–208.

Whiteley, P. (2004): Developmental, behavioural and somatic factors in pervasive developmental disorders: preliminary analysis. *Child. Care Health Dev.* **30**, 5–11.

Wolff, M., Weiskopf, N., Serra, E., Preissl, H., Birbaumer, N. & Kraegeloh-Mann, I. (2005): Benign partial epilepsy in childhood: selective cognitive deficits are related to the location of focal spikes determined by combined EEG/MEG. *Epilepsia* **46** (Suppl. 10), 1661–1667.

Chapter 11

Language disorders in cerebellar pathology

Daria Riva, Chiara Vago, Federica Aggio, Chiara Pantaleoni, Stefano D'Arrigo, Arianna Usilla, and Sara Bulgheroni

Developmental Neurology Division, National Neurologic Institute 'C.Besta', Via Celoria 11, 20133 Milan, Italy
driva@istituto-besta.it

Summary

The role of the cerebellum in organising higher brain functions has been confirmed in numerous studies on adults. More recently, this role has been acknowledged in the developmental age as well. Congenital cerebellar disorders, especially those affecting the vermis (generalized or selective hypoplasia, involving any of its lobes) or the cerebellar hemispheres, are a frequent finding in paediatric neurological disorders. These anatomical lesions are associated with neuropsychological impairment or various types of developmental disorder, and particularly with more or less severe mental deficiencies, severe language disorders, and behavioural changes, even to the point of autism.
Acquired cerebellar lesions (especially tumours and stroke) in children of normal intelligence have allowed the identification of different neuropsychological profiles, depending on the site involved: lesions of the vermis coincide with behavioural problems and verbal production deficiencies, in the sense of both impaired speech and genuine language disorders, while lesions of the cerebellar hemispheres are associated with side-specific cognitive impairment patterns.

Introduction

In recent years, the functions of the cerebellum have been profoundly reassessed and numerous studies have extended its role to the regulation and processing of non-motor abilities. Motor control can be highly sophisticated and precise and can be divided into two main activities: on the one hand, it allows the precise temporal interplay between different sets of muscles through the cerebellar circuits; on the other, it ensures that these movements can take place with extraordinary speed. The non-motor abilities include language, procedural memory, executive functions, visuospatial abilities, and emotional and social behaviour.

For some time now, there have been reports of adults with CNS pathology involving the cerebellum suffering from various types of neuropsychological disorder. Many clinical observations on groups and individual patients, and several more sophisticated neuropsychological studies (mainly involving patients with degenerative cerebellar diseases) have unexpectedly revealed a vast range of neuropsychological deficits, and that these deficits can even be differentiated depending on whether the ability being tested is processed by the frontal (Luria,

1966; Stuss et al., 1986), parietal, or occipital areas – the associative areas (Beyerman, 1917) with which the cerebellum has the greatest number of connections (Ghez & Fahn, 1985).

Studies have been conducted on patients with agenesis or hypoplasia of the cerebellum (Bond, 1895) and on those with primary cerebellar disorders, and the deficits described have varied considerably in extent. Patients with Friedreich's ataxia have visuospatial difficulties, a low IQ, and emotional problems (Hart et al., 1985); patients with olivopontocerebellar atrophy (Kish et al., 1988; Kluin et al., 1988) show different degrees of deficiency in verbal and non-verbal intelligence, frontal functions, and memory (Bond, 1895; Rubinstein & Freeman, 1940); patients with ataxia-telangiectasia have low intelligence (Bond, 1895).

In the human brain, several phylogenetically new parts have evolved and increased in size, with a concomitant increase and evolution of the associative areas in the cerebral cortex. Anatomical and clinical evidence has already suggested that this expansion contributes not only to the control and learning of highly complex motor functions, but also to sensory, cognitive, linguistic, and emotional aspects of human behaviour.

The anatomical evidence stems from the modularity of the cerebellum, whose cortical cells are organized in longitudinal micromodules arrayed perpendicularly to the surface of the cortex and parallel to one another. The increase in the dimensions of the cerebellum coincides with an increase in its computational capacity. This derives from the principles of information processing according to which, if modules of individually low processing power are assembled in parallel, the resulting network can acquire an extraordinary computational capacity, which can be used in cooperation with different areas of the cerebral cortex to which the cerebellum sends its signals (Ghez & Fahn, 1985).

Cerebellar outputs and inputs convey signals through the thalamus to the cerebral cortex in segregated communication channels, thus preserving the cerebellum's modularity (Leiner et al., 1993). Through these channels, the modules of the lateral neocerebellum can send signals to the supratentorial cortexes of language and other functions, such as the Broca area in the prefrontal cortex.

Having the opportunity for such an ample evolution, and consequently for developing the capacity to process a given type of function, means that – given the constraints imposed by the dimensions of the skull – natural selection ought to particularly favour the areas that process functions which are especially beneficial to the human being; thus, in an evolutionistic perspective, this would mean that the cerebellum must process crucially important functions. When the cerebellum increases in size, the number of its neurons seems to exceed the number of neurons in the supratentorial cortex. Moreover, the connections shown between the cerebellum and the supratentorial structures enable the former to access the processing of functions of a higher order and to subserve a great variety of human brain functions (Ghez & Fahn, 1985).

The reciprocal links connecting the cerebellum to these structures have been elucidated in a large number of studies (Schmahmann & Sherman, 1998): reciprocal connections between the cerebellum and cortical areas (here we shall consider only the frontal and prefrontal areas and the limbic regions) have been demonstrated from the frontal cortex to the cerebellum through the pons (Schmahmann & Pandya, 1995; Schmahmann & Pandya, 1997a) and *vice versa* through the thalamus (Schmahmann & Pandya, 1990; Middleton & Strick, 1994, 1997; Schmahmann & Pandya, 1997b), and reciprocal anatomical connections have also been found between the parahippocampal structures (Schmahmann & Pandya, 1993), the cingulate gyrus (Vilensky & Van Hoesen, 1981), and the hypothalamus (Snider, 1950; Haines & Dietrichs, 1984).

It is also important to bear in mind that these cerebellar–cerebral connections cross over, as shown by positron emission tomography studies that have identified a crossed cerebellar diaschisis (that is, a metabolic depression in the cerebellar hemisphere contralateral to a supratentorial lesion and *vice versa*) (Ishihara et al., 1999; Jansen et al., 2005) and by functional magnetic resonance imaging (fMRI) studies that will be discussed later on.

As for the mechanisms of action, given the extremely uniform organisation of the cerebellum, all the areas have a similar operational capacity, but each area also processes different functions depending on the different types of afferent/efferent connections.

In conclusion, the cerebellum is not needed for the basic perception of the components of the functions it helps to process; its principal activity lies in adjusting the internal and external inputs to 'central information', so it works as an associative area (Leiner et al., 1991; Leiner et al., 1993).

The close correlation between the cerebellum and the supratentorial structures is confirmed by the fact that, during the course of neurogenesis, the neocerebellum and prefrontal areas have a parallel phylogenetic development and, from the ontogenetic point of view, they are the two areas of the brain with the slowest growth (Chiesielki et al., 1997). This long maturation time would expose the cerebellum to a greater risk of becoming the site of various pathologies originating in early ontogeny than other earlier-maturing brain structures. Within the cerebellum, moreover, the latest areas to develop should be more severely affected than those developing earlier. This would explain the frequent involvement of the cerebellum in many paediatric neurological diseases, and particularly why, within the cerebellum, the vermis may be hypoplastic more often than the hemispheres, and some of the vermian lobes may be hypoplastic while others are normal.

The mechanisms used by the cerebellum for regulating and learning even highly complex motor tasks are the same as those responsible for regulating and learning cognitive processes, assuring them the necessary speed, coherence, and consistency. The mechanisms for the regulation and timing of the interplay between different sets of muscles in motor actions also guarantee a rapid, online, and consistent interplay between the components and subcomponents of the cognitive and neuropsychological systems, and particularly in the sphere of language discussed in this chapter.

This processing has been demonstrated in numerous studies on adults concerning procedural memory (Corsi, 1972; Molinari et al., 1997a), executive functions (Grafman et al., 1992; Daum & Ackerman, 1997; Lalonde & Botez-Marquard, 2000), and visuospatial abilities (Botez & Botez, 1992; Fabbro et al., 2004).

More recently, in adults suffering from various types of cerebellar pathology, Schmahmann coherently formalized the previously described deficiencies in what the author called a *cognitive-affective* syndrome (Schmahmann & Sherman, 1998), represented by an executive dysfunction (planning, verbal fluency, and working memory), visuospatial disorganisation (including memory), various types of language deficiency (agrammatism, mild anomia, dysprosodia), and personality changes (disinhibited or otherwise uncontrolled behaviour) (Schmahmann, 1997).

This processing would have a quite clearly defined topography: while lesions of the cerebellar hemispheres would be associated mainly with cognitive processing disorders, lesions of the vermis correlate mostly with emotional disorders and problems in social relationships (Schmahmann & Sherman, 1998).

Language

Studies have particularly focused on the role of the cerebellum in processing language since data were published about research conducted on adult patients with focal lesions.

A right cerebellar lesion has been associated with both expressive (agrammatism) and expressive-receptive language deficiency syndromes (Silveri *et al.*, 1994; Marien *et al.*, 1996; Molinari *et al.*, 1997b; Zettin *et al.*, 1997). This seems to be caused by a dissociation between the cerebellar and frontal areas involved in processing language, because of the so-called 'crossed cerebello-cerebral diaschisis' phenomenon, which describes a more or less severe temporary disactivation of the frontal areas secondary to a lesion of the contralateral cerebellar areas. As mentioned earlier, the cerebellum has extensive two-way input and output connections with the frontal lobes (Asanuma *et al.*, 1983; Stanton *et al.*, 1993; Schmahmann & Pandya, 1993; Middleton & Strick, 1994). It receives high-level multisensorial information, arriving from the frontal and parietal supratentorial associative areas through the pontine nuclei ('mossy fibres') and the red nucleus/inferior olive system ('climbing fibres'). Its output is conveyed to the frontal and prefrontal cortex (Brodmann areas 45 and 44, and the Broca area) through the thalamus, and particularly through the ventrolateral nucleus (Leiner *et al.*, 1991). This complex system of afferent and efferent connections justifies the relation between the cerebellum and the language areas, and the former's involvement in language processing.

The above considerations are confirmed by functional studies showing that the cerebellum has a direct role in sustaining language: patterns of activation of the cortex (Broca's area and the supplementary motor area) and cerebellum are associated with word and rhyme generation tasks (Klein *et al.*, 1995; Marien *et al.*, 2001).

More recent fMRI studies in healthy adults have documented the activation of the areas of language and of the contralateral cerebellum using various verbal tasks, Stowe *et al.* (2004) showing that the right cerebellar hemisphere is activated for the comprehension of ambiguous and unambiguous sentences. In right-handed and left-handed adults, Hubrich-Ungureanu *et al.* (2002) demonstrated that the crossed-activation pattern is maintained in different dominance conditions for language. Kassubeck *et al.* (2004) further extended the demonstration of the crossed activation pattern to the American Sign Language used by the deaf. Few studies have been conducted in normal children (for obvious reasons), but a study by Wood *et al.* (2004) on 48 children using a word-generation test and orthographic lexical retrieval showed that the left side was more activated in 85 per cent of cases, and that the typical areas of activation were the frontomedial gyri (96 per cent), followed by the inferior (94 per cent), medial (92 per cent), temporoinferior (85 per cent), and superior gyri (65 per cent), and the cerebellum (67 per cent).

Type and extent of contribution to language

An important query relates to the real nature of the cerebellum's contribution to the processing of functions of a higher order in general, and of language in particular. It remains to be determined whether the cerebellum's contribution to cognitive acts is operational rather than one of direct processing – that is, whether or not these functions are represented in the cerebellum.

As mentioned earlier, the cerebellum is arranged in parallel modules lying perpendicular to the cortical surface and forming a network that, with the successive recruitment of the modules, achieves a sophisticated and extremely rapid computational capacity (Leiner *et al.*, 1991; Loritz, 1991). This means that, if the cerebellum's contribution to the frontal system consists only in its afferent/efferent connections being segregated together in a system oriented specifically towards the frontal lobe, then the representation of language functions (and other cognitive functions) is confined to the known neocortical linguistic structures. This leaves the cerebellum the role of orchestrator and modulator by means of very rapid online processing, providing an interface between different cognitive systems. The aphasic pictures (such as agrammatism) seen in patients with cerebellar lesions would thus be caused by an inadequate contribution of the cerebellum to this specific operational cooperation, represented by the timing of the interplay of grammatical and syntactic features, with the inclusion of critical particles in the right place at the right time (Silveri et al., 1998). In this case, the role of the cerebellum would consequently be 'peripheral' (Fabbro et al., 2004), a role that we prefer to define as operational, because it differs from that of the classic language areas but is nonetheless fundamental and 'specific' in its own way; its malfunctioning gives rise to the same type of symptom, secondary to the malfunctioning of a supratentorial area for language representation. We consequently do not take a minimalistic or reductive view of the role of the cerebellum: it is not just an extraordinary gadget for speeding up a process, it is an irreplaceable part of a complex and remarkable system that processes the multicomponent system of language.

Side-specific language deficiencies have been described in relation to lesions of the right cerebellar hemisphere (Riva, 2000a; Marien et al., 2001), as if there were a specialization within the cerebellum, like in the cerebral hemispheres, but language disorders have also been found after left cerebellar lesions (Fabbro, 2000; Riva & Giorgi, 2000).

Developmental studies are more rare, but seem to confirm the important role of the cerebellum in cognitive and affective development. In infancy, cerebellar anomalies are fairly frequent in genetic and congenital diseases. Conversely, numerous studies have been published on children with cerebellar disease who showed more or less severe mental retardation and neuropsychological, language, and behavioural disorders in various combinations. Reports of disturbances of the higher functions in children with acquired cerebellar disease are relatively more rare (partly because of the genuine rarity of acquired pathology in children). Concerning the former, it should be stressed first of all that – given the frequent, often severe mental retardation accompanying the syndromes or diseases involving a congenital cerebellar hypoplasia – any cognitive assessment is often limited to administering development scales or, where these are unfeasible, to direct observation of the child. Together with their more or less severe mental insufficiency, these children also tend to have widely variable behaviour disorders. It is only recently, thanks also to our growing understanding of the cerebellum, that highly sophisticated studies on patients with acquired focal cerebellar lesions have prompted the application of such methods to the examination of children as well, wherever possible.

Numerous hereditary degenerative disorders involving the cerebellum have been extensively described in childhood (Connor et al., 1993). Degenerative ataxias with tapetoretinal lesions are accompanied by a variety of intellectual disturbances (Dooley et al., 1992; Di Mauro et al., 1993); children suffering from carbohydrate-deficient glycoprotein syndrome (Jensen et al., 1995) have variable degrees of decline in IQ (sometimes only very mild); children with Friedreich's disease have visuospatial deficiencies, a low IQ, and emotional problems (Fehrenbach et al., 1984); and paediatric patients with olivopontocerebellar atrophy have varying degrees of deficiency in verbal and non-verbal intelligence, frontal functions, and memory (Kish et al., 1988). Patients with Louis Barr syndrome (ataxia-telangiectasia) also have a limited intelligence (Aguillar et al., 1968). Autosomal recessive congenital cerebellar atrophy is accompanied by moderate intellectual impairment, but the damage is more evident in the more complex planning tests, with a greater delay in information processing (Guzzetta et al., 1993).

Many genetic syndromes are associated with cerebellar alterations (such as Joubert's syndrome) (Kendall *et al.*, 1990) and many others with different chromosome deletions, duplications, or unbalanced translocations (Arts *et al.*, 1995) – for example, Williams, Down, and Rett syndromes. All these syndromes entail more or less severe intellectual deficiencies, associated with varying degrees of behavioural and emotional changes. In fragile-X syndrome (Mostofsky *et al.*, 1998) there is a marked reduction in the volume of the posterior vermis, which is accompanied by a picture of mental insufficiency of variable severity, and more or less frankly autistic behavioural characteristics.

In all these pathologies, the altered intelligence is accompanied by language disorders of greater or lesser severity, which are sometimes peculiar to a given condition, as in Williams syndrome.

In our series of 52 children with congenital cerebellar alterations (unpublished data), 30 per cent have no diagnosis, 10 patients have hypoplasia of the vermis [Joubert syndrome, type VI orofaciodigital or Varadi syndrome, cerebellar vermis hypoplasia, oligophrenia, congenital ataxia, coloboma and hepatic fibrosis (COACH) syndrome, Moebius syndrome, and autosomal recessive vermis hypoplasia with tapetoretinal degeneration and cerebral palsy], 13 patients have hypoplasia of the vermis and cerebellar hemispheres (cardiofaciocutaneous syndrome, Coffin-Siris syndrome, PEHO-like syndrome, hypomelanosis of Ito, and cerebral palsy), two patients have type II pontocerebellar hypoplasia, and 27 patients have cerebellar atrophy (carbohydrate deficient glycoprotein syndrome type Ia, ataxia-telangiectasia, Cockayne syndrome, infantile neuroaxonal dystrophy, methylmalonic aciduria with homocystinuria, mitochondrial encephalopathy, congenital cerebellar ataxia, and disequilibrium syndrome).

We distinguished the cerebellar alterations as hypoplasia or atrophy or forms of the two in combination, localized to the cerebellar vermis alone, or to the vermis and the hemispheres. Global intellectual, neuropsychological, and behavioural assessment identified a more marked mental retardation in the forms that affected the cerebellum extensively, with a more severe deterioration in language than in other functions. No significant behavioural changes were apparent.

Acquired cerebellar disease

Acquired cerebellar disease undeniably provides an extraordinary study opportunity, because the lesion is usually circumscribed and not part of a condition likely to involve a diffuse dysgenic or metabolic disease affecting the whole brain (even if it escapes detection using routine radiological investigation techniques).

Few studies have been published so far concerning premature children (Allin *et al.*, 2001) and children operated for tumours of the posterior fossa (Levisohn *et al.*, 2000; Riva & Giorgi, 2000; Scott *et al.*, 2001; Catsman-Berrevoets *et al.*, 2003; Steinlin *et al.*, 2003).

The cases of stroke reported so far refer mainly to post-acute mutism, except for those we ourselves described as practically post-surgical neoplastic lesions (Riva, 2000b).

In the past 20 years, a whole constellation of symptoms – represented mainly by mutism and occasionally by behavioural disorders – has been combined under the umbrella term of 'posterior fossa syndrome', observed in subjects operated for various type of cerebellar lesion. The first case of mutism was reported incidentally in 1972 by Stein *et al.* (1972). Some years later, Hirsch *et al.* (1979) reported on children with mutism associated with various neuropsychological deficiencies after the resection of extensive tumours of the vermis. Since then, approximately 205 cases of post-surgical mutism have been described and 93 per cent of these also had emotional or inhibition problems, or both. Alongside the surgical aetiopathogenesis, other vascular causes (Frim & Ogilvy, 1995; Koh *et al.*, 1997; Al-Anazi *et al.*, 2001; Turkel *et al.*, 2004), post-traumatic causes (Ersahin *et al.*, 1997; Koh *et al.*, 1997; Miyakita *et al.*, 1999), and infectious causes (Drost *et al.*, 2000; Mewasingh *et al.*, 2003; Papavasiliou *et al.*, 2004) have also been described.

There is a general consensus concerning the characteristics of the syndrome: after surgery, symptoms are preceded by a brief period of normal emotional and language functioning, which may vary from a few hours to approximately two days. The emotional disorders can vary from depressed mood, agitation, and irritability (Turkel *et al.*, 2004), to emotional instability (Pollack *et al.*, 1995) and apathy (Siffert *et al.*, 2000), to eating disorders (Pollack, 1997).

In addition to mutism, Pollack *et al.* (1995) found pseudobulbar signs and emotional changes, and a decreased initiation of voluntary movements. The causes of these findings are thought to be a transient bilateral dysfunction of the afferent or efferent dentate/thalamic pathways, or their cells of origin, owing to bilateral oedema of the brachium pontis (Van Dongen *et al.*, 1994).

Our series of children with acquired cerebellar lesions included one 4-year-old girl with viral cerebellitis whose mutism was not followed by dysarthria, and she had no genuine language disorder (as is commonly described), but she developed agrammatical language. She also had a dramatic inability to place actions and symbolic activities in sequence, and was very slow in completing all the tests administered. However, given the viral aetiopathogenesis, some co-involvement of the supratentorial structures could not be ruled out, though none was apparent on MRI (Riva, 1998). Nonetheless, only by the assessment of children with posterior fossa tumours in various locations of the vermis and cerebellar hemispheres has it been possible to correlate neuropsychological deficiency patterns with different lesion sites (Riva & Giorgi, 2000).

In children operated on for tumours of the vermis, we were able to distinguish two different pictures, one represented by disturbed social and emotional behaviour of varying severity, the other by disorders of verbal production, both developing with mutism after surgery (Riva & Giorgi, 2000).

The *behavioural disorders* included minor problems with socialization and generally with communication, the most salient aspects of which were a certain tendency for isolation, intolerance of people in close proximity, and a marked emotional lability. These children also tended to speak very little, but when prompted their language was normal.

After near-total demolition of lobes VI and VII, a 9-year-old girl suffering from medulloblastoma of the cerebellar vermis became frankly autistic; she would avert her gaze, would tolerate nobody near her, not even members of her family, strongly sought solitude, and hated to be touched. She also showed signs of complex behavioural stereotyping, and her language was reduced to echolalia with iterative repetitions of bizarre expressions, and sometimes of obscenities. After the acute stage, her language became telegraphic, frequently omitting functional words and using phrases with the verb in the infinitive. The picture was very similar to the agrammatism described in aphasic adults. When the child could be tested thoroughly, frontal function deficiencies also came to light. The situation improved after a few months, with a satisfactory recovery of the child's social and cognitive activities, albeit with a persistent tendency for isolation and a reduced empathy in relation to others.

The *verbal production disorders*, on the other hand, were represented by post-surgical mutism, the evolution of which enabled us to identify two clearly distinct types of disorder.

In the first type, patients were perfectly capable of understanding language and providing clear linguistic responses immediately after surgery but, within a period of 3 to 5 days, none of them could produce any sounds, although there were no signs of any cranial nerve deficiency and their brain-stem evoked responses were normal. They all had normal involuntary palatal, lip, and tongue movements, but none of them could imitate tongue or lip movements on command. After about a month, they recovered the ability to emit sounds, first by phonating when they laughed or cried, and then by producing single words; after 5 to 6 weeks, they were able to produce grammatically correct but highly dysarthric sentences. The children fully recovered their ability to use expressive language 3 to 6 months after the operation, but their speech patterns continued to be dysarthrically monotonous. Over the subsequent 6 to 24 months, they all completely re-acquired their normal speech.

The second type of mutism evolved instead towards a genuine language disorder. After recovering word production, their language was not dysarthric, but slow and monotonous, lacking normal prosody. Despite a normal tendency to communicate and the absence of dysarthria, these children made use of a telegraphic language, often structured in the form of simple noun/verb sentences that frequently omitted grammatical elements and often included uninflected verbs. Their language was reminiscent of the agrammatical language frequently encountered in aphasic patients (including children) with acquired left frontal lesions.

Surgical lesions of the cerebellar hemispheres were associated instead with a variety of neuropsychological deficiencies that tend to be side-specific (Riva & Giorgi, 2000). Tumours of the right cerebellar hemisphere correlated with an altered processing of verbal intelligence and complex language tasks; those of the left cerebellar hemisphere coincided with a diminished capacity to process non-verbal tasks and, in some cases, an impaired prosodic intonation. Regardless of the side of the lesion, some difficulties were encountered with the processing of executive and time-based attention tests, as shown in our previous study (Riva et al., 1989). None of the children had frank behavioural problems. In the group with hemispheric tumours, the deficits tended to be hemisphere-specific and were similar to those observed in children with acquired one-sided cerebral hemisphere lesions (Aram & Whitaker, 1988; Riva et al., 1991). The left/right distinction also had a certain tendency to apply to the deficit in frontal executive test scores: sequential auditory memory deteriorated in patients with right cerebellar lesions, while sequential visual memory was impaired in those with left cerebellar lesions (Marlow, 1992).

It seems clear from the above considerations that the cerebellum is indispensable in constructing mental organization in children, and that the intrinsic fragility attached to its lengthy neurogenesis exposes it to the risk of damage. Given the frequency of cerebellar pathologies, alone or as part of more complex pictures, mental organization and language suffer damage that is all the more important in that it takes effect from the very beginning of the maturation process of the functions. This explains why children with congenital cerebellar disease almost always present a complex picture, in which cognitive deficiencies (usually defined as mental insufficiency of variable degree) are associated with language and behavioural disorders that exacerbate their condition.

Studying patients with acquired lesions has enabled us to identify a possible intracerebellar functional topography. Schmahmann (1991) proposed a topographical model of the cerebellum that was confirmed in his studies on adults (Schmahmann & Sherman, 1998), where the vermis is a structure geared to process emotional behaviour, while the cerebellar hemispheres (and the posterior parts in particular) would be involved in processing cognitive functions. Studies in children with neoplastic lesions (and stroke) seem to confirm this topography and reveal an even more complex picture: behavioural changes to the point of autism would occur in the case of damage to the superior/inferior lobes of the vermis, in association with language disorders not only of anarthric, but also of agrammatical type. The girl with autistic symptoms also had an agrammatical type of language disorder, however, suggesting that the problem must be rather more complex. Side-specific neuropsychological impairments seem to be associated with cerebellar hemispheric lesions.

It is important not to forget that, after the same type of surgery for the same pathology, many children presented no such behavioural or cognitive changes, or so mild as to go undetected. This means that the problem must be very complex and that more or less dramatic reactions to cerebellar lesions, with problems of diaschisis from other supratentorial associative structures, may also depend on a neuronal organization that differs genetically from one subject to another.

Changes in cognitive and social behaviour correlating with cerebellar pathology imply that such lesions have a causal link with the generation of deficiencies. The close-knit network of connections that includes the cerebellum in an extremely complex system would justify the finding that a cerebellar lesion can be accompanied by different types of impairment and, as suggested by Schmahmann & Sherman (1998), the role of the cerebellum in this flow of information is to make the end result of processing by the network harmonious and integrated – just as the result of motor programming and processing is harmonious and integrated. Even more where language is concerned, the cerebellum uses its formidable capacity to interface the various components and produce a fluent and coherent end product.

References

Aguillar, M.J., Kamoshita, S., Landing, B.H., Boder, E. & Sedgwick, R.P. (1968): Pathological observations in ataxia-telangiectasia: a report on five cases. *J. Neuropathol. Exp. Neurol.* **27**, 659–676.

Al-Anazi, A., Hassounah, M., Sheik, B. & Barayan, S. (2001): Cerebellar mutism caused by arteriovenous malformation of the vermis. *Br. J. Neurosurg.* **15**, 47–50.

Allin, M., Matsumoto, H., Santhouse, A.M., Nosarti, C., AlAsady, M.H., Stewart, A.L., Rifkin, L. & Murray, R.M. (2001): Cognitive and motor function and the size of the cerebellum in adolescents born very pre-term. *Brain* **124**, 60–66.

Aram, D.M. & Whitaker, H.A. (1988): Cognitive sequelae of unilateral lesions acquired in early childhood. In: *The developmental implications of brain lateralization*, eds. D.L. Molfese & S. Segalowitz, pp. 156–178. New York: Guildford Press.

Arts, W.F.M., Hofstee, Y., Drejer, G.F., Beverstock, G.C. & Oosterwijk, J.C. (1995): Cerebellar and brain-stem hypoplasia in a child with a partial monosomy for the short arm of chromosome 5 and partial trisomy for the short chromosome 10. *Neuropediatrics* **26**, 41–44.

Asanuma, C., Thach W.T. & Jones E.G. (1983): Distribution of cerebellar terminations and their relation to other afferent terminations in the ventral lateral thalamic region in the monkey. *Brain Res.* **5**, 237–265.

Beyerman, W. (1917). Über angeborene Kleinhirnstörungen [On congenital cerebellar disorders]. *Archiv für Psychiatrie* **57**, 610–658.

Bond, H. (1895): Atrophy and sclerosis of the cerebellum. *J. Ment. Sci.* **174**, 409–420.

Botez, T.H. & Botez, M.I. (1992): Unilateral and bilateral cerebellar lesions: neuropsychological performances. *Neurology* **42**, 290.

Catsman-Berrevoets, C.E., Van Dongen, H.R., Aarsen, F.K. & Paquier, P.F. (2003): Transient cerebellar eye closure and mutism after cerebellar tumor surgery: long-term clinical follow-up of neurologic and behavioral disturbances in a 14-year-old girl. *Pediatr. Neurosurg.* **38**, 122–127.

Chiesielski, K.T., Harris, R.J., Hart, B.L. & Pabst, H.F. (1997): Cerebellar hypoplasia and frontal lobe cognitive deficits in disorders of early childhood. *Neuropsychologia* **35**, 643–655.

Connor, K.E. & Rosenberg, R.N. (1993): The hereditary ataxias. In: *The molecular and genetic basis of neurological disease*, eds. R.N. Rosenberg, S.B. Prusiner, S. DiMauro, R.L. Barchi & L.M. Kunkel, pp. 56–86. Boston MA: Butterworth-Heinemann.

Corsi, P.M. (1972): *Human memory and the medial temporal region of the brain*. Montreal: McGill University. [Ph.D thesis.]

Daum, I. & Ackerman, H. (1997): Neuropsychological abnormalities in cerebellar syndromes – facts or fiction? *Int. Rev. Neurobiol.* **41**, 455–471.

Di Mauro, R.L., Barchi, L.M., Kunkel, B.H., Matthews, K.D., Affi, A.K. & Hanson, J.W. (1993): Autosomal recessive cerebellar hypoplasia. *J. Child Neurol.* **4**, 189–194.

Dooley, J.M., Laroche, G.R., Tremblay, F. & Riding, M. (1992): Autosomal recessive cerebellar hypoplasia and tapetoretinal degeneration: a new syndrome. *Pediatr. Neurol.* **8**, 232–234.

Drost, G., Verrips, A. & Thijssen, H.O. & Gabreels. (2000): Cerebellar involvement as a rare complication of pneumococcal meningitis. *Neuropediatrics* **31**, 97–99.

Ersahin, Y., Mutluer, S., Saydam, S. & Barcin, E. (1997): Cerebellar mutism: report of two unusual cases and review of the literature. *Clin. Neurol. Neurosurg.* **99**, 130–134.

Fabbro, F. (2000): Introduction to language and cerebellum. *J. Neurolinguistics* **13**, 83–94.

Fabbro, F., Tavano, A., Corti, S., Bresolin, N., De Fabritiis, P. & Borgatti R. (2004): Long-term neuropsychological deficits after cerebellar infarctions in two young adult twins. *Neuropsychologia* **42**, 536–545.

Fehrenbach, R.A., Wallesch, C.W. & Claus, D. (1984): Neuropsychological findings in Friedreich's ataxia. *Arch. Neurol.* **41**, 306–308.

Frim, D.M. & Ogilvy, C.S. (1995): Mutism and cerebellar dysarthria after brain-stem surgery: case report. *Neurosurgery* **36**, 854–857.

Grafman, J., Litvan, I., Massaquoi, S., Stewart, M., Sirigu, A. & Hallett, M. (1992): Cognitive planning deficit in patients with cerebellar atrophy. *Neurology* **42**, 1493–1496.

Ghez, C. & Fahn, S. (1985): The cerebellum. In: *Principles of neural science*, eds. E.R. Kandel & J.H. Schwartz, pp. 503–522. New York: Elsevier Science.

Guzzetta, F., Mercuri, E., Bonanno, S., Longo, M. & Spano, M. (1993): Autosomal recessive congenital cerebellar atrophy: a clinical neuropsychological study. *Brain Dev.* **15**, 439–445.

Haines, D.E. & Dietrichs, E. (1984): An HRP study of hypothalamo-cerebellar and cerebello-hypothalamic connections in squirrel monkey (Saimiri sciureus). *J. Comp. Neurol.* **229**, 559–575.

Hart, R.P., Kwentus, J.A., Leshner, R.T. & Frazier R. (1985): Information processing speed in Friedreich's ataxia. *Ann. Neurol.* **17**, 612–614.

Hirsch, J.F., Renier, D., Czernichow, P., Benveniste, L. & Pierre-Kahn, A. (1979): Medulloblastoma in childhood: survival and functional results. *Acta Neurochir.* **48**, 1–15.

Hubrich-Ungureanu, P., Kaemmerer, N., Henn, F.A. & Braus, D.F. (2002): Lateralized organization of the cerebellum in a silent verbal fluency task: a functional magnetic resonance imaging study in healthy volunteers. *Neurosci. Lett.* **319**, 91–94.

Ishihara, M., Kumita, S., Mizumura S. & Kumazaki, T. (1999): Crossed cerebellar diaschisis: the role of motor and premotor areas in functional connections. *J. Neuroimaging* **9**, 30–33.

Jansen, A., Floel, A., Van Randenborgh, J., Konrad, C., Rotte, M., Forster, A.F., Deppe, M. & Knecht, S. (2005): Crossed cerebro-cerebellar language dominance. *Hum. Brain Mapp.* **24**, 165–172.

Jensen, P.R., Hansen, F.J. & Skovby, F. (1995): Cerebellar hypoplasia in children with the carbohydrate-deficient glycoprotein syndrome. *Neuroradiology* **37**, 328–330.

Kassubek, J., Hickok, G. & Erhard, P. (2004): Involvement of classical anterior and posterior language areas in sign language production, as investigated by 4 T functional magnetic resonance imaging. *Neurosci. Lett.* **364**, 168–172.

Kendall, B., Kingsley, D., Lambert, S.R., Taylor, D. & Finn, P. (1990): Joubert syndrome: a clinico-radiological study. *Neuroradiology* **31**, 502–506.

Kish, S.J., El-Awar, M., Schut, L., Leach, L., Oscar-Beramn, M. & Freedman, M. (1988): Cognitive deficits in olivopontocerebellar atrophy: implications for the cholinergic hypothesis of Alzheimer's dementia. *Ann. Neurol.* **24**, 200–206.

Klein, D., Milner, B., Zatorre, R.J., Meyer, E. & Evans, A.C. (1995): The neural substrates underlying word generation: a bilingual functional-imaging study. *Proc. Natl. Acad. Sci. USA* **92**, 2899–2903.

Kluin, K.J., Gilman, S., Markel, D.S., Koeppe, R.A., Rosenthal, G. & Junck, L. (1988): Speech disorders in olivopontocerebellar atrophy correlate with positron emission tomography findings. *Ann. Neurol.* **23**, 547–554.

Koh, S., Turkel, S.B. & Baram, T.Z. (1997): Cerebellar mutism in children: report of six cases and potential mechanisms. *Pediatr. Neurol.* **16**, 218–219.

Lalonde, R. & Botez-Marquard, T. (2000): Neuropsychological deficits of patients with chronic or acute cerebellar lesions. *J. Neurolinguistics* **13**, 117–128.

Leiner, H.C., Leiner, A.L. & Dow, R.S. (1991): The human cerebro-cerebellar system: its computing, cognitive, and language skills. *Behav. Brain Res.* **44**, 113–128.

Leiner, H.C., Leiner, A.L. & Dow R.S. (1993): Cognitive and language functions of the human cerebellum. *Trends Neurosci.* **16**, 444–447.

Levisohn, L., Cronin-Golomb, A. & Schmahmann, J.D. (2000): Neuropsychological consequences of cerebellar tumour resection in children: cerebellar cognitive affective syndrome in a paediatric population. *Brain* **123**, 1041–1050.

Loritz, D. (1991): Cerebral and cerebellar models of language learning. *Applied linguistics* **12**, 299–318.

Luria, A.R. (1966): *Higher cortical functions in man.* New York: Basic Books.

Marien, P., Saerens, J., Nanhoe, R., Moens, E., Nagels, G., Pickut, B.A., Dierckx, R.A. & De Deyn, P.P. (1996): Cerebellar induced aphasia: case report of cerebellar induced prefrontal aphasic language phenomena supported by SPECT findings. *J. Neurol. Sci.* **144**, 34–43.

Marien. P., Engelborghs, S., Fabbro, F. & De Deyn, P.P. (2001): The lateralized linguistic cerebellum: a review and a new hypothesis. *Brain Lang.* **79**, 580–600.

Marlowe, W.B. (1992): The impact of a right frontal lesion on the developing brain. *Brain Cogn.* **20**, 205–213.

Mewasingh, L.D., Kadhim, H., Christophe, C., Christiaens, F.J. & Dan, B. (2003): Nonsurgical cerebellar mutism (anarthria) in two children. *Pediatr. Neurol.* **28**, 59–63.

Middleton, F.A. & Strick, P.L. (1994): Anatomical evidence for cerebellar and basal ganglia involvement in higher cognitive function. *Science* **266**, 458–461.

Middleton, F.A. & Strick, P.L. (1997): Cerebellar output channels. In: *The cerebellum and cognition. International review of neurobiology*, ed. J.D. Schmahmann, vol. 41, pp. 61–82. San Diego: Academic Press.

Miyakita, Y., Taguchi, Y., Sakakibara, Y., Matsuzawa, M. & Kitagawa, H. (1999): Transient mutism resolving into cerebellar speech after brain stem infarction following a traumatic injury of the vertebral artery in a child. *Acta Neurochir.* **141**, 209–213.

Molinari, M., Leggio, M.G., Solida, A., Corra, R., Misciagna, S., Silveri, M.C. & Petrosini, L. (1997a): Cerebellum and procedural learning: evidence from focal cerebellar lesions. *Brain* **120**, 1753–1762.

Molinari, M., Leggio, M.G. & Silveri, M.C. (1997b): Verbal fluency and agrammatism. *Int. Rev. Neurobiol.* **41**, 325–329.

Mostofsky, S.H., Mazzocco, M.M.M., Aakalu, G., Warsofsky, I.S., Denkla, M.B. & Reiss, A.L. (1998): Decreased cerebellar posterior vermis size in fragile X syndrome. *Neurology* **50**, 121–130.

Papavasiliou, A.S., Kotsalis, C. & Trakadas, S. (2004): Transient cerebellar mutism in the course of the acute cerebellitis. *Pediatr. Neurol.* **30**, 71–74.

Pollack, I.F. (1997): Posterior fossa syndrome. *Int. Rev. Neurobiol.* **41**, 411–432.

Pollack, I.F., Polinko, P., Albright, A.L., Towbin, R. & Fitz, C. (1995): Mutism and pseudobulbar symptoms after resection of posterior fossa tumors in children: incidence and pathophysiology. *Neurosurgery* **37**, 885–893.

Riva, D. (1998): The cerebellar contribution to language and sequential functions: evidence from a child with cerebellitis. *Cortex* **34**, 279–287.

Riva, D. (2000a): Cerebellar contribution to behaviour and cognition in children. *J. Neurolinguistics* **13**, 215–225.

Riva, D. (2000b): The cerebellum contributes to higher cognitive and social behaviour in childhood: evidence from acquired cerebellar lesions. In: *Localization of brain lesions and developmental functions*, Mariani Foundation Paediatric Neurology Series, vol. 9, eds. D. Riva & A. Benton, pp. 151–160. London: John Libbey.

Riva, D. & Giorgi, C. (2000): The cerebellum contributes to higher functions during development: evidence from a series of children surgically treated for posterior fossa tumours. *Brain* **123**, 1051–1061.

Riva, D., Pantaleoni, C., Milani, N. & Fossati Bellani, F. (1989): Impairment in neuropsychological functions in children with medulloblastomas and astrocytomas of the posterior fossa. *Childs Nerv. Syst.* **5**, 107–110.

Riva, D., Pantaleoni, C., Milani, N. & Devoti, M. (1991): Late sequelae of right versus left hemispheric lesions. In: *Acquired aphasia in children: acquisition and breakdown of language in the developing brain*, eds. I.P. Martins, A. Castro-Caldas, H.R. Van Dongen & A. Van Hout. Amsterdam: Kluwer Academic Publishers.

Rubinstein, H.S. & Freeman, W. (1940): Cerebellar agenesis. *J. Nerv. Merit. Dis.* **92**, 489–502.

Schmahmann, J.D. (1991): An emerging concept: the cerebellar contribution to higher function. *Arch. Neurol.* **48**, 1178–1187.

Schmahmann, J.D. (1997): Rediscovery of an early concept. *Int. Rev. Neurobiol.* **41**, 3–27.

Schmahmann, J.D. & Pandya, D.N. (1990): Anatomical investigation of projections from the thalamus to the posterior parietal cortices in the rhesus monkey. *J. Comp. Neurol.* **295**, 299–326.

Schmahmann, J.D. & Pandya, D.N. (1993): Prelunate, occipitotemporal, and parahippocampal projections to the basis pontis in rhesus monkey. *J. Comp. Neurol.* **337**, 94–112.

Schmahmann, J.D. & Pandya, D.N. (1995): Prefrontal cortex projections to the basilar pons in rhesus monkey: implications for the cerebellar contribution to higher function. *Neurosci. Lett.* **199**, 175–178.

Schmahmann, J.D. & Pandya, D.N. (1997a): Anatomic organization of the basilar pontine projections to the basilar pons from prefrontal cortices in rhesus monkeys. *J. Neurosci.* **17**, 438–458.

Schmahmann, J.D. & Pandya, D.N. (1997b): The cerebrocerebellar system. *Int. Rev. Neurobiol.* **41**, 31–60.

Schmahmann, J.D. & Sherman, J.C. (1998): The cerebellar cognitive affective syndrome. *Brain* **121**, 561–579.

Scott, R.B., Stoodley, C.J., Anslow, P., Paul, C., Stein, J.F., Sugden, E.M. & Mitchell, C.D. (2001): Lateralized cognitive deficits in children following cerebellar lesions. *Dev. Med. Child. Neurol.* **43**, 685–691.

Siffert. J., Poussaint, T.Y., Goumnerova, L.C., Scott R.M, LaValley, B., Tarbell, N.J. & Pomeroy, S.L. (2000): Neurological dysfunction associated with postoperative cerebellar mutism. *J. Neurooncol.* **48**, 75–81.

Silveri, M.C., Leggio, M.G. & Molinari, M. (1994): The cerebellum contributes to linguistic production: a case of agrammatic speech following a right cerebellar lesion. *Neurology* **44**, 2047–2050.

Silveri, M.C., Di Betta, A.M., Filippini, V., Leggio, M.G. & Molinari, M. (1998): Verbal short-term store-rehearsal system and the cerebellum. Evidence from a patient with a right cerebellar lesion. *Brain* **121**, 2175–2187.

Snider, R.S. (1950): Recent contributions to the anatomy and physiology of the cerebellum. *Arch. Neurol. Psychiatry* **64**, 196–219.

Stanton, G.B., Goldenberg, M.E. & Bruce, C.J (1993): Frontal eyefield efferents in the macaque monkey II: topography of terminal fields in midbrain and pons. *J. Comp. Neurol.* **271**, 493–506.

Stein, B.M., Fraser, R.A.R. & Tenner, M.S. (1972): Normal pressure hydrocephalus: complication of posterior fossa surgery in children. *Pediatrics* **49**, 50–58.

Steinlin, M., Imfeld, S., Zulauf, P., Boltshauser, E., Lovblad, K.O., Ridolfi Luthy, A., Perrig, W. & Kaufmann, F. (2003): Neuropsychological long-term sequelae after posterior fossa tumour resection during childhood. *Brain* **126**, 1998–2008.

Stowe, L.A., Paans, A.M., Wijers, A.A. & Zwarts, F. (2004): Activations of 'motor' and other non-language structures during sentence comprehension. *Brain Lang.* **89**, 290–299.

Stuss, D.T., Benson, D.F., Clermont, R., Della Malva, C.L., Kaplan, E.F. & Weir, W.S. (1986): Language functioning after bilateral prefrontal leukotomy. *Brain Lang.* **28**, 66–70.

Turkel, S.B., Shu Chen, L., Nelson, M.D., Hyder, D., Gilles, F.H., Woodall, L., Braslow, K. & Tavare, C.J. (2004): Case series: acute mood symptoms associated with posterior fossa lesions in children. *J. Neuropsychiatry Clin. Neurosci.* **16**, 443–445.

Van Dongen, H., Catsman-Berrevoets, C.E. & Van Mourik, M. (1994): The syndrome of cerebellar mutism and subsequent dysarthria. *Neurology* **44**, 2040–2046.

Vilensky, J.A. & Van Hoesen, G.W. (1981): Corticopontine projections from the cingulate cortex in the rhesus monkey. *Brain Res.* **205**, 391–395.

Wood, A.G., Harvey, A.S., Wellard, R.M., Abbott, D.F., Anderson, V., Kean, M., Saling, M.M. & Jackson, G.D. (2004): Language cortex activation in normal children. *Neurology* **63**, 1035–1044.

Zettin, M., Cappa, S., D'Amico, A., Rago, R., Perino, C., Perani, D. & Fazio, F. (1997). Agrammatic speech production after a right cerebellar haemorrhage. *Neurocase* **3**, 375–380.

Chapter 12

Cortical specialization for language in childhood: evidence from negative cases

Isabel Pavão Martins

Language Research Laboratory, I.M.M., Lisbon Faculty of Medicine, Hospital de Sta Maria, 1600 Lisbon, Portugal
labling@fm.ul.pt

Summary

Acquired aphasia in childhood has provided models to study the role of specific brain areas for language at different ages, yet it does not investigate the possibility of language sparing after lesions of the language cortex, nor the effects of lesions remote from the classical language areas on verbal capacities. In the present study we analysed a series of 'negative cases' – that is, left hemispheric lesions without aphasia – to identify brain areas with no clinical impact on language during childhood, and to explore their effects on specific verbal tasks.

Fifteen cases, seven boys and eight girls ranging from 4 to 15 years of age, with lesions of the left hemisphere without aphasia, were selected from a series of children with acquired brain lesions. Eleven had static lesions (stroke or trauma) and four suffered from primary intracranial tumours. Clinical observations from the acute stage and formal language assessments were obtained in all patients. Brain images (computed tomography or magnetic resonance imaging) were analysed for lesion localization and the involvement of the classical language areas.

Although none of the children had ever been aphasic, nine had subclinical impairment of oral or written language. Most patients (13 of 15) had lesions outside the language areas, involving the medial prefrontal cortex, medial temporal, or the occipital lobes. Only two cases had partial lesions of Broca's area with no impairment of spoken language.

These cases are complementary to those of acquired aphasia, showing that regions remote from the classical language areas do not cause aphasia. However, they participate in different aspects of language during normal development.

Introduction

Cerebral regions responsible for language were identified during the 19th century through the neuropathological examination of aphasic patients, a corpus of knowledge that was corroborated by imaging studies undertaken 150 years later (Cannestra *et al.*, 2000; Kreisler *et al.*, 2000; Papathanassiou *et al.*, 2000). Language is supported by an implementation system localized in the perisylvian region of the left hemisphere which is specialized in decoding, analysing, and programming speech sounds, and is interconnected to a large-scale conceptual system through mediating neuronal networks (Dronkers *et al.*, 2000).

Acquired childhood aphasia, although rare, has been taken as a model for studying the stability of the neural organization for language with increasing age and cognitive development. The theoretical assumptions underlying this inference are first, that a biological manipulation (a lesion) of a specific brain area will impair functions subserved by the corresponding neuroanatomical network; and second, that there is an analogy with the adult brain. If similar lesions produce identical patterns of dysfunction at different ages, we may assume that the functional organization for language does not change with age.

In the past 20 years, with the development of neuroimaging, studies of acquired aphasia have shown that under normal circumstances language has an identical organization in adults and children, suggesting a genetically determined basis for its functional architecture. This evidence comes from three main foci of research: the frequency of crossed aphasia, the clinical presentation of language impairments and anatomoclinical studies in different age groups, and genetic studies in developmental language disorders. The prevalence of aphasia following right hemisphere lesions (crossed aphasia) is identical in children and adults, indicating an early lateralization of language to the left hemisphere (Carter *et al.*, 1982; Marien *et al.*, 2001), a finding confirmed by functional activation patterns of healthy children performing verbal tasks (Balsamo *et al.*, 2002; Dahaene-Lambertz *et al.*, 2002; Ahmad *et al.*, 2003). As for the clinical presentation of language impairments, all types of aphasia described in adults have been reported in children (Rapin, 1995; Paquier & Van Dongen, 1996; Nass *et al.*, 1998) and their neuroanatomical correlations resemble those described in adult aphasics (Cranberg *et al.*, 1987; Martins & Ferro, 1993; Martins, 2000). This suggests a relative stability of language networks and thus of the intrahemispheric functional organization with age. Finally, the identification of a gene responsible for a familial form of specific language impairment gave support to a genetic basis for the development of language (Vargha-Khadem *et al.*, 1998).

However, there are also differences between age groups. One of these is the high prevalence of mutism and non-fluent types of speech in children (Martins & Ferro, 1993), which might suggest that the areas subserving speech initiation and programming require larger neuronal networks than in adults. This is in agreement with functional imaging studies carried out in healthy subjects showing that identical verbal tasks – namely verbal fluency tasks – produce a more extensive activation of the left hemisphere in children than in adults (Gaillard *et al.*, 2000; Gaillard *et al.*, 2003), and that the degree of language lateralization increases with age (Holland *et al.*, 2001). This indicates that the neuronal networks sustaining speech production may become more restricted and lateralized as language becomes more efficient or automatized. This hypothesis is in accordance with the observation that as a brain region becomes functional there is a reduction in its numbers of synapses (Huttenlocher & Dabholkar, 1997). It is therefore possible that the limits of the language areas are less well defined in the child's brain.

In addition to this, there is some evidence that left hemisphere regions outside the language cortex may play a crucial role in language recovery after early brain damage (eventually more than in adults) – either directly, by taking up language functions, or indirectly, by promoting language reorganization in the other cerebral hemisphere. This has been demonstrated by cortical electrical stimulation (Duchowny *et al.*, 1996), by the amytal test (De Vos *et al.*, 1995), and by functional magnetic resonance imaging or positron emission tomography studies (Muller *et al.*, 1999; Liégeois *et al.*, 2004) in children with static or progressive lesions overlying the language areas, and in children with epilepsy secondary to left hemispheric lesions. One of those studies (Liégeois *et al.*, 2004) pointed to the hypothetical participation of the hippocampus in recovery, a region remote from the language areas but crucial for learning. Furthermore, longitudinal studies of children with perinatal lesions have suggested that the areas involved in the early stages of language development are different from those underlying its subsequent automatization (Bates *et al.*, 1999). Those differences concern both interhemispheric and intra-hemispheric organization.

In summary, although lesion studies in children replicate the results found in adults with aphasia, functional imaging and longitudinal studies suggest a higher participation of other areas, remote from the language cortex, during recovery or during the early stages of language acquisition. Consequently, the investigation of the verbal impact of cortical areas outside the classical language cortex is theoretically justified and may be of practical relevance in determining prognostic factors for aphasia recovery at different ages. However, there is little information about this. Although there are reports of large series of patients with early brain lesions unbiased for their clinical manifestations (that is, including negative cases) (Vargha-Khadem *et al.*, 1985; Aram, 1988; Riva *et al.*, 1991; Chapman *et al.*, 2003; Max, 2004), most of these included cases with perinatal pathology, where the acute effects on language could not be assessed or were not described. On the other hand, most studies of neuroanatomical correlations are based on positive cases – that is, children with clinical aphasia.

To evaluate the primary role of the extrasylvian cortex in language, and thus the boundaries of the language cortex in childhood, we analysed language functions and lesion localization in a series of children with clinically intact oral language following a left hemisphere lesion. Our aim was to determine first, whether classical language areas were spared in those cases, explaining the lack of language impairment and corroborating an identical organization of language in children and adults, or whether they were involved, which would suggest that language organization depends upon wider or different neuronal networks in children and adults, which could compensate for a lesion in the classical language areas; and second, to determine whether any specific localization has a systematic effect on verbal tasks.

Methods

Patients included in this report were children referred to our centre for neuropsychological assessment following an acquired brain lesion. As our laboratory is part of an acute care hospital, most of the patients were first observed in the acute stage of their illness.

From a prospective study on acquired hemispheric lesions in childhood which has been ongoing in our centre for several years (Martins, 2004), we selected for the present analysis all cases fulfilling the following criteria:

- presence of a focal brain lesion sustained after some normal language acquisition (that is, after 18 to 24 months) and before 15 years of age;
- absence of aphasia, documented since lesion onset (or first manifestations in progressive lesions) by clinical history (from family), clinical records from the acute stage, and formal language evaluations undertaken in our laboratory;
- left hemispheric lesion documented by neuroimaging examinations [computed tomography (CT) or magnetic resonance imaging (MRI)];
- previous right handedness;
- no clinical history (or imaging evidence) of previous brain lesion, or history of developmental language disorder.

Aphasic seizures, or transient post-epileptic (post-critical) aphasia, were not criteria for patient exclusion, as they could result from generalization of the epileptic activity to neighbouring areas involved in language. Similarly, acquired disorders of reading and writing did not constitute criteria for patient exclusion, as they can be observed in adults with lesions outside the language cortex. Different aetiologies were included, namely stroke, trauma, and tumours. Time post-onset – that is, timing of formal language evaluation in relation to lesion onset – cannot be estimated in tumours, as their exact onset is not known; therefore, in those cases we refer the evaluations to the time since the first symptoms occurred and not to lesion onset.

Procedures

Clinical and biographic data were recorded in all cases by a standard semistructured interview with the parents (undertaken by a neurologist), which included age at first symptoms, clinical manifestations (namely any language impairment or regression of previous linguistic skills), the type and frequency of epilepsy, data regarding the perinatal period and developmental milestones (language and handedness in particular), and previous school achievement. Clinical notes from the acute period of illness were reviewed for any description of language impairment during the acute stage. A neurological examination was carried out.

Formal language assessment included: rating for the severity of aphasia (Goodglass & Kaplan, 1983); analysis of spontaneous speech for fluency (speech rate, prosody, articulation, effort, word-finding difficulties) and positive signs (paraphasias, perserveration, circumlocutions); confrontation naming of objects and line drawings; word, digit, and sentence repetition; lexical comprehension (object identification by name and the British Picture Vocabulary Scale (Dunn et al., 1982)); comprehension of simple verbal commands; and a short version of the Token Test (De Renzi & Vignolo, 1962). Most of these tests form part of the Lisbon Aphasia Battery (Castro-Caldas, 1979) or the ELOLA battery (Agostini et al., 1998). Children younger than 7 years were also assessed by the Reynell Developmental Language Scales (Reynell, 1977). Children who had completed the first degree of primary school were evaluated with reading and writing tests.

Visuo-spatial abilities were tested by a battery that included the following: spontaneous drawing, the Line Orientation Test (Benton et al., 1983), the Visual Retention Test (Benton et al., 1967), and a crossing-out screening test for neglect. IQ was determined by the Raven Coloured Matrices (Raven et al., 1986) or the WISC (Wechsler, 1949). Test scores below mean for age by 2 or more standard deviations were considered pathological, while those ranging from -1.5 to -2 SD were considered mildly impaired.

To exclude the possibility of language organization in the right hemisphere, data on language lateralization (results of the sodium amobarbital test, occurrence of aphasic seizures or post-epileptic aphasia), and the presence of simultaneous lesions of the right hemisphere were sought and recorded.

Imaging analysis

CT and MRI scans were analysed by two independent observers according to standard brain maps (Matsui & Hirano, 1978; Damasio, 1995). The following regions of interest in the left hemisphere were analysed for the presence or absence of lesions: Broca's and Wernicke's area (cortical and subcortical), insula, supramarginal and angular gyrus (Broadman areas 40 and 39) of the parietal cortex, subcortical white matter, and basal ganglia. Lesion localization outside those areas was described. The inter-judge reliability for the regions of interest was calculated by the Cronbach α index. Areas of disagreement were reviewed by both observers and discussed until agreement was reached.

Results

Clinical data and language lateralization

Of 73 patients with left hemisphere lesions (62 cases with a single unilateral lesions and 11 with bilateral lesions), 20 (27.4 per cent) were never aphasic and there were no data concerning the occurrence of aphasia in the acute stage in another case. Fifteen cases of those 20 had brain imaging studies documenting a left hemisphere lesion and were included in this study (Table 1).

There were eight girls and seven boys. Seven patients suffered from strokes (intracranial haemorrhages attributed to arteriovenous malformations in four, intracerebral haematomas of undetermined aetiology in two, and ischaemic infarction in one case), four had traumatic brain injury and four children had primary intracranial tumours (astrocytoma or ependymoma). Average age at the time of lesion onset ranged between 1 year, 5 months and 14 years in patients with static lesions. Patients with tumours had their first symptoms between 4 and 13 years of age. All children with established handedness were right handed. Three children had not began formal education at the time of the lesion, one patient (patient 6) had repeated one school grade before lesion onset, and another child (patient 2) had been diagnosed as having developmental dyslexia and dysgraphia (with two grade repetitions) before the onset of stroke.

There is information confirming language lateralization to the left hemisphere in seven patients. Three patients with tumours (patients 13, 14, and 15) had focal dysphasic seizures and postictal aphasia, with an EEG focus lateralized to the left hemisphere. In three patients (patients 4, 5, and 6, patient 4 being described below in detail), selective amytal testing produced aphasia when injected into branches or the trunk of the left internal carotid artery; and patient 1 became transiently aphasic when a balloon was inflated to occlude a left middle cerebral artery aneurysm (transient ischaemic attack). Three cases with traumatic aetiology (patients 9, 10, and 11) had bilateral lesions, the right hemispheric lesion being located on the right prefrontal cortex.

Case description, patient 4

S.R., an 8-year-old, right handed girl, was admitted because of a sudden headache with vomiting. Observed in the emergency room, she had no language impairment or focal neurological signs. MRI showed an extensive left frontal haematoma involving the prefrontal cortex (orbito-frontal and dorsolateral regions) including Broca's area. A bedside language evaluation, on the 10th day post-onset, and formal full language testing carried out 3 months later were both normal (spoken language, reading, praxis, visuo-spatial abilities, and written calculation), except for a mild writing difficulty (slow writing with orthographic and syntactic errors). Her IQ was within the normal range (FSIQ = 123, VIQ = 129, PIQ = 114). Angiography showed a frontal arteriovenous malformation (AVM) fed by anterior branches of the left middle cerebral artery, which was occluded by an endovascular approach. To determine language lateralization and to detect eloquent areas supplied by AVM feeding branches, sodium amytal was injected in the left middle cerebral artery, producing a transient non-fluent aphasia (word-finding difficulties, poor speech initiation). Injection into the right middle cerebral artery did not produce a language disorder, showing that language was lateralized to the left hemisphere. The AVM was later removed surgically with no sequelae.

Neuropsychological evaluation (Table 2)

Formal evaluations were carried out at variable times post-onset. Most children (seven) with static lesions were evaluated within the first 3 months from symptom onset (five during the

Table 1. Patients: clinical features

Patient number	Age at onset years:months	Sex	School grade	Aetiology	Acute neurological impairment				Evidence language lateralization
					Acute seizures or epilepsy	Motor defect	Visual field defect	Somatosensory defect	
1	10:03	f	5	infarction	–	R	–	–	TIA
2	10:04	m	2	ich**	–	R	–	–	–
3	08:06	f	2	ich-avm	seizures	R	–	–	–
4	08:11	f	4	ich-avm	–	–	–	–	amytal
5	11:00	f	6	ich-avm	–	R	R hemianopia	–	amytal
6	14:00	m	7	ich-avm	–	R	R sensory	–	amytal
7	06:11	m	1	ich**	–	–	–	–	–
8	10:07	m	5	trauma	–	–	–	–	–
9	04:03	f	pre school	trauma	seizures	–	–	–	–
10	13:10	m	8	trauma	–	–	–	–	–
11	01:05	f	pre school	trauma	–	L	–	–	–
12	4:07*	m	pre school	tumour	–	R	–	–	–
13	13:00*	m	10	tumour	seizures	–	R sensory	–	postictal
14	9:00*	f	3	tumour	epilepsy	–	–	–	postictal
15	7:00*	f	1	tumour	epilepsy	–	–	–	postictal

f = female, m = male, ich = intracranial haematoma; avm = arteriovenous malformation.
* age of first symptoms; ** undetermined aetiology.
TIA = transient ischaemic attack with aphasia, during balloon inflation.

Table 2. Formal language assessment

Patient No	Time pos onset	Age (y) at evaluation	Positive signs in spontaneous speech							Visual naming	Sentence repetition	Digit span	Token test	Reading writing
			Word-finding difficulties	Para phasias	Circum locutions	Slow speech rate	Dysarthria					
1	2 m	10	–	–	–	–	+	N	N	N	N	N
2	7 d	10	–	–	–	–	–	N	impaired	N	impaired	dyslexia
3	18 d	8.5	–	–	–	–	–	N	N	impaired	impaired	N
4	10 d	8.9	–	–	–	–	–	N	N	N	N	N
5	2 y	13	–	–	–	–	–	N	N	N	N	N
6	45 d	14	–	–	–	–	–	N	N	N	N	Impaired
7	4 d	6.9		–	–	–		N	N	impaired	impaired	impaired
8	3.5 m	10	–	–	–	–	–	N	impaired	N	N	N
9	5 y	9	–	–	–	–	–	N	N	N	N	N
10	1 y	15	–	–	–	+	–	impaired	N	N	N	impaired
11	3 y	4	–	–	–	–	–	N	na	na	na	na
12	3 m*	5	–	–	–	–	–	N	na	na	na	na
13	2 y*	15.5	–	–	–	–	–	N	N	impaired	N	N
14	2 y*	11	–	–	–	–	–	N	N	N	N	N
15	11 m*	7.9	–	–	–	–	–	impaired	N	N	N	N

* Time since first symptoms, d = days, m = months, y = years. N = normal; na = not applicable.

first 2 weeks), and four in the chronic period. Among children with tumours, only one was observed within 3 months of first symptoms. In all children clinical information (from clinical records and family interview) confirmed that they had no evident language impairment in the acute stage.

Language evaluation

None of the patients presented any impairment of conversational speech (speech fluency, rate, prosody), or word-finding difficulties, grammatical errors, or paraphasias. All had normal scores in tests of lexical comprehension and word repetition. Seven patients had mild subclinical impairments on one or two (at maximum) verbal oral tasks: confrontation naming (n = 2), sentence repetition (n = 2), digit span forward (n = 3), or the Token Test (n = 3). An additional case, a preschool child (patient 11), had a mild impairment on the comprehension subscale of the Reynell scales (scoring − 1.8 below the mean for age). Three children (patients 6, 7, and 10) scored below the normal range for age on reading (word-reading aloud or comprehension of a written text) or writing to dictation. Another case (patient 2) had a previous history of dyslexia, so the impairment could not be attributed to the focal brain lesion. Altogether, nine patients had an impairment of oral of written language, though the disturbance was mild in all cases.

Visuo-spatial evaluation

All children except one (patient 10, with an IQ of 73) had IQ scores within the normal range (above 85 on the WISC and above the 25th centile on the Raven Coloured Matrices). None of the patients had neglect of the right hemispace on a crossing out task, copy of geometric figures, reading or writing tasks, or spontaneous drawing. There were no abnormal scores on the line orientation test.

Lesion localization

The localization of the lesions is shown in Table 3. Inter-judge reliability for involvement of regions of interest was 0.88. The majority of children (13 of 15) had lesions outside the classical cortical language areas of the left hemisphere and in none did the lesion involve Wernicke's area. In two patients (patients 4 and 14) the lesions involved Broca's area. One of these (patient 4), described above, had a ruptured frontal AVM, and the other (patient 14) had a frontal tumour overlying that area and suffered transient post-epileptic aphasia, suggesting language lateralization to the left hemisphere. None of the children had any spoken language impairment. Four children (patients 1, 2, 5, and 12) had lesions localized to the basal ganglia and subcortical white matter, namely the lenticular nucleus, the posterior limb of the internal capsule, and the left thalamus. In two of these patients (patients 1 and 5) the lesion extended to the insula. The other patients had lesions sparing the classical language areas. They involved the prefrontal cortex in four cases (patients 3, 6, 8, 9, and 10), including the dorsolateral prefrontal cortex but sparing Broca's area (patient 10), the frontal pole (patient 9), or the medial frontal and anterior cingulus (patients 3, 6, and 8). One boy (patient 12) had a superior parietal/rolandic glioma, another (patient 7) had a stroke involving the occipital lobes, patient 5 had a posterior subcortical AVM which bled twice (into the occipital lobe the first time and into the basal ganglia the second time), and patient 15 had a medial temporal tumour involving the hippocampus.

Table 3. Lesion localization in the left hemisphere

Patient number	Brain imaging	Outside language cortex	Cortical language areas — Broca's cortical	Broca's sc	Insula	Temporal BA41,42	Wernicke's area B/W	Wernicke's area I	Wernicke's area W	Wernicke's area sc	Angular/ supra-marginal	Caudate nucleus	Lenticular nucleus	Globus pallidus	Internal capsulae	Corona radiata	Thalamus
1	CT	–	–	–	+	–	–	–	–	–	–	–	+	–	–	–	–
2	CT	–	–	–	–	–	–	–	–	–	–	–	–	–	post limb	–	–
3	CT	ant cingulus	–	–	–	–	–	–	–	–	–	–	–	–	–	–	–
4	MRI	orbitofrontal	+	+	–	–	–	–	–	–	–	–	–	–	–	–	–
5	CT	occipital	–	–	+	–	–	+	–	–	–	–	+	+	post limb	–	+
6	MRI	ant cingulus	–	–	–	–	–	–	–	–	–	–	–	–	–	–	–
7	CT	occipital	–	–	–	–	–	–	–	–	–	–	–	–	–	–	–
8	CT	ant cingulus	–	–	–	–	–	–	–	–	–	–	–	–	–	–	–
9	CT	frontal pole	–	–	–	–	–	–	–	–	–	–	–	–	–	–	–
10	CT	dorsolateral PFC	–	–	–	–	–	–	–	–	–	–	–	–	–	–	–
11	CT	subcortical frontal	–	–	–	–	–	–	–	–	–	–	–	–	–	–	–
12	CT	–	–	–	–	–	–	–	–	–	–	–	–	–	–	–	+
13	CT	postcentral	–	–	–	–	–	–	–	–	–	–	–	–	–	–	–
14	CT	dorsolateral PFC	+	–	–	–	–	–	–	–	–	–	–	–	–	–	–
15	MRI	internal temporal	–	–	–	–	–	–	–	–	–	–	–	–	–	–	–

sc = subcortical, B/W = CT slice where Broca's and Wernicke's areas are both visualized; I = temporal isthmus, W = CT slice including Wernicke's area. BA = corresponding to Brodman areas; PFC = prefrontal cortex.

Case description, patient 1

P.S., a 10-year-old right handed girl, had a subarachnoid haemorrhage following the rupture of a giant aneurysm of the left middle cerebral artery. There were no focal neurological signs. During endovascular occlusion, the first attempt to inflate the balloon produced a transient occlusion of the left middle cerebral artery and transient aphasia (speech arrest followed by anomia and literal paraphasias on confrontation naming) which resolved as the balloon was collapsed, thus demonstrating language lateralization to the left cerebral hemisphere. Some hours later she became dysarthric with a right hemiplegia owing to a left subcortical infarct. She had no language impairment, either acutely or on formal follow-up evaluations carried out 2 months and 4, 5, and 8 years later. She recovered motor function but developed mild spasticity of the right upper limb and became left handed. Four years later her IQ was within the normal range (FSIQ = 102, VIQ = 103, PIQ = 101). Seven years later she developed focal aphasic seizures which were controlled with antiepileptic drugs. An EEG showed epileptic activity localized to the left frontotemporal region.

Children with normal oral language evaluations had either language cortex sparing (n = 4) or part involvement (n = 3), if we consider the temporal isthmus and the insula as part of that cortex. The two patients with lesions involving Broca's area had normal examinations.

Of the eight cases with low scores on any oral language task, none had involvement of the cortical language regions and one had a lesion of the posterior limb of the internal capsule. There was no significant association between damage to the prefrontal cortex and impairment in any verbal test, since of eight patients with frontal lobe lesions four had language impairment, and of seven patients without frontal involvement, four had language impairment.

Discussion

In this report we investigate the neuroanatomical basis of language acquisition by analyzing a series of 'negative' cases: children who suffered acquired lesions of the left cerebral hemisphere but did not became aphasic. Our aim was to contribute to defining the anatomical boundaries of the language cortex in children. Our hypothesis, based on published positive cases, was that the lesions should spare the classical language areas of the left hemisphere. If the reverse was found it would suggest either that the participation of those areas in language is not as fundamental as observed in adults, or that these children had atypical types of hemispheric specialization (either intrahemispheric or interhemispheric).

In accordance to our hypothesis, we found that in the majority of cases lesions spared the classical language areas of the left hemisphere. In none of the patients did the lesion involve Wernicke's area, a region that has been identified as essential for language acquisition (Bates et al., 1999) and recovery (Martins, 2004) in other clinical studies. Broca's area was affected in two patients, and four had subcortical involvement.

Of the two cases with Broca's area involvement, one suffered from an AVM and the other had a tumour. In both cases language could have been displaced to the right hemisphere, explaining the lack of language symptoms – as described in some adult patients with frontal AVMs (Lazar et al., 2000), or in children with tumours overlying Broca's area, although rare (De Vos et al., 1995; Thiel et al., 2005). However, in both cases there was evidence (by the amytal test in the patient with AVM, and the occurrence of postictal aphasia in the case with tumour) that language was lateralized to the left hemisphere and not the right, making that explanation unlikely. Postictal aphasia has been shown to indicate hemispheric dominance for language

(Loddenkemper & Kotagal, 2005). Therefore the more probable hypothesis for language sparing was its localization to the neighbourhood of Broca's area, as observed in series of patients with early lesions (De Vos *et al.*, 1995; Liégeois *et al.*, 2004). In addition, it is also known that the occurrence of a Broca's type of aphasia requires more extensive damage than to Broca's area alone (Mohr *et al.*, 1978).

In relation to subcortical and thalamic lesions of the left hemisphere, it has been shown that these may cause aphasia in adults and in children (Alexander *et al.*, 1987; Kirk & Kertez, 1994; Martins, 2000) depending on their exact location, extension, and the metabolic effects on the overlying cortex (Radanovic & Scaff, 2003), but they may also produce impairment on verbal tests – especially those related to frontal lobe functions – without clinical aphasia, as observed in our patients. It is not unusual for them to spare language.

The most frequently involved region in this series of patients was the anterior cingulus, the medial frontal and the dorsolateral prefrontal region, sparing Broca's area. Medial frontal lesions in adults may impair language initiation and can produce transient mutism followed by a transcortical motor aphasia, particularly if they extend to the supplementary motor area (Bogous-slavsky & Regli, 1990), but that area was spared in the present cases.

Thus our results are a mirror image of those of acquired childhood aphasia, where it has been shown that the lesion site determines the pattern of linguistic impairment. However, we also found that most cases had subtle language impairments that were not associated with clinical aphasia. Those deficits involved more complex language tasks, syntactic comprehension, sentence and digit repetition (requiring phonological memory), and confrontation naming. There was no systematic association between a particular area and any language impairment. In addition, some cases had acquired disorders of reading and writing. These findings show the effect on language of a more extensive network involving accessory areas necessary to mediate between a conceptual system and an operational language system. None of the children presented symptoms of neglect, the most common cognitive manifestation of lesions of the right hemisphere, showing they had no reverse pattern of dominance and no 'crowding effect' of any possible language reorganization (especially in chronic progressive lesions).

In conclusion, our analysis corroborates by its negative perspective the findings from acquired childhood aphasia of an early intrahemispheric organization of language. However, we must point out some limitations of the study that restrict the generalization of the results. The sample of patients was small and may have been biased, because referral to our centre is mainly for language disorders. Second, the timing of the patients' evaluation was not uniform and some patients were only evaluated formally in the chronic period, when aphasia might no longer be evident. We tried to overcome this problem by excluding patients about whom there were no data on the acute period of illness. Third, this series involved different aetiologies which may have different recovery mechanisms and be associated with different processes of functional reorganization (Anderson *et al.*, 1990). To clarify this issue a larger and more homogeneous series of patients is required, as well as a systematic study of cortical regions outside the language cortex.

Acknowledgments: I would like to thank Professor J. M. Ferro for his contribution to the analysis of lesion localization.

References

Agostini, M.D., Metz-Lutz, M.N., Van Hout, A., Chavance, M., Deloche, G., Pavão-Martins, I. & Dellatollas, G. (1998): Batterie d'évaluation du langage oral de l'enfant aphasique (ELOLA): standardization française (4–12 ans). *Rev. Neuropsychol.* **8**, 319–367.

Ahmad, Z., Balsamo, L.M., Sachs, B.C., Xu, B. & Gaillard, W.D. (2003): Auditory comprehension of language in young children: neural networks identified with fMRI. *Neurology* **60**, 1598–1605.

Alexander, M.P., Naeser, A. & Palumbo, C.L. (1987): Correlations of subcortical CT lesions sites and aphasia profiles. *Brain* **110**, 961–991.

Anderson, S.W., Damasio, H. & Tranel, D. (1990): Neuropsychological impairments associated with lesions caused by tumor or stroke. *Arch. Neurol.* **47**, 397–405.

Aram, D.M. (1988): Language sequelae of unilateral brain lesions in children. In: *Language, communication and the brain*, ed. F. Plum, pp. 171–197. New York: Raven Press.

Balsamo, L.M., Xu, B., Grandin, C.B., Petrella, J.R., Braniecki, S.H., Elliott, T.K. & Gaillard, W.D. (2002): A functional magnetic resonance imaging study of left hemisphere language dominance in children. *Arch. Neurol.* **59**, 1168–1174.

Bates, E., Vicari, S. & Trauner, D. (1999): Neural mediation of language development: perspectives from lesion studies of infants and children. In: *Neurodevelopmental disorders*, ed. H. Tager-Fluberg, pp. 533–581. Cambridge, MA: The MIT Press.

Benton, A.L., Spreen, O., Fangman, M.W. & Carr, D.L. (1967): Visual retention test. Administration C: norms for children. *J. Spec. Educ.* **1**, 151–156.

Benton, A.L., Hamsher, K.S., Varney, N.S. & Spreen, O. (1983): *Judgement of line orientation, form H. Contributions to neuropsychological assessment.* New York: Oxford University Press.

Bogousslavsky, J. & Regli, F. (1990): Anterior cerebral artery territory infarction in the Lausanne stroke registry. clinical and etiologic patterns. *Arch. Neurol.* **47**, 144–150.

Cannestra, A.F., Bookheimer, S.Y., Pouratian, N., O'Farrell, A., Sicotte, N., Martin, N.A., Becker, D., Rubino, G. & Toga, A.W. (2000): Temporal and topographical characterization of language cortices using intraoperative optical intrinsic signals. *Neuroimage* **12**, 41–54.

Carter, R.L., Hohennegger, M.K. & Satz, P. (1982): Aphasia and speech organization in children. *Science* **218**, 797–799.

Castro-Caldas, A. (1979): *Diagnóstico e evolução das afasias de causa vascular* [Tese de Doutoramento]. Lisboa: Faculdade de Medicina de Lisboa.

Chapman, S.B., Max, J.E., Gamino, J.F., McGlothlin, J.H. & Cliff, S.N. (2003): Discourse plasticity in children after stroke: age at injury and lesion effects. *Pediatr. Neurol.* **29**, 34–41.

Cranberg, L.D., Filley, C.M., Hart, E.J. & Alexander, M.P. (1987): Acquired aphasia in childhood: clinical and CT investigations. *Neurology* **37**, 1165–1172.

Dahaene-Lambertz, G., Dahene, S. & Hertz-Pannier, L. (2002): Functional neuroimaging of speech perception in infants. *Science* **289**, 213–215.

Damasio, H. (1995): *Human brain anatomy in computerized images.* Oxford: Oxford University Press.

De Renzi, E. & Vignolo L. A. (1962): The Token Test: a sensitive test to detect receptive disturbances in aphasics. *Brain* **85**, 665–678.

De Vos, K. J., Wyllie, E., Geckler, C., Kotagal, P. & Comair, Y. (1995): Language dominance in patients with early childhood tumors near left hemisphere language areas. *Neurology* **45**, 349–356.

Dronkers, N.F., Pinker, S. & Damasio, A. (2000): Language and the aphasias. In: *Principles of neural science*, 4th edition, eds. E.R. Kandel, J.H. Schwartz & T.M. Jessell, pp. 1169–1198. New York: McGraw-Hill.

Duchowny, M., Jayakar, P., Harvey, A.S., Resnick, T., Alvarez, L., Dean, P. & Levin, B. (1996): Language cortex representation: effects of developmental versus acquired pathology. *Ann. Neurol.* **40**, 31–38.

Dunn, L.M., Dunn, L.M., Whetton, C. & Pintilie, D. (1982): *British Picture Vocabulary Scale, short form.* Windsor: NFER-Nelson.

Gaillard, W., Hertz-Pannier, L., Mott, S., Barnett, A., LeBihan, D. & Theodore, W. (2000): Functional anatomy of cognitive development fMRI of verbal fluency in children and adults. *Neurology* **54**, 180–185.

Gaillard, W., Sachs, B., Whitnah, J., Ahmad, Z., Balsamo, L., Petrella, J., Braniecki, S., McKinney, C., Hunter, K., Xu B. & Grandin, C. (2003): Developmental aspects of language processing: fMRI of verbal fluency in children and adults. *Hum. Brain Mapp.* **18**, 176–185.

Goodglass, H. & Kaplan, E. (1983): *The assessment of aphasia and related disorders.* Philadelphia: Lea and Fabiger.

Holland, S., Plante, E., Byars, A., Strawsburg, R., Schmisthorst & Ball, W. (2001): Normal fMRI brain activation patterns in children performing a verb generation task. *Neuroimage* **14**, 837–843.

Hunttenlocher, P.R. & Dabholkar, A.S. (1997): Regional differences in synaptogenesis in human cerebral cortex. *J. Comp. Neurol.* **387**, 167–178.

Kirk, A. & Kertesz, A. (1994): Cortical and subcortical aphasias compared. *Aphasiology* **8**, 65–82.

Kreisler, A., Godefroy, O., Delmaire, C., Debachy, B., Leclercq, M., Pruvo, J.P. & Leys, D. (2000): The anatomy of aphasia revisited. *Neurology* **54**, 1117–1123.

Lazar, R.M., Marshall, R.S., Pile-Spellman, J., Duong, H.C., Mohr, J.P., Young, W.L., Solomon, R.L., Perera, G.M. & De La Paz, R.L. (2000): Interhemispheric transfer of language in patients with left frontal cerebral arteriovenous malformation. *Neuropsychologia* **38**, 1325–1332.

Liégeois, F., Connelly, A., Cross, J.H., Boyd, S.G., Gadian, D., Vargha-Khadem, F. & Baldweg, T. (2004): Language reorganization in children with early onset lesions of the left hemisphere: an fMRI study. *Brain* **127**, 1229–1236.

Loddenkemper, T. & Kotagal, P. (2005): Lateralizing signs during seizures in focal epilepsy. *Epilepsy Behav.* **7**, 1–17.

Marien, P., Paquier, P., Engelborghs, S. & Deyn, P.P. (2001): Acquired crossed aphasia in dextral children revisited. *Brain Lang.* **79**, 426–443.

Martins, I.P. (2000): Basal ganglia lesions, language and neuropsychological dysfunction. In: *Localization of brain lesions and developmental functions*, Mariani Foundation Paediatric Neurology Series, vol. 9, eds. D. Riva & A. Benton, pp. 57–65. Eastleigh: John Libbey.

Martins, I.P. (2004): Persistent acquired childhood aphasia. In: *Neurogenic language disorders in children*, ed. F. Fabro, pp. 231–251. Amsterdam: Elsevier.

Martins, I.P. & Ferro, J.M. (1993): Acquired childhood aphasia: a clinicoradiological study of 11 stroke patients. *Aphasiology* **7**, 489–495.

Matsui, T. & Hirano, H. (1978): *An atlas of the human brain for computerized tomography*. New York: Igaku-Shoin.

Max, J.E. (2004): Effect of side of lesion on neuropsychological performance in childhood stroke. *J. Int. Neuropsychol. Soc.* **10**, 698–708.

Mohr, J.P., Pessin, M.S., Finkelstein, S., Funkenstein, H.H., Duncan, G.W. & Davis, K.R. (1978): Broca aphasia: pathologic and clinical. *Neurology* **28**, 311–324.

Muller, R.A., Rothermel, M.D., Behen, M.E., Muzik, O., Chakraborty, P.K. & Chugani, H.T. (1999): Language organization in patients with early and late left hemisphere lesions: a PET study. *Neuropsychologia* **37**, 545–557.

Nass, R., Leventhal, F., Levine, B., Lebron, D., Maxfield, C., McCaul, P., George, A. & Allen, J. (1998): Conduction aphasia in a 3 year old with a left posterior cortical/subcortical abscess. *Brain Lang.* **62**, 70–88.

Papathanassiou, D., Etard, O., Mellet, E., Zago, L., Mazoyer, B. & Tzourio-Mazoyer, N. (2000): A common language network for comprehension and production: a contribution to the definition of language epicenters with PET. *Neuroimage* **11**, 347–357.

Paquier, P. & Van Dongen H. R. (1996): Review of research on the clinical presentation of acquired childhood aphasia. *Acta Neurol. Scand.* **93**, 428–436.

Radanovic, M. & Scaff, M. (2003): Speech and language disturbances due to subcortical lesions. *Brain Lang.* **84**, 337–352.

Rapin, I. (1995): Acquired aphasia in children. *J. Child Neurol.* **10**, 267–270.

Raven, J.C., Court, J.H. & Raven, J. (1986): *Raven's Progressive Matrices and Raven's Coloured Matrices*. London. H.K. Lewis.

Reynell, J K. (1977): *Manual for the Reynell Developmental Language Scales (Revised)*. Windsor: NFER Publishing Co.

Riva, D., Pantaleoni, C., Milani, N. & Devoti, M. (1991): Late sequelae of right versus left hemispheric lesions. In: *Acquired aphasia in children*, eds. I.P. Martins, A. Castro-Caldas, H.R. Van Dongen & A. van Hout, pp. 213–224. Dordrecht: Kluwer, Academic Publishers.

Thiel, A., Habedank, B., Winhuisen, L., Herholz, K., Kessler, J., Haupt, W.F. & Heiss, W.D. (2005): Essential language function of the right hemisphere in brain tumor patients. *Ann. Neurol.* **57**, 128–131.

Vargha-Khadem, F., O'Gorman, A.M. & Watters, G.V. (1985): Aphasia and handedness in relation to hemispheric side, age at injury and severity of cerebral lesion during childhood. *Brain* **108**, 677–696.

Vargha-Khadem, F., Watkins, K.E., Price, C.J., Ashburner, J., Alcock, K.J., Connelly, A., Frackowiak, R.S., Friston, K.J., Pembrey, M.E., Mishkin, M., Gadian, D.G. & Passingham, R.E. (1998): Neural basis of an inherited speech and language disorder. *Proc. Natl. Acad. Sci. USA* **95**, 12695–12700.

Wechsler, D. (1949): *Wechsler Intelligence Scale for Children. Manual*. New York: New York University School of Medicine.

Chapter 13

Language in Italian children with Williams syndrome

Virginia Volterra[*], Olga Capirci[*] and Arianna Bello[°]

[*] *Institute of Cognitive Sciences and Technologies-CNR, via Nomentana 56, 00161 Rome, Italy;*
[°] *Center for Research on Child Neurocognitive Diseases, University of Parma, via Volturno 39, 43100 Parma, Italy*
virginia.volterra@istc.cnr.it

Summary

Williams syndrome is a genetic disorder characterized by clinical anomalies and a special cognitive and behavioural profile. Facility for language has been claimed to be unusually advanced for the degree of mental retardation normally found.
In the first section of this chapter we summarize the early studies conducted on the linguistic abilities of Italian-speaking children with Williams syndrome compared with typically developing children. The main finding is that language in children with Williams syndrome is far from intact and does not appear, for the most part, ahead of non-verbal mental age. In the second section, we report recent studies comparing early stages of language development in children with Williams syndrome and Down syndrome. Our findings suggest that the apparent sparing of linguistic abilities of Williams syndrome children is in part an artefact of comparisons made with children with Down syndrome, whose morphosyntactic abilities are more affected in relation to their non-verbal mental age and their lexical repertoire.
In the final section we present studies actually carried out by our laboratory on the relation between gesture and speech in young and older children with Williams syndrome. Preliminary results indicate that despite their motor difficulties, children with Williams syndrome use gesture to communicate, supporting recent theories on the role of co-verbal gesturing in speech production. Taken together, the results reported show the theoretical relevance of these studies and provide useful indications for clinicians.

Introduction

Williams syndrome, sometimes also called Williams-Beuren syndrome, is a rare syndrome (incidence is estimated to be 1 in 25,000 live births) associated with a microdeletion on chromosome 7q11.23 (Ewart *et al.*, 1993; Frangiskakis *et al.*, 1996; Pérez Jurado *et al.*, 1996).

Children with Williams syndrome usually present with several severe clinical anomalies, including facial dysmorphology (elfin-like face with heavy orbital ridge, stellate iris pattern, temporal dimples, full cheeks, retroussé nose, flared nostrils, flat nasal bridge, prominent and wide mouth, and irregular dentition), and abnormalities of the cardiovascular, renal, musculoskeletal, endocrine, and other organ systems. Williams syndrome children also suffer from hyperacusis – an unusual sensitivity to certain environmental sounds (Klein *et al.*, 1990; Miani *et al.*, 2001). Mental retardation (ranging from mild to severe) together with facial dysmorphology are the most common features of Williams syndrome.

Williams syndrome has received special attention for the particular cognitive and linguistic profile that has been described by some investigators. Older children and adolescents with Williams syndrome were described as showing unusual linguistic abilities despite their poor performance in various visuospatial tasks. A facility for language is rarely observed in other populations with the same degree of mental retardation. For this reason, it has been suggested that Williams syndrome may provide evidence for the independence of language from cognition (Maratsos & Matheny, 1994; Pinker, 1994 and 1999 for discussion). The hypothesized dissociation between language and non-verbal cognition seemed to emerge most clearly when the performance of children with Williams syndrome was compared with that of children with Down syndrome on the same verbal and non-verbal tasks (Bellugi & St. George, 2001, for a review).

In the last 10 years, our laboratory at CNR (Institute of Psychology, now Institute of Cognitive Sciences and Technologies), in collaboration with the Children's Hospital Bambino Gesù (Department of Neurology and Rehabilitation at Santa Marinella), has conducted various studies on language in children with Williams syndrome. In this chapter we briefly review these studies from a chronological perspective and with a focus on the more recent studies.

Review of early studies on language in Italian children with Williams syndrome

In our first study (Volterra *et al.*, 1996), the linguistic abilities of Italian children with Williams syndrome were investigated. We explored the lexical and morphosyntactic abilities in 17 individuals with Williams syndrome aged between 4.10 and 15.3 years. The mean mental age of these individuals with Williams syndrome was 5.2 years (range 3.8 to 6.8), reflecting a mean IQ of 56 (range 38 to 90). In all the relevant language measures, children with Williams syndrome were compared with a sample of 116 typically developing children whose chronological age corresponded to the mental age range of the children with Williams syndrome. The language measures that were used included both lexical and grammatical measures. Comprehension was evaluated by the Peabody Picture Vocabulary Test (PPVT) and the Test for Reception of Grammar (TROG). Production was evaluated by the Boston Naming Test (BNT), the Category Test for Semantic Fluency (WF category), the Phonological Fluency Test (WF phonology), the Sentence Repetition Test (SRT), and three story description tasks.

Results of the comparison showed that the two groups did not differ on the PPVT for lexical comprehension, on the WF category for semantic fluency, or on mean length of utterance (MLU) calculated from the story descriptions. However, individuals with Williams syndrome did obtain significantly poorer results than normal controls on the TROG, the BNT, and the SRT; in contrast, they performed significantly better than controls on the WF phonology.

Our main conclusion was that the language produced by individuals with Williams syndrome in this age range was for the most part not ahead of their mental age, and that our data offered very little evidence for a dissociation between language and cognition. Furthermore, the language produced by children with Williams syndrome was unusual from several points of view. By investigating language development in such children when exposed to Italian, we were able to see certain patterns that would be difficult to detect in English. In particular, our children with Williams syndrome produced some grammatical errors that were qualitatively different from anything that has usually been reported for typically developing children acquiring Italian, including errors of gender agreement and verb conjugation, and substitutions of prepositions and function words. We also found word order inversions that have rarely been reported for children acquiring Italian or English.

To explore whether these qualitative deviations were determined by a different rate of language acquisition, we conducted a detailed longitudinal study of the first stages of cognitive and linguistic development of an Italian girl with Williams syndrome, followed through weekly observations from 18 months to 58 months of age and systematically tested every 2 months (Capirci *et al.*, 1996). The results of the study confirmed a delayed and partially atypical profile of language development in children and adolescents with Williams syndrome. Despite an initial delay which appeared less marked than is usually reported for children with this syndrome, Elisa's rate and sequence of development seemed to be similar to those observed in control children. However, in contrast to children with typical development, she displayed an uneven pattern of within-domain dissociations. She showed fluent vocabulary and proficient use of syntax, at least in some contexts, but failed with simple grammatical agreement. Thus she made several kinds of grammatical errors (gender agreement between article and noun and pronominalization) that are rarely made by children at the same syntactic level.

In a subsequent paper we explored the question of variability in performance between individuals within the group with Williams syndrome. Comparing Italian children and adolescents with Williams syndrome with a group of younger typically developing children on the same visuo-spatial and linguistic tasks, our results suggested that children with Williams syndrome do not have a single cognitive profile. Instead, considerable variability across individuals with Williams syndrome was found. In the four individual cases we examined in detail, each of the children showed a different pattern of sparing and impairment on the linguistic and visual-spatial tasks. However, in all four cases a particular difficulty in visuo-motor construction test was recognized (Pezzini *et al.*, 1999).

In another study reporting a case of dizygotic twins, one boy with Williams syndrome and one typically developing girl, our goal was to verify whether the child with Williams syndrome had a cognitive profile unique to the syndrome (Volterra *et al.*, 1999). This special case gave us a unique opportunity to compare in more detail the neuropsychological profile of a child with Williams syndrome with that of a normal control, matched for age and family background. Several tests designed to assess visuo-perceptual, visuo-motor, linguistic, and memory abilities were administered to both children when they were aged 10 years 9 months. Compared with his sister, the boy with Williams syndrome showed a developmental delay in many non-verbal and verbal abilities. He achieved a level of performance similar to his sister only in facial recognition, phonological word fluency, and memory for phonologically similar words. However, despite the overall delayed performance of the boy, both twins displayed a cognitive profile characterized by strength in lexical comprehension and relative weakness in visuomotor abilities.

In a more recent study (Volterra *et al.*, 2001), two distinct lines of investigation were presented: linguistic competence in the written language of deaf children and adults, and linguistic development in children and adolescents with Williams syndrome. Italian deaf people have selective difficulties in aspects of grammatical morphology that play a syntactic rather than a semantic function. Italian people with Williams syndrome displayed a particular asymmetric fragmentation within linguistic abilities: a profile of strength in phonological abilities, but serious deficits in semantic and morphosyntactic aspects of language. These two very different populations provided us with important clues for investigating which aspects of language, and specifically of grammar, are influenced by modality of perception.

Review of recent studies on language in Italian children with Williams syndrome

From the above section, it is clear that our first studies were conducted on subjects with Williams syndrome compared with typically developing children, whose chronological age corresponded to the mental age of children with Williams syndrome. Their linguistic performance was never directly compared on the same tasks with that of children with genetic syndromes of different aetiology, and mental retardation. In the present section, we will summarize two recent studies directly comparing Italian-speaking children with Williams syndrome and Italian-speaking children with Down syndrome of comparable global cognitive level (Vicari *et al.*, 2002; Volterra *et al.*, 2003).

Children with Down syndrome usually show impairment in language acquisition – although there are rare exceptions (Vallar & Papagno, 1993; Rondal, 1995). Problems in morphology and syntax are frequently reported (Fowler, 1990; Miller, 1992; Chapman, 1995; Fowler, 1995; Shaner-Wolles, 2000). Various studies conducted on Italian children with Down syndrome by our laboratory, in collaboration with the Children's Hospital Bambino Gesù, have confirmed these findings (Caselli *et al.*, 1997; Fabbretti *et al.*, 1997; Caselli *et al.*, 1998; Iverson *et al.*, 2003).

The goal of our first comparative study (Vicari *et al.*, 2002) was to gather more detailed data on language acquisition in Italian-speaking children with Williams syndrome and in children with Down syndrome of comparable global cognitive level (that is, matched for chronological and mental age) and in typically developing children matched for mental age. In particular, we wished to investigate whether infants with Williams syndrome are as proficient in language processing during infancy as they are reported to be in adolescence and adult life. Another aim of the study was to explore whether language development in atypical populations is merely delayed, in comparison with the developmental stages followed by typically developing children, or whether it follows a different developmental trajectory.

The sample consisted of 12 children with Williams syndrome (chronological age 58.2 months; mental age 34 months) matched on the basis of mental age with a group of 12 children with Down syndrome (chronological age 67.2 months; mental age 32.2 months) and a group of 12 typically developing children (chronological age 29.7 months; mental age 30 months). In all three groups, mental age was assessed using the Brunet-Lezine scale or the Leiter intelligence performance scale. The Primo Vocabolario del Bambino (PVB) questionnaire – the Italian version of the Bates MacArthur Communicative Development Inventory – was adopted for assessing lexical and grammatical competence. The Words and Sentences Form used consists of a section on vocabulary production (670 words) and a section on grammatical complexity (37 pairs of sentences). Typically developing children produced an average of 488 different words (SD±116.4), while children with Williams syndrome and Down syndrome produced an average of 452±157.3 and 457±125.4 different words, respectively. There was no significant difference between the three groups of children. Differences emerged when the performances of the three groups were considered in the section of the questionnaire referring to grammatical complexity. The three groups of children, with equivalent vocabularies, differed in the type of sentences used. Children with Down syndrome used more simple and telegraphic sentences (mean 14.9±11.8) than typically developing controls (3.2±3.5). Children with Williams syndrome used a smaller number of telegraphic sentences than children with Down syndrome, but a larger number than typically developing controls (7.6±9.7). Typically developing children produced more complete sentences (28.8±8.1) than children with Williams syndrome (21.9±13.4) or Down syndrome (13.1±10.4).

Comprehension was assessed by a verbal comprehension test (VCT) which explores children's ability to understand increasingly complex phrases. Specifically, the child was asked to perform a requested action correctly. Children with Down syndrome scored lower (mean 29.9±4.7) than typically developing controls (33.7±1.6) or children with Williams syndrome (31.9±2.4).

Samples of spontaneous production (about 20 minutes per child) were collected and videotaped. In order to compute the mean length of the utterance in words (MLU-w), the spontaneous conversation of each child was orthographically transcribed. Computation of MLU-w in the three groups showed that children with Williams syndrome had a significantly longer utterance length in their spontaneous production (mean 3.1±0.8) than children with Down syndrome (2.4±0.5). Typically developing controls (2.9±0.7) did not differ statistically from Williams syndrome ($F_{(1,31)} = 0.7$) or from Down syndrome individuals. These results for MLU-w are in agreement with results for the grammatical complexity scale on the PVB, relative to the proportion between telegraphic/incomplete and complete sentences.

A phrase repetition test was used to ascertain the children's ability to imitate verbal stimuli, particularly phrases and sentences of different lengths. The evaluation consisted of the total number of phrases repeated correctly out of the total number of phrases repeated. Children with Down syndrome repeated a smaller number of phrases more accurately (mean 23.6±18.6) than the typically developing controls group (57.1±19.9) or the children with Williams syndrome (54.01±32.8). No difference was found between Williams syndrome and typically developing controls.

In a second study (Volterra et al., 2003) we concentrated our attention on a qualitative analysis of linguistic repetitions of a small number of young children with Williams syndrome, comparing their performance with that of children with Down syndrome and typically developing children. The sample consisted of six children with Williams syndrome, who were individually matched on the basis of chronological and mental age and productive vocabulary size to six children with Down syndrome, and six typically developing children matched on the basis of mental age and vocabulary size. We conducted a detailed analysis of their performance in the phrase repetition test, evaluating the total number of phrases repeated correctly out of the total number of phrases repeated, the total number of errors, and the type of error produced (omission, lexical substitution, error of bound morphology, addition of new elements, word order inversions). The children with Down syndrome repeated fewer sentences (mean 36.5) than the children with Williams syndrome and the typically developing children (47.5 and 41.0, respectively). More evident was the difference in the mean of correct sentences repeated by children with Down syndrome (mean 10) and by the other two groups (28.7 for the children with Williams syndrome and 25.3 for the typically developing children). Sentences correctly repeated, but in which one or more words were added, were counted as correct sentences. Sentences with additions were produced by the children with Williams syndrome and were very rarely observed in the other two groups. The total number of additions for children with Williams syndrome was 44 (25 final additions and 19 local additions), only 4 and 3 for children with Down syndrome and typically developing children, respectively. Examples of additions produced by children with Williams syndrome were: target sentence 'Il bimbo va a casa' (the child goes home) was repeated with a local addition as 'Il bimbo va a guardare la casa' (the child goes to look the house); target sentence 'Il topo' (the mouse) was repeated as 'Il topo mangia il formaggio' (the mouse eats the cheese).

Finally, we considered the total number of errors produced by the children, counting the following: each element omitted or substituted (the child repeated the target sentence omitting or substituting one or more elements – article, name, verb, preposition, and so on – in the sentence repeated); each morphological modification of a word (the child used a different morphological form of the same word in the repeated sentence – a singular form instead of a plural one, a feminine instead of a masculine form, and so on); each repetition with word order inversion (a different order of one or more elements in the sentence repeated). The mean number of errors produced was very similar for children with Williams syndrome and typically developing children. The mean number of errors produced by children with Down syndrome was almost twice that produced by children with Williams syndrome and typically developing children.

In order to analyse in more detail the types of errors produced from a qualitative perspective, the proportions of the different types of error produced by the three groups of children were examined. Omissions were proportionally the most frequent error produced by all groups of children. In the children with Williams syndrome, the percentage of omissions was lower (71 per cent) compared with both children with Down syndrome (87 per cent) and typically developing children (87 per cent). Errors in bound morphology were present in an appreciable proportion both in children with Williams syndrome and in those with Down syndrome (10 per cent and 4 per cent, respectively), but they were almost absent in the typically developing children (0.5 per cent). Only children with Williams syndrome and Down syndrome produced sentences with incorrect agreement between article and noun (for example, target sentence 'I cani' (the dog) was repeated as 'Le cani' – feminine plural article 'le' instead of masculine plural article 'i').

Lexical substitutions were proportionally produced more frequently by children with Williams syndrome (15 per cent) than by children with Down syndrome (7 per cent) and by typically developing children (4 per cent). Lexical substitutions produced by typically developing children were on nouns, while lexical substitutions produced by children with Williams syndrome and Down syndrome were also on articles, prepositions, and verbs. Finally, word order inversions were produced in a higher proportion by typically developing children (8 per cent), in an appreciable percentage by Williams syndrome children (4 per cent), and in a smaller proportion by Down syndrome children (2 per cent). All the word order inversions produced were at the sentence level (not noun-phrase internal); only children with Williams syndrome and Down syndrome produced sentences in which the order inversion generated semantically or grammatically unacceptable sentences (for example, target sentence 'Maria mette la bambola a letto' (Maria puts the doll to bed) was repeated as 'Maria mette il letto a bambola' (Maria puts the bed to doll).

Gestures and words in children with Williams syndrome

While we have devoted many years to the study of the relation between language and gesture in typically developing children, deaf children, and children exposed to a signed input, we are only beginning to study the nature and development of gesture in children with atypical patterns of language and cognitive development.

Relatively few studies have examined the relation between gesture and developing language in children with Williams syndrome, and such studies have often focused on a limited set of gestures. It has been reported that children with Williams syndrome have a delay in starting to produce gestures (Bertrand et al., 1998), and that they show a limited use of gestures with either a declarative or an instrumental function (Laing et al., 2002).

A study conducted by Capirci and collaborators (Capirci *et al.*, 2001) aimed to clarify similarities and differences in the use of gestures and words by typically developing children and children with Williams syndrome and Down syndrome. Three preschool children with Williams syndrome (chronological age range 39 to 51 months; mental age range 26 to 36 months) were individually matched with three children with Down syndrome (chronological age range 36 to 50 months; mental age range 26 to 39 months) and with three typically developing children matched for mental age (chronological age range 24 to 34 months; mental age range 25 to 37 months). All nine children examined had already reached the two-word stage. The children were observed at home, in 40-minute free play interactions with their mothers (20 minutes), and with an unfamiliar adult (20 minutes). All interactions were videotaped and all of the children's verbal and gestural communicative productions were fully transcribed and analysed as described below. The children's utterances were categorized in three major classes: (1) vocal only (utterances consisting only of spoken words); (2) gestural only (utterances consisting only of gestures); and (3) mixed, or vocal-gestural utterances (consisting of speech accompanied by gestures). The children's gestures were classified as follows:

- pointing gestures;
- conventional gestures: hands or body movements, or both, that are known to be used within Italian culture and are associated with stable meaning (for example, rotating the index finger on the cheek for GOOD);
- iconic gestures: hands and body movement referring to objects, people, places, or events by some idiosyncratic representation of their form or function (for example, flapping the hands for BIRDIE, or raising the arms high for TALL);
- beats: gestures without a clear and stable meaning that serve to highlight or emphasize aspects of discourse structure or the content of accompanying speech (comparable to those that in Iverson *et al.*'s 1999 study were classified as 'emphatic' gestures).

Mixed utterances were further coded according to the information conveyed by the gestural elements, and were distinguished into three major types: *reinforcing* (for example, waving the hand in the gesture meaning 'hello' while saying 'hello'); *disambiguative* (for example, pointing to a ball while saying 'this one is mine'); *additive* (for example, waving the hand in the gesture meaning 'hello' while saying 'mommy').

The results showed that all the children observed produced a greater amount of vocal than gestured utterances. However, the children with Down syndrome produced more utterances containing gestures than the children in the other two groups. With respect to the type of gestures produced, it was found that almost all the children produced pointing more than other gestures. However, children with Down syndrome produced more iconic gestures than children with Williams syndrome and typically developing children. The information conveyed by gestures in the utterances produced by the two groups of children with genetic syndromes was on the whole comparable to that observed in typically developing children: gestures were used mainly to reinforce the meaning of verbal utterances, even though gestures with 'disambiguative' and 'additive' functions were also observed. Children with Williams syndrome thus appeared to be similar to typically developing children with respect to the frequency, type, and function of gestures produced, and this result does not support the indications provided by previous studies on a more limited use of gestures by children with Williams syndrome. In contrast, children with Down syndrome produced more and different types of gestures compared with both the Williams syndrome group and the typically developing children. This is in agreement with earlier indications of a possible enhancement of gestural communication in children with Down syndrome, as provided by the studies of Caselli *et al.* (1998) and Singer-Harris *et al.* (1997), and as often reported by clinicians (Abrahamsen, 2000).

A very recent study conducted in our laboratory focused on the role of gestures in older children with Williams syndrome (Bello et al., 2004). This study investigated lexical organization and lexical retrieval in children with Williams syndrome by examining both naming accuracy and the use of accompanying gestures in a picture naming task such as the BNT. This test consists of 60 line drawings representing different objects that children are requested to name. Ten children with Williams syndrome (mean chronological age 10 years, 11 months; mean mental age 5 years, 11 months) were given the test. These children's performance, and their use of gestures during the task, were compared with those of two distinct groups of typically developing children: 10 matched for chronological age (mean chronological age 10 years, 8 months) and 10 matched by mental age (mean mental age 6 years). It was found that the overall naming accuracy of children with Williams syndrome was compatible with their mental age. However, compared with both their mental age-matched and chronological age-matched typically developing children, the children with Williams syndrome showed a greater overall rate of gesture production, a richer gestural repertoire than typically developing children, and used a significantly larger number of iconic gestures. The majority of iconic gestures noted in all children (Williams syndrome and typically developing alike) appeared to represent the function rather than the form of the object depicted (for example, a child produced a gesture meaning 'brush' moving the extended index finger in the air, as though mimicking the movement of a painting brush). There were few cases of iconic gestures reproducing the form of the represented object (such as, for 'globe' a child traced a circle in the air with the index finger). In all three groups of children, iconic gestures tended to co-occur with circumlocutions. Analysis of these circumlocutions and of the gestures co-occurring with them indicated that, when the children could not provide the name for an object, they sought the word in the appropriate semantic space, and this appeared to be at least partially expressed or codified in the gesture produced. This result seems to confirm McNeill's hypothesis (McNeill, 2000), according to which the gesture often does not map neatly into a single word but has some unique semiotic properties, in particular 'the synthetic property'.

The use of gesture during attempts at lexical retrieval does not necessarily mean that gestures help in lexical retrieval, but rather that gestures produced during circumlocution reflect activation of a conceptual space that words and gestures share, as well as activation of the motor programmes (visual-manual as well as acoustic-articulatory) associated with the objects and events represented in this shared conceptual-semantic space.

Conclusions

Studies conducted by our laboratory have shown that children with Williams syndrome have, in the presence of well preserved phonological processes, slightly impaired lexical-semantic and morphosyntactic abilities, challenging the popular view that such children show a peculiar and marked dissociation between relatively preserved linguistic abilities and visuo-spatial deficits. A complex pattern of spared and impaired functions, both in the linguistic and the visuo-spatial domains, is the emerging picture for the mental architecture of children with Williams syndrome, replacing the previous interpretation of a dichotomy between language and visuo-spatial abilities (Karmiloff-Smith et al., 1997).

Recent studies conducted with younger children confirm and extend previous findings in older children and adolescents with Williams syndrome. They confirm that linguistic ability is not ahead of mental age in the Williams population in this early age range, in accordance with a revised view of Williams syndrome that has already been suggested by research within the older age range explored in previous studies (Volterra et al., 1996). Our data further suggest that the apparent sparing of linguistic abilities in Williams syndrome children is in part an artefact of comparisons made with children with Down syndrome, whose morphosyntactic abilities are more compromised in comparison to their non-verbal mental age and to their lexical repertoire. Children with Williams syndrome do not speak like their normally developing peers at the same chronological age; their expressive lexical repertoire and use of sentences resemble those of younger typically developing children at a comparable level of non-verbal abilities. In addition, they often produce – as do children with Down syndrome – sentences that are unacceptable semantically or pragmatically, and are very rarely produced by typically developing children. Thus these differences compared with typically developing children could be related to cognitive impairment and not to a specific syndrome.

Nevertheless, there are intriguing qualitative differences between the groups at a more detailed level, including a tendency for children with Williams syndrome to produce errors that are rarely observed in children with Down syndrome or in typically developing children at any age. In particular, children with Williams syndrome have a tendency to add material not present in the model. In many cases, the material added was not consistent with the picture shown at that time, but was present in a target sentence presented previously. In the case of children with Williams syndrome, their spared ability to hear and store speech sounds may allow them to acquire some aspects of language that are especially difficult for children with Down syndrome, but this ability is not enough to guarantee productive control over all semantic and grammatical aspects of language.

Regarding the use of gesture, we note that the tight relation between language and gesture and the intricate relation between gesture and lexical retrieval reported above, especially for children with Williams syndrome, are all compatible with recent discoveries on the shared neural substrates of language and gesture. Specifically, Rizzolatti and colleagues (1996) have shown that hand and mouth representations overlap in a broad frontal-parietal network that they have called the 'mirror neuron system,' activated during both perception and production of familiar and meaningful manual gestures and mouth movements.

The main hypothesis underlying much current work on the interplay between gesture and speech is that there is a continuity between an earlier 'preverbal' and a subsequent, somehow functionally 'equivalent' linguistic form, and that the use of gesture is a robust developmental phenomenon, with similar features across different children and cultures. The output systems of speech and gesture may draw on underlying brain mechanisms common to both language and motor functions (Iverson & Thelen, 1999). Within this broad framework, evidence on children with atypical patterns of language and cognitive development, such as those with Williams syndrome, may be particularly relevant in assessing the resilience of gesture as a developmental phenomenon. In addition, such findings could be extremely relevant in clinical practice for the implementation of new intervention programmes in which motor, gestural, and linguistic abilities are considered as a whole.

Acknowledgments: Some of the research reported in this chapter on older children was funded by FIRB/MIUR (grant RBNE01SZB4), some of the research on younger children was part of the European Science Foundation EUROCORES Programme OMLL, supported by funds from the CNR and the EC Sixth Framework Programme under Contract no. ERAS-CT-2003-980409.

Some portions of this chapter have been published in Volterra, V., Capirci, O., Caselli, M.C. & Vicari, S. (2004): Language in preschool Italian children with Williams and Down syndromes. In: *Williams syndrome across languages*, eds. S. Bartke & J. Siegmueller, pp. 163–185. Amsterdam: John Benjamins Publishing Company.

References

Abrahamsen, A. (2000): Explorations of enhanced gestural input to children in the bimodal period. In: *The signs of language revisited: an antology to honor Ursula Bellugi and Edward Klima*, eds. K. Emmorey & H. Lane, pp. 357–399. Mahwak: Erlbaum.

Bello, A., Capirci, O. & Volterra, V. (2004): Lexical production in children with Williams syndrome: spontaneous use of gesture in a naming task. *Neuropsychologia* **42**, 201–213.

Bellugi, U. & St. George, M., ed. (2001): *Journey from cognition to brain to gene. Perspectives from Williams syndrome*. Cambridge MA: MIT Press.

Bertrand, J., Mervis, C.B. & Neustat, I. (1998): Communicative gesture use by preschoolers with Williams syndrome: a longitudinal study. Paper presented at the *International Conference of Infant Studies*. Atlanta, USA.

Capirci, O., Sabbadini, L. & Volterra, V. (1996): Language development in Williams syndrome: a case study. *Cogn. Neuropsychol.* **13**, 1017–1039.

Capirci, O., Iverson, J.M., Pirchio, S., Spampinato, K. & Volterra, V. (2001): Speech and gesture in discourse produced by children with Williams syndrome and children with Down syndrome. 10th European Conference on Developmental Psychology, Uppsala University, Sweden.

Caselli, M.C., Longobardi, E. & Pisaneschi, R. (1997). Gesti e parole in bambini con sindrome di Down. *Psicologia Clinica e dello Sviluppo* **1**, 45–63.

Caselli, M.C., Vicari, S., Longobardi, E., Lami, L., Pizzoli, C. & Stella, G. (1998): Gestures and words in early development of children with Down syndrome. *J. Speech Lang. Hear. Res.* **41**, 1125–1135.

Chapman, R.S. (1995): Language development in children and adolescents with Down syndrome. In: *The handbook of child language*, eds. P. Fletcher & B. MacWinney, pp. 641–663. Oxford: Blackwell.

Ewart, A.K., Morris, C.A., Atkinson, D., Jin, W., Sternes, H., Spallone, P., Stock, A.D., Leppert, M. & Keating, M.T. (1993): Hemizygosity at the elastin in a developmental disorder, William syndrome. *Nat. Genet.* **5**, 11–16.

Fabbretti, D., Pizzuto, E., Vicari, S. & Volterra, V. (1997): A story description task with Down syndrome: lexical and morphosyntactic abilities. *J. Intellect. Disabil. Res.* **41**, 165–179.

Fowler, A.E. (1990): Language abilities in children with Down syndrome: evidence for a specific delay. In: *Children with Down syndrome: a developmental perspective*, eds. D. Cicchetti & M. Beeghley. Cambridge, UK: Cambridge University Press.

Fowler, A.E. (1995): Language variability in persons with Down syndrome. In: *Down syndrome: living and learning in the community*, eds. L. Nadel & D. Rosenthal. New York: Wiley-Liss.

Frangiskakis, J.M., Ewart, A.K., Morris, C.A., Mervis, C.B., Bertrand, J., Robinson, B.F., Klein, B.P., Ensing, G.J., Everett, L.A., Green, E.D., Pröschel, C., Gutowski, N.J., Noble, M., Atkinson, D.L., Odelberg, S.J. & Kating, M.T. (1996): LIM-kinase 1 hemizygosity implicated in impaired visuo-spatial constructive cognition. *Cell* **86**, 59–69.

Iverson, J.M. & Thelen, E. (1999): Hand, mouth and brain. The dynamic emergence of speech and gesture. *J. Consc. Stud.* **6**, 19–40.

Iverson, J.M., Longobardi, E. & Caselli, M.C. (2003): The relationship between gestures and words in children with Down syndrome and typically-developing children in the early stages of communicative development. *Int. J. Lang. Commun. Disord.* **38**, 179–197.

Karmiloff-Smith, A., Grant, J., Berthoud, I., Davies, M., Howlin, P. & Udwin, O. (1997): Language and Williams syndrome: how intact is 'intact'? *Child Dev.* **68**, 246–262.

Klein, A.J., Armstrong, B.L., Gree, M. K. & Brown, F.R. (1990): Hyperacusis and otitis media in individuals with Williams syndrome. *J. Speech Hear. Disord.* **55**, 339–344.

Laing, E., Butterworth, G., Ansari, D., Gsodl, M., Longhi, E., Paterson, S. & Karmiloff-Smith, A. (2002): Atypical development of language and social communication in toddlers with Williams syndrome. *Dev. Sci.* **5**, 233–246.

Maratsos, M. & Matheny, L. (1994): Language specificity and elasticity: brain and clinical syndrome studies. *Annu. Rev. Psychol.* **45**, 487–516.

Miani, C., Passon, P., Bracale, A.M., Barotti, A. & Panzolli, N. (2001): Treatment of hyperacusis in Williams syndrome with bilateral conductive hearing loss. *Eur. Arch. Otorhinolaryngol.* **258**, 314–344.

McNeill, D. (2000): *Language and gesture*. New York: Cambridge University Press.

Miller, J.F. (1992): Development of speech and language in children with Down syndrome. In: *Clinical care for persons with Down syndrome*, eds. J.Y. Lott & E.E. McLoy, pp. 39–50. Cambridge, MA: MIT Press.

Pérez Jurado, L.A., Peoples, R., Kaplan, P., Hamel, B. & Francke, U. (1996): Molecular definition of the chromosome 7 in Williams syndrome end parent of origin on growth. *Am. J. Hum. Genet.* **59**, 781–792.

Pezzini, G., Vicari, S., Volterra, V., Milani, L. & Ossella, M.T. (1999): Children with Williams Syndrome: is there a single neuropsychological profile? *Dev. Neuropsychol.* **15**, 141–155.

Pinker, S. (1994): *The language instinct: how the mind creates language.* New York: William Morrow.

Pinker, S. (1999). *Words and rules.* London: Weidenfeld & Nicholson.

Rondal, J.A. (1995). *Exceptional language development in Down syndrome.* Cambridge, UK: Cambridge University Press.

Rizzolatti, G., Fadiga, L., Gallese, V. & Fogassi, L. (1996): Premotor cortex and the recognition of motor actions. *Cogn. Brain Res.* **3**, 131–141.

Shaner-Wolles, C. (2000): Within-language dissociations in mental retardation: Williams-Beuren and Down Syndrome. In: *BUCLD 24*: *Proceedings of the 24th annual Boston University Conference on Language Development*, eds. S.C. Howell, S.A. Fish & T. Keith-Lucas, vol. 2, pp. 633–644. Somerville, MA: Cascadilla Press.

Singer Harris, N., Bellugi, U., Bates, E., Jones, W. & Rossen, M. (1997): Contrasting profiles of language development in children with Williams and Down syndromes. *Dev. Neuropsychol.* **13**, 345–370.

Vallar, G. & Papagno, C. (1993): Preserved vocabulary acquisition in Down syndrome children: the role of phonological short-term memory. *Cortex* **29**, 467–483.

Vicari, S, Caselli, M.C., Gagliardi, C., Tonucci, F. & Volterra, V. (2002): Language acquisition in special populations: a comparison between Down and Williams syndromes. *Neuropsychologia* **40**, 2461–2470.

Volterra, V., Capirci, O., Pezzini, G., Sabbadini, L. & Vicari, S. (1996): Linguistic abilities in Italian children with Williams syndrome. *Cortex* **32**, 663–677.

Volterra, V., Longobardi, E., Pezzini, G., Vicari, S. & Antenore, C. (1999): Visuo-spatial and linguistic abilities in a twin with Williams Syndrome. *J. Intellect. Disabil. Res.* **43**, 294–305.

Volterra, V., Capirci, O. & Caselli M.C. (2001): What atypical populations can reveal about language development: the contrast between deafness and Williams syndrome. *Lang. Cogn. Process.* **16**, 19–239.

Volterra, V., Caselli, M.C., Capirci, O., Tonucci, F. & Vicari, S. (2003): Early linguistic abilities of Italian children with Williams syndrome. *Dev. Neuropsychol.* **23**, 33–58.

Chapter 14

Verbal and non-verbal communication disorders in children with bilateral perisylvian polymicrogyria

Veronica Saletti, Sara Bulgheroni and Daria Riva

Developmental Neurology Division, National Neurologic Institute 'C.Besta', via Celoria 11, 20133 Milan, Italy
driva@istituto-besta.it

Summary

The bilateral perisylvian polymicrogyria (BPP) is a relative common malformation of cortical development, frequently associated with pseudobulbar palsy and subsequent severe dysarthria or anarthria, epilepsy and variable degree of mental retardation.
A clinical and radiological variability of BPP has been widely reported.
Neurocognitive functions of patients with BPP have been little studied, probably because severe dysarthria or anarthria and mental retardation are major obstacles to assessment. The main neuropsychological information available often concerns the intelligence quotient (IQ), which is reportedly slightly lower than normal in the majority of cases, and related to the extent of the cortical malformation. Recently poor expressive and receptive language skills have been described and related to a specific dysfunction of perisylvian language regions and not just to the global cognitive deficits or to the oromotor defect resulting from the severity of the pseudobulbar palsy.
In this chapter, after a brief summary of the few published cognitive studies conducted on subjects affected by BPP, we present our preliminary data of a study of six children of age 7 years 9 months to 12 years 4 months, with BPP of variable extent on MRI.
We investigated intelligence, receptive and expressive language skills. In addition, and in view of the recent findings of a close relationship between word and gesture, we also examined praxic abilities and communicative use of gesture.
Our results were consistent with previous studies on cognitive function in BPP patients. Furthermore we found that the lack of verbal language was not compensated by the spontaneous use of symbolic gesture, and ideomotor (*i.e.* symbolic-communicative) praxis was more disorganized than ideative praxis. In the final section we discuss the theoretical and clinical importance of these findings that reinforce the close relation between word and gesture.

Polymicrogyria

Polymicrogyria is a malformation of cortical development in which the brain surface is irregular and the normal gyral pattern is replaced by an excessive number of small, partly fused gyri separated by shallow sulci (Friede, 1989; Barth, 1987; Jansen & Andermann, 2005).

The term polymicrogyria thus refers to the macroscopic appearance of the dysplastic cortex, which is also characterized by an anomalous arrangement of the cortical cell layers. Microscopically, two types of polymicrogyria are recognized: unlayered type and four-layered type.

In unlayered polymicrogyria, which is presumably the result of an early disruption of normal neuron migration (from 6–7 weeks to 20–24), the external molecular layer is continuous and fails to follow the profile of the circumvolutions, and the underlying neurons have a radial or vertical distribution but no laminar organization. The simplified, 4-layered polymicrogyria may be the outcome of a late disorder of neuron migration, or of a disruption of cortical organization (from week 16 into postnatal life). The two types of polymicrogyria may occur together in contiguous cortical areas, indicating that they form a continuum rather than distinct malformations (Barth, 1987; Robain, 1996; Jansen & Andermann, 2005).

For a long time, polymicrogyria was believed to be an exclusively acquired condition due to foetal cerebral ischaemia (placental perfusion failure or twin-twin transfusion) or viral infections such as intrauterine cytomegalovirus (CMV) infection (Barkovich *et al.*, 1995; Barkovich & Lindan, 1994; Sugama & Kusano, 1994). Pre- and peri-natal ischaemic risk factors are not always found in the history of subjects suffering from polymicrogyria, however, and the distribution of the malformation does not always coincide with the vascularization territories or the boundaries of the main cerebral arteries (Guerrini *et al.*, 2000). There is now an increasing body of evidence that genetic factors are involved in its pathogenesis. The association of polymicrogyria with several genetically determined syndromes, *e.g.* Zellweger, Aicardi, and Walker-Warburg syndrome, the finding of polymicrogyria in patients with chromosomal abnormalities, and the occurrence of familial cases of polymicrogyria all strongly support a genetic component in its development (Jansen & Andermann, 2005). Studies to delineate the genetic basis of the polymicrogyria have just begun during the past few years. A gene whose mutation is responsible for a polymicrogyria syndrome has recently been identified: this is the *GPR56* gene, which is essential to human cerebral cortex development and patterning (Piao *et al.*, 2004). Analyzing the pattern of this gene's expression suggests that polymicrogyria may be the result of mutations in genes involved in the regional patterning of the cerebral cortex in early stages of development. These findings imply that polymicrogyria is the end-point of different aetiological processes, not necessarily occurring at the same time in cortical development (Jansen & Andermann, 2005).

The incidence of polymicrogyria is not known. The difficulty in obtaining accurate data on its incidence and prevalence derives largely from its clinical and aetiological heterogeneity. Advances in imaging studies have improved the diagnosis and classification of this condition, which now appears to be relatively common (Jansen & Andermann, 2005).

The diagnosis of polymicrogyria can derive from the detection of an irregularity of the cortex/white-matter junction on thin-section magnetic resonance imaging (MRI) (Raybaud *et al.*, 1996). In some patients, the polymicrogyric cortex appears thicker and in others thinner than normal on T2-weighted images: this is probably the result of myelination in subcortical and intracortical fibers (Takanashi & Barkovich, 2003).

Polymicrogyria may be focal or diffuse, unilateral or bilateral. The extent of polymicrogyria varies from focal polymicrogyria in an otherwise normal brain, to diffuse polymicrogyria with associated multiple brain abnormalities. The topographical distribution of polymicrogyria does not always appear to be completely random. Several distinct region-specific patterns of bilateral polymicrogyria have been described, including frontal, frontoparietal, perisylvian, lateral parietal, parasagittal parieto-occipital, and generalized polymicrogyria; unilateral polymicrogyria has also been reported (Barkovich et al., 2001).

The symptoms naturally correlate with the cortical regions affected by the malformation and vary from severe encephalopathy with refractory epilepsy to selective cognitive deficiencies in otherwise normal individuals (Jansen & Andermann, 2005).

Bilateral perisylvian polymicrogyria

Bilateral perisylvian polymicrogyria (BPP) was the first bilateral polymicrogyria syndrome to be described (Kuzniecky et al., 1993) and is the most common form of polymicrogyria (Jansen & Andermann, 2005).

In BPP, MRI and pathological studies have shown that the cerebral cortex on the borders and deep within the Sylvian fissure is thickened and abnormally infolded; compared with normal controls, the Sylvian fissure is often deeper, wider and more vertically oriented, and it extends more posteriorly up to the parietal lobes; the opercula are hypoplasic and fail to cover the underlying insula. The abnormality is usually symmetrical, but varies in extent among different patients (Kuzniecky et al., 1993). The majority of patients with BPP have the clinical phenotype initially defined in 1993 as congenital bilateral perisylvian syndrome (CBPS) with pseudobulbar palsy, epilepsy and a variable degree of mental retardation (Kuzniecky et al., 1993).

Pseudobulbar palsy or facial, pharyngeal, glossal and masticatory muscle paresis results in restricted tongue movements, drooling, feeding problems, and dysarthria. Voluntary and emotional facial movements can be dissociated (Kuzniecky et al., 1993). Similar symptoms and signs due to bilateral anterior opercular infarctions were described in 1926 by Foix, Chavany and Marie. The congenital form of pseudobulbar paresis was first described by Worster-Drought in 1956, but there was no mention of any mental retardation or epilepsy, both common features of CBPS. It was only in 1986 that the first patients, two 41-year-old monozygotic twins with the clinical and radiological characteristics of CBPS (then called Foix-Chavany-Marie congenital syndrome) were described (Graff-Radford et al., 1986).

Epilepsy is a very frequent symptom in patients with BPP. Infantile spasms may be the presenting seizure type (Kuzniecky et al., 1994a), but seizures generally develop only towards the end of the first decade, or even in the second decade of life. Seizures commonly consist of atypical absence, atonic/tonic and generalized tonic-clonic seizures. Most patients develop multiple seizure types, and seizure control may be poor (Kuzniecky et al., 1994b).

Clinical manifestations of BPP also include pyramidal signs of variable severity and associated malformations (e.g. arthrogryposis, club foot and micrognathia) (Gropman et al., 1997; Kuzniecky et al., 1993).

CBPS was initially only diagnosed in patients presenting the severe form, but the description of familial cases of CBPS has since broadened its phenotypic spectrum (Guerreiro et al., 2000; Jansen & Andermann, 2005). Indeed, systematic investigations on family members of patients with the classical clinical signs of CBPS have led to the identification of individuals with neuroimaging evidence of polymicrogyria restricted to the posterior aspects of the parieto-occipital regions, and with a history of speech delay in early childhood or mild dysarthria (Montenegro et al., 2001). Thus a considerable inter- and intra-familial variability has been reported in clinical and radiological aspects of BPP.

Several familial cases have been reported and different patterns of inheritance have been suggested, illustrating the genetic heterogeneity of BPP, but most of the families provided evidence compatible with an X-linked transmission (Guerreiro et al., 2000).

Neuropsychological features of bilateral perisylvian polymicrogyria

Review of the previous studies

Neurocognitive functions have not been studied much to date in subjects with perisylvian polymicrogyria.

In the majority of cases, the only neuropsychological information available concerns the intelligence quotient (IQ), which is reportedly slightly lower than normal in the majority of cases (Kuzniecky et al., 1993).

The shortage of neuropsychological studies is only partially justified by the relative rarity of the condition. In fact, the diffusion and widespread use of magnetic resonance imaging (MRI) have led to reports on numerous series, some concerning a considerable number of patients (Kuzniecky et al., 1993; Gropman et al., 1997).

It is more likely that the patients' dysarthria or anarthria and any associated motor impairments prove an important obstacle to neuropsychological assessment. In fact, these patients are often labeled as severely retarded because of their severe dysarthria or mutism (Jansen et al., 2005).

In the first large-scale case series consisting of 31 patients with BPP described in The Lancet by Kuzniecky in 1993, intellectual assessment showed that 75 per cent of these patients had mild to moderate cognitive impairments, with a mean full-scale intelligence quotient (FSIQ) of 70, while the remainder had low to average intelligence (FSIQ 82–91). Neuropsychological assessment of speech and language showed variable non-fluent speech difficulties with normal visual and tactile naming. Considering the degree of mental impairment, verbal comprehension was normal for words and short phrases, but some patients had difficulty understanding lengthy and grammatically complex sentences. The variable verbal production difficulties were basically considered a word production/articulation defect due to the severity of the pseudobulbar palsy.

Other studies have emphasized the language difficulties, which were more severe than might have been expected judging from the severity of the facial, pharyngeal, glossal and masticatory muscle paresis, or the cortical pseudobulbar palsy. For instance, the identical twins with what would now be called CBPS, studied by Graff-Radford et al. (1986), failed to respond to speech therapy and were unable to learn sign language, reading or writing. In a study comparing cognitive function in subjects with CBPS and early-acquired opercular syndrome, moreover, CBPS patients were more severely impaired in their language abilities (both comprehension and production) than in their visuo-perceptive or visuo-motor abilities, suggesting that the language defect was the result of a massive dysfunction of the cortical areas responsible for language (Sans & Fernandez-Alvarez, 1996).

In 2002, Guerreiro et al. described a series of 15 children aged 4 to 14 years with a diagnosis of developmental language disorder (DLD) and involved in a neuroimaging study to identify any neuroanatomical substrate for their language disorder. In 12 cases, brain MRI identified BPP, which was limited to the posterior parietal cortex in 6 and spread along the whole sylvian fissure in the other 6. The 12 children's average performance intelligence quotient (PIQ) was 89. Although none of these cases were mentally retarded (because the study had ruled out children with an IQ below 70), there was evidence of a correlation between extent of polymicrogyria and severity of PIQ. In addition, a positive correlation emerged between extent of cortical polymicrogyria and severity of clinical signs, *i.e.* patients with diffuse polymicrogyria around the entire Sylvian fissure and extending to the inferior frontal regions did not speak at all, or they had severe dysarthria and mixed phonological-syntactic deficits, whereas the children whose polymicrogyria was limited to the posterior aspects of the parietal regions (without involving the anterior two-thirds of the sylvian fissure and frontal lobe) had milder or no dysarthria and only phonological programming deficits.

Jansen *et al.* (2005) recently reported the first detailed neuropsychological profile of a series of 14 adults with BPP. The neuropsychological assessment considered verbal and performance intelligence, verbal and visual memory, receptive and expressive language, frontal lobe function and handedness. Intelligence testing revealed a mean full IQ of 77, a verbal IQ (VIQ) of 77, and a performance IQ (PIQ) of 80. Only 4 patients were mentally retarded, with a FSIQ of less than 70; most patients had borderline or low-to-average intelligence. The PIQ correlated negatively with the extent of the cortical malformation while the VIQ (which was lower than the mean PIQ) did not correlate with the neuroimaging results, suggesting that BPP affects VIQ regardless of the severity of the cortical disorganization observable on imaging. In addition, early age at seizure onset correlated positively with PIQ scores and negatively with the extent of cortical lesion, reflecting that patients with more severe BPP are more likely to have early seizure onset, resulting in greater interference with ongoing cognitive development. Receptive and expressive language skills were equally poor and no significant correlations were found between the scores on tests of receptive or expressive language and the extent of cortical disorganization. Most patients had average or low-to-average memory abilities with no specific memory impairment, and a relatively well-preserved frontal function. The authors suggested that these cognitive profiles were related, at least in part, to specific areas of cortical dysfunction (*i.e.* in the perisylvian language regions) and not just to a global dysfunction.

Preliminary results of our study

We studied a sample of six children with BPP, three females and three males, aged between 7.9 and 12.4 years.

On brain MRI, the polymicrogyria affected bilaterally the whole of the Sylvian fissures in four patients, the anterior two thirds in one and the posterior portion in one. The signs of pseudobulbar palsy were evident in all cases, and were severe in four, moderate in one and mild in one. Epileptic seizures, well controlled by antiepileptic theraphy, were observed in four children. Pyramidal signs of variable severity were present in all children.

All patients underwent the same neuropsychological assessment of intelligence evaluated by the Leiter International Performance Scale (Leiter, 1979), lexical comprehension evaluated by the Peabody Picture Vocabolary test – Revised (PPVT-R) (Stella *et al.*, 2000), and grammatical comprehension evaluated by an Italian linguistic comprehension test (Prove di valutazione della comprensione linguistica, Rustioni, 1994). We also videotaped the children at play for an hour to assess spontaneous expressive abilities which were verbal in two children and only gestural in the four anarthric children. The Italian version of the MacArthur Communicative Developmental Inventory: now Bates' Inventory was also used to determine the number of acquired verbal and gestural labels (Caselli & Casadio).

The play observation and Bates' Inventory results were used to assign a communication age equivalent to the stage of language development in tipically developing children.

We also assessed ideomotor and ideative praxic abilities using a shortened version of the De Renzi tests (1980; 1988).

We found that the severity of the dysarthria, up to the point of anarthria, correlated directly with the bilateral involvement of the frontal opercula; in fact, bilateral involvement of the frontal opercula was associated with severe pseudobulbar palsy and no speech at all.

Intellectual impairment, that was mild in four children, moderate in one and severe in one, correlated with the overall extent of cortical malformation.

Language comprehension was more impaired than expected on the basis of mental age in all patients, without correlations with the neuroimaging. Language production was severely affected in all cases and impaired verbal expression was accompanied by a limited use of gestural communication. The communication age was in all cases inferior to the mental age and correlated negatively with the extent of cortical disorganization. Ideomotor (*i.e.* symbolic-communicative) praxis was more disorganized than ideative praxis.

Our results are consistent with previous studies on cognitive function in BPP and further reinforce the close association between word and gesture.

Like previous studies, we confirm: the clinical and radiological variability of BPP; the association between a symmetrical bilateral involvement of the insular opercula and pseudobulbar features; the correlation between the intellectual impairment and the extent of cortical malformation; and the severely impaired expressive and receptive language skills (Guerreiro *et al.*, 2002; Jansen *et al.*, 2005).

The degree of oromotor dysfunction does not correlate with the extent of the malformations on MRI, but does depend on their symmetrical distribution: patients with asymmetrical opercular and insular abnormalities tend to have milder forms of dysarthria (Guerreiro *et al.*, 2002; Jansen *et al.*, 2005).

The language disorder, both productive and receptive, is worse than might be expected on the basis of the intellectual impairment and cannot be explained simply by the articulatory defect. Some authors believe that the phonatory-articulatory dysfunction interferes with language learning because word production would be fundamental for the purposes of its correct representation. Studies on normal language development attribute a crucial role to babbling in language learning because it enables the child to connect the articulatory patterns with the acoustic features of the sound, and the verbal sounds would be recognized by coupling the acoustic input with the articulatory configurations of the sounds (Liberman *et al.*, 1967; Liberman & Mattingly, 1985). The lack of articulatory praxis would consequently interfere with the development of adequate language abilities (Goodstein,1968). It has been demonstrated, however, that subjects with infantile cerebral palsy and congenital anarthria can acquire adequate verbal comprehension skills (Fourcin, 1975; Bishop & Robson, 1989).

We also found deficiencies in the concurrent/compensatory use of gesture for communication, contributing further data to support the strict interdependence between gesture and word (for a review see Bates & Dick, 2002) in children with abnormal development.

There is now a considerable body of evidence that language and gesture are strictly interdependent, forming part of one and the same communication system.

In children who develop language normally, there is a strict relationship between early language development and several aspects of manual activity, such as communicative and symbolic gestures. For instance the spontaneous acquisition of gestures precedes and predicts the emergence of the first words, and the combination of gestures and words heralds the emergence of word associations (Volterra *et al.*, 2005). Adults in all cultures use gestures to accompany verbal production. Congenitally blind people use gestures very similar to those used by the normally sighted, both when they speak to people who can see and when they communicate among themselves, though they cannot have had any visual models to imitate, indicating that gestures are an integral part of speaking and may reflect, or even facilitate, the thinking that underlies speech (Iverson & Goldin-Meadow, 1998).

Studies conducted in conditions of disease, in both adults and children, have also confirmed the strict interdependence between language and gesture.

In adults, there is a known association between aphasic and apraxic disorders, particularly for gestures with a strong symbolic value, in cases of acquired left hemisphere lesions (Heath *et al.*, 2001) or Alzheimer's disease (Glosser *et al.*, 1998).

Recent studies have shown that a poor use of communicative gestures in the early years of life in children with language delay may predict a specific language impairment (Thal & Tobias, 1992), providing further proof of the close relationship between gesture and speech. Other studies that examined the role of co-verbal gesturing in speech production in mentally retarded children with Williams syndrome found that these children made more use of gestures, in particular of iconic gestures (pictographic representations of the use or shape of the object) in naming tests than controls matched for mental age and chronological age. Iconic gestures were used while the children were producing circumlocutious descriptions and evidently having difficulty accessing their lexicon. The analysis of iconic gestures and circumlocutions indicated the activation of the common conceptual space and motor programs associated with naming the object (Bello, *et al.*, 2004).

Cognitive psychologists believe that speech and gestures share common cognitive processes. According to the lexical retrieval hypothesis (Krauss *et al.*, 2000), gestures and words are linked at the phonological coding stage of language development. In the event of lexical retrieval difficulties, the gestures produced take on the spatial and dynamic characteristics of the concept being expressed, thereby facilitating access to the mental lexicon and leading to the articulation of the required word or phrase. According to the information packaging hypothesis (Kita, 2000), gestures are also involved in the conceptual planning of a thought to verbalize: the implication is that gestures serve not only as aids to lexical recovery, but are also involved more pervasively in cognitive activity. Gestures produced during lexical retrieval activate a common semantic conceptual space of gestures and words, and thus the manual-visual and acoustic-articulatory motor programs associated with the object or event represented in the semantic conceptual space (Bello *et al.*, 2004).

These cognitive hypotheses are supported by recent findings that gesture and speech share common neural substrates. Rizzolatti and Arbib (1998) demonstrated in monkeys and humans that the representations of the hand and the mouth overlap over large areas of a fronto-parietal network that is called the 'mirror neuron system' because it discharges during both observation and production of similar manual gestures and mouth movements. This mirror system includes area F5 in the monkey, which is thought to be the phylogenetic precursor of Broca's area: in fact, both are located in the inferior part of area 6, have a similar cell architecture, and are concerned with controlling oro-laryngeal, oro-facial, and arm-hand movements.

Recent fMRI (Tanaka and Inui, 2002; Grezes *et al.*, 2003; Buccino *et al.*, 2004) and PET (Schlaug *et al.*, 1994) studies have shown that Broca's area is activated not only during speech, but also during the execution, imitation and observation of hand-arm movements and gestures.

Very recent behavioral studies in humans have demonstrated that observation of upper limb actions influences speech production and that words and gestures influences each other when emitted simultaneously, providing evidence that spoken word and symbolic gesture are coded as a single signal by a unique communication system mediated by Broca's area (Bernardis & Gentilucci, 2006; Gentilucci *et al.*, 2004).

Considering these recent advances in our knowledge of the neuron system involved in processing words and gestures, the verbal and gestural 'communication' disorders of BPP patients are presumably attributable to a dysfunction of the cortical areas responsible for processing the communication system, *i.e.* for the different aspects and different language properties in different representation modalities.

Despite the considerable plasticity of the brain in developmental age, the bilateral nature of the cortical malfunction prevents language from being reorganized in the areas remaining anatomically intact. As demonstrated by recent PET (Van Bogaert *et al.*, 1998) and fMRI (Janszky *et al.*, 2003), studies, moreover, the dysplastic cortex maintains its functional identity.

For the time being, our understanding of how the malformed cortex functions is not enough to support any clinical-anatomical interpretation of neuropsychological function. In any event, it is worth repeating that brain MRI must have a place in the routine investigation of children with language disorders, and that further studies are needed to better define the neuropsychological features of perisylvian polymicrogyria, also with a view to programming suitable rehabilitation measures.

References

Barkovich, A.J. & Lindan, C.E. (1994): Congenital cytomegalovirus infection of the brain: imaging analysis and embryologic considerations. *Am. J. Neuroradiol.* **15**, 703–715.

Barkovich, A.J., Kuzniecky, R.I., Jackson, G.D., Guerrini, R. & Dobyns, W.B. (2001): Classification system for malformations of cortical development: update 2001. *Neurology* **57**, 2168–2178.

Barkovich, A.J., Rowley, H.A. & Bollen, A. (1995): Correlation of prenatal events with the development of polymicrogyria. *Am. J. Neuroradiol.* **16**, 822–827.

Barth, P.G. (1987): Disorders of neuronal migration. *Can. J. Neurol. Sci.* **14**, 1–16.

Bates, E. & Dick, F. (2002): Language, gesture, and the developing brain. *Dev. Psychobiol.* **40**, 293–310.

Bello, A., Capirci, O. & Volterra, V. (2004): Lexical production in children with Williams syndrome: spontaneous use of gesture in a naming task. *Neuropsychologia* **42**, 201–213.

Bernardis, P. & Gentilucci, M. (2006): Speech and gesture share the same communication system. *Neuropsychologia* **44**, 178–190.

Bishop, D.V. & Robson, J. (1989): Accurate non-word spelling despite congenital inability to speak: phoneme-grapheme conversion does not require subvocal articulation. *Br. J. Psychol.* **80**, 1–13.

Buccino, G., Lui, F., Canessa, N., Patteri, I., Lagravinese, G., Benuzzi, F. Porro, C.A. & Rizzolatti, G. (2004): Neural circuits involved in the recognition of actions performed by nonconspecifics: an fMRI study. *J. Cogn. Neurosi.* **16**, 114–126.

Caselli, M.C. & Casadio, P. (1995): Il primo vocabolario del bambino. Guida all'uso del questionario MacArthur per la valutazione della comunicazione e del linguaggio nei primi anni di vita. Milano: FrancoAngeli.

De Renzi, E., Motti, F. & Nichelli, P. (1980): Imitating gestures. A quantitative approach to ideomotor apraxia. *Arch. Neurol.* **37**, 6–10.

De Renzi, E. & Lucchelli, F. (1988): Ideational apraxia. *Brain* **111**, 1173–1185.

Foix, C., Chavany, J. & Marie, J. (1926): Diplégie facio-linguo-masticatrice d'origine cortico-sous-corticale sans paralysie des membres. *Rev. Neurol.* **33**, 214–219.

Fourcin, A. (1975): Language development in the absence of espressive speech. In: *Foundations of language development*, eds. E.H. Lenneberg & E. Lenneberg, vol. 1. New York: Academic press.

Friede, R.L. (1989): Dysplasias of cerebral cortex. In: *Developmental Neuropathology* (2nd ed.), pp. 330–346. New York: Springer-Verlag.

Gentilucci, M., Stefanini, S., Roy, A.C. & Santunione, P. (2004): Action observation and speech production: study on children and adults. *Neuropsychologia* **42**, 1554–1567.

Goodstein, L.D. (1968): Psychosocial aspects of cleft palate. In: *Cleft palate and communication*, eds. D.C. Spriestersbach & D. Sherman. New York: Academic Press.

Glosser, G., Wiley M.J. & Barnoski, E.J. (1998): Gestural communication in Alzheimer's disease. *J. Clin. Exp. Neuropsychol.* **20**, 1–13.

Graff-Radford, N.R., Bosch, E.P., Stears, J.C. & Tranel, D. (1986): Developmental Foix-Chavany-Marie sindrome in identical twins. *Ann. Neurol.* **20**, 632–635.

Grezes, J., Armony, J.L., Rowe, J., Passingham, R.E. (2003): Activations related to 'mirror' and 'canonical' neurones in the human brain: an fMRI study. *Neuroimage* **18**, 928–937.

Gropman, A.L., Barkovich, A.J., Velina, L.G., Conry, J.A., Dubovsky, E.C. & Packer, R.J. (1997): Pediatric congenital bilateral perisylvian syndrome: clinical and MRI features in 12 patients. *Neuropediatrics* **28**, 198–203.

Guerreiro, M.M., Andermann, E., Guerrini, R., Dobyns, W.B., Kuzniecky, R., Silver, K., Van Bogaert, P., Gillain, C., David, P., Ambrosetto, G., Rosati, A., Bartolomei, F., Parmeggiani, A., Paetau, R., Salonen, O., Ignatius, J., Borgatti, R., Zucca, C., Bastos, A.C., Palmini, A., Fernandes, W., Montenegro, M.A., Cendes, F. & Andermann, F. (2000): Familial perisylvian polymicrogyria: a new familial syndrome of cortical maldevelopment. *Ann. Neurol.* **48**, 39–48.

Guerreiro, M.M., Hage, S.R., Guimaraes, C.A., Abramides, D.V., Fernandes, W., Pacheco, P.S., Piovesana, A.M., Montenegro, M.A. & Cendes, F. (2002): Developmental language disorder associated with polymicrogyria. *Neurology* **59**, 245–250.

Guerrini, R., Barkovich A.J., Sztriha, L. & Dobyns, W.B. (2000): Bilateral frontal polymicrogyria. A newly recognized brain malformation syndrome. *Neurology* **54**, 909–913.

Heath, M., Roy, E.A., Black, S.E. & Westwood, D.A. (2001): Intransitive limb gestures and apraxia following unilateral stroke. *J. Clin. Exp. Neuropsychol.* **23**, 628–642.

Iverson, J.M. & Goldin-Meadow, S. (1998): Why people gesture when they speak. *Nature,* **396**, 228.

Jansen, A. & Andermann, E. (2005): Genetics of the polymicrogyria syndromes. *J. Med. Genet.* **42**, 369–378.

Jansen, A.C., Leonard, G., Bastos, A.C., Esposito-Festen, J.E., Tampieri, D., Watkins, K., Andermann, F. & Andermann, E. (2005): Cognitive functioning in bilateral perisylvian polymicrogyria (BPP): clinical and radiological correlations. *Epilepsy Behav.* **6**, 393–404.

Janszky, J., Ebner, A., Kruse, B., Mertens, M., Jokeit, H., Seitz, R.J., Witte O.W., Tuxhorn, I. & Woermann, F.G. (2003): Functional organization of the brain with malformations of cortical development. *Ann. Neurol.* **53**, 759–767.

Kita, S. (2000): How representational gestures help speaking. In: *Language and gesture*, ed. D. McNeill, pp. 162–185. New York: Cambridge University Press.

Krauss, R., Chen, Y. & Gottesman, R. (2000): Lexical gestures and lexical access: a process model. In: *Language and gesture*, ed. D. McNeill, pp. 261–283. New York: Cambridge University Press.

Kuzniecky, R., Andermann, F. & Guerrini, R. (1993): Congenital bilateral perisylvian syndrome: study of 31 patients. The CBPS multicenter collaborative study. *Lancet* **341**, 608–612.

Kuzniecky, R., Andermann, F. & Guerrini, R. (1994a): Infantile spasms: an early epileptic manifestation in some patients with the congenital bilateral perisylvian syndrome. *J. Child. Neurol.* **9**, 420–423.

Kuzniecky, R., Andermann, F. & Guerrini, R. (1994b): CBPS multicenter collaborative study. The epileptic spectrum in the congenital bilateral perisylvian syndrome. *Neurology* **44**, 379–385.

Leiter, R.G. (1979): Leiter International Performance Scale. Chicago: Stoelting Co.

Liberman, A.M., Cooper, F.S., Shankweiler, D.P. & Studdert-Kennedy, M. (1967): Perception of the speech code. *Psychol. Rev.* **74**, 431–461.

Liberman, A.M. & Mattingly, I.G. (1985): The motor theory of speech perception revised. *Cognition* **21**, 1–36.

Montenegro, M.A., Guerreiro, M.M., Lopes-Cendes, I. & Cendes, F. (2001): Bilateral posterior parietal polymicrogyria: a mild form of congenital bilateral perisylvian sindrome? *Epilepsia* **42**, 845–849.

Piao, X., Hill, R.S., Bodell, A., Chang, B.S., Basel-Vanagaite, L., Straussberg, R., Dobyns, W.B., Qasrawi, B., Winter, R.M., Innes, A.M., Voit, T., Ross, M.E., Michaud, J.L., Descarie, J.C., Barkovich, A.J. & Walsch, C.A. (2004): G protein-coupled receptor-dependent development of human frontal cortex. *Science,* **303**, 2033–2036.

Raybaud, C., Girare, N., Canto-Moreira, N. & Poncet, M. (1996): Hight-definition magnetic resonance imaging identification of cortical dysplasias: micropolygyria *versus* lissencephaly. In: *Dysplasias of cerebral cortex and epilepsy*, eds. R. Guerrini, F. Andermann, R. Canapicchi, J. Roger, B.G. Zifkin & P. Pfanner, pp.131–143. Philadelphia: Lippincott-Raven.

Rizzolatti, G. & Arbib, M.A. (1998): Language within our grasp. *TINS*, **21**: 188–194.

Robain, O. (1996): Introduction to the pathology of cerebral cortical dysplasia. In: *Dysplasias of cerebral cortex and epilepsy*, eds. R. Guerrini, F. Andermann, R. Canapicchi, J. Roger, B.G. Zifkin & P. Pfanner, pp. 1–9. Philadelphia: Lippincott-Raven.

Rustioni Metz Lancaster, D. (1994): *Prove di valutazione della comprensione linguistica*. Firenze: Organizzazioni Speciali.

Sans, A. & Fernandez-Alvarez, E. (1996): Neuropsychological findings in congenital bilateral perisylvian syndrome *versus* early acquired opercular syndrome. In: *Dysplasias of cerebral cortex and epilepsy*, eds. R. Guerrini, F. Andermann, R. Canapicchi, J. Roger, B.G. Zifkin & P. Pfanner, pp. 279–283. Philadelphia: Lippincott-Raven.

Schlaug, G., Knorr, U. & Seitz, R.J. (1994): Inter-subject variability of cerebral activations in acquiring a motor skill: a study with positron emission tomography. *Exp. Brain. Res.* **98**, 523–534.

Stella, G. (2000): *Peabody – Test di vocabolario recettivo*. Torino: Omega.

Sugama, S. & Kusano, K. (1994): Monozygous twin with polymicrogyria and normal co-twin. *Pediatr. Neurol.* **11**, 62–63.

Takanashi, J. & Barkovich, A.J. (2003): The changing MR imaging appearance of polymicrogyria: a consequence of myelination. *Am. J. Neuroradiol.* **24**, 788–793.

Tanaka, S. & Inui, T. (2002): Cortical involvement for action imitation of hand/arm postures *versus* finger configurations: an fMRI study. *Neuroreport* **13**, 1599–1602.

Thal, D.J. & Tobias, S. (1992): Communicative gestures in children with delayed onset of oral expressive vocabulary. *J. Speech Hear. Res.* **35**, 1281–1289.

Van Bogaert, P., David, P., Gillain, C.A., Wikler, D., Damhaut, P., Scalais, E., Nuttin, C., Wetzburger, C., Szliwowski, H.B., Metens, T. & Goldman, S. (1998): Perisylvian dysgenesis. Clinical, EEG, MRI and glucose metabolism features in 10 patients. *Brain* **121**, 2229–2238.

Volterra, V., Caselli, M.C., Capirci, O. & Pizzuto, E. (2005): Gesture and the emergence and development of language. In: *Beyond nature-nurture: essays in honor of Elizabeth Bates*, eds. M. Tomasello & D.I. Slobin, pp. 3–40. Mahwah, NJ: Lawrence Erlbaum.

Worster-Drought, C. (1956): Congenital suprabulbar paresis. *J. Laryngol. Otol.* **70**, 453–463.

Development language disorders (DLD)

Chapter 15

Specific language impairment: definition and diagnostic criteria

Giovanna Zardini

National Neurologic Institute 'C. Besta', via Celoria 11, 20133 Milan, Italy
giovanna.zardini@libero.it

Summary

The term *specific language impairment* (SLI) refers to a number of clinical conditions featuring a significant limitation in the development of language ability, in the absence of factors usually accompanying language learning problems, including hearing impairment, low nonverbal intelligence test scores, diagnosable neurological damage, and so forth.

The category of SLI includes both cases of language delay and of language impairment. Language production and comprehension may be variably affected, with varying degrees of impairment in the different areas of language, including phonetics-phonology, morpho-syntax, and lexicon-semantics. This results in heterogeneous language profiles that, sometimes irrespective of therapeutic-rehabilitation treatments, may present with a different clinical evolution.

The diagnosis of SLI is achieved applying criteria negative exclusion and positive inclusion of both. The presence of hearing problems, low nonverbal intelligence test scores, neurological disorders, abnormalities of oral structure and/or function, and of a definite pervasive developmental disorder formally exclude a diagnosis of SLI. In this scenario, selected exclusion criteria, such as those of low nonverbal IQ and of the impairment in reciprocal social interaction and communication, are still a matter of study and debate. Inclusion criteria are the impairment of language abilities, documented by standardized tests evaluating production as well as comprehension and covering different areas of language, and data obtained from the analysis of language abilities derived from samples of the child's spontaneous speech.

The study of SLI across different languages has allowed the identification of some common features, present in all children with SLI, and some other features proper of the language that a particular child with SLI is acquiring.

Introduction

The term *specific language impairment* (SLI) refers to a number of clinical conditions featuring a significant limitation in the development of language ability, in the absence of other factors usually accompanying language learning problems, including hearing impairment, low nonverbal intelligence test scores, diagnosable neurological damage, psychiatric disorders, and severe deprivation.

The early descriptions of SLI date back to the first half of the nineteenth century. As reported by Leonard (1998), Gall in 1822 published a description of seemingly normal children who had clear problems in expressive language, but did not display difficulties in comprehension nor other disturbances. This clinical characterization advanced the definition of 'developmental dysphasia' that was formulated in the following century on the base exclusion criteria.

Over the first half of the twentieth century, a remarkable number of studies were carried out by authors from different countries. These authors described children with an extremely limited speech output, but apparently normal nonverbal intelligence and seemingly good comprehension. Different terms were applied to these children: 'congenital aphasia', 'hearing mutism', 'infantile aphasia', 'developmental aphasia' and, in the 1960s, 'developmental dysphasia'. Since the 1960s, other terms have appeared in the literature, including 'infantile speech', 'specific language deficit', and so forth.

The term *specific language impairment* was introduced by Fey and Leonard in 1983, and is the most widely adopted term at present, especially in the English literature. French authors still prefer the term 'dysphasia'. Chevrie-Muller (2000) applies the term *troubles spécifiques du développement du langage* to selected language disorders identified by exclusion, reserving the term *dysphasie* to the most severe forms of SLI.

According to Leonard (1998), there are two different reasons for such changes in terminology. First, 'aphasia' and 'dysphasia' both have a neurological connotation. The second reason rests on the effort to characterize the linguistic features of these children's speech, according to the new theories of generative-transformational grammar, which has had such a great impact on the study of language development in normal and abnormal conditions. Leonard points out that, as late as the early 1960s, children with postnatal brain injury were still included in the category of developmental dysphasia. The new theories, besides the characterization of the speech deficit, allow formulating a hypothesis on the nature of this deficit.

The main feature of children with SLI is that they do not acquire language as rapidly and effortlessly as the normal children. SLI is quite a frequent condition, the prevalence of which ranges from 4 to 7 per cent according to the different studies, the language considered, and the mean age of the case series. As for other developmental disorders, SLI is more likely to be seen in males than in females, and children with SLI are more likely than other children to have parents and/or siblings with a history of language learning problems.

Children with SLI share some common features, but the heterogeneity of the language profiles and the possible evolution of this disorder with age are, nevertheless, remarkable. Therapeutic-rehabilitation treatments and age usually improve these children's learning problems, but the deficits in language may persist in adolescence and into adulthood (van der Lely, 1997). Children with SLI are also at risk for reading-writing disorders and more general learning difficulties when they reach school age (Bishop & Adams, 1990; Bird et al., 1995). Adults who had been diagnosed with SLI and successfully treated, often score lower on tests of language production and comprehension than same-age peers with no such history (Tomblin et al., 1992). Moreover, adults with a history of SLI tend to achieve a lower academic success and less remunerated employments (Records et al., 1992).

The category of SLI includes deficits of language production and deficits involving both production and comprehension. The different areas of language may be variably affected, including phonetics-phonology, morpho-syntax, and lexicon-semantics.

The clinical diagnostic criteria in the main international classifications of diseases diverge on some points with respect to language disorders. The *Diagnostic and Statistical Manual of*

Mental Disorders, Third Edition (DSM-III) (American Psychiatric Association, 1980) and the *International Classification of Diseases, Tenth Revision* (ICD-10) (WHO, 1992) employ the term 'specific developmental language disorders', and separate SLI from mental impairment and pervasive developmental disorders (PDD). Mentally impaired and PDD children, however, may feature language profiles similar to those of SLI. Despite this, the language disorders seen in these children occur within a different context and differ from a developmental perspective. Both the DSM and ICD classifications distinguish between disorders of word articulation, and 'expressive' and 'mixed receptive/expressive' developmental language disorders. The ICD-10 classification also includes the Landau-Kleffner syndrome among language disorders; this syndrome however, featuring language disruption associated with a convulsive disorder or an epileptiform EEG without clinical seizures, cannot be considered a SLI *per se*. It must be noted that the DSM-III and the ICD-10 classifications make no difference between language delay and language impairment, that is between a functional and a structural disorder of language (Gerard, 2003). Functional disorders refer to children with difficulties in the development of a linguistic competence that is potentially present. In structural disorders, by contrast, it is linguistic competence that is primarily impaired.

The *Diagnostic and Statistical Manual of Mental Disorders, Fourth Edition* (DSM-IV) (American Psychiatric Association, 1994) employs the term 'specific disorder of oral communication'; this term appears to be ambiguous, as it does not distinguish disorders of word articulation and verbal language from those disorders affecting nonverbal language and communication.

Diagnostic criteria

The diagnosis of SLI is based on etiopathogenic exclusion criteria, which distinguish SLI from other disabling conditions featuring language impairment among other symptoms, and inclusion criteria defining the main features of the language profile.

The exclusion criteria for SLI are the following:

1. Hearing problems, either sensorineural or conductive. The diagnosis of SLI requires that the child must have a normal hearing threshold at standard audiometric screening (20 dB threshold at frequencies in the 500–4000 Hz range). Many authors agree that recurrent episodes of otitis media, occurring between 9 months and 2 years of age and possibly leading to conductive hearing losses of variable degree, may interfere with normal phonology at a time that is crucial for the development of perceptive abilities and phonemic discrimination.
2. Low nonverbal intelligence test scores. A most fundamental criterion in the diagnosis of SLI is a score on nonverbal intelligence measures within age-appropriate levels. Children must score a nonverbal IQ of at least 85. The ICD-10 classification, however, admits a nonverbal score as low as 70.
3. Neurological disorders. Several neurological conditions, possibly leading to language disorders, must be ruled out before a diagnosis of SLI is appropriate. There should be no evidence of seizure disorders, cerebral palsy, or focal brain lesions. A period of febrile convulsions during infancy, including complicated febrile seizures chronically treated with antiepileptic drugs, is not considered as an exclusionary criterion. Also not exclusionary are other specific developmental disorders, including the attention deficit-hyperactivity disorder (ADHD) and the specific developmental disorders of motor function, such as clumsiness.
4. Abnormalities of oral structure and/or function, including harelip and cleft palate, but also impaired volitional movements. Children with SLI in the form of a global expressive disorder, however, often also display features of oral dyspraxia.

5. Impaired reciprocal social interaction and communication, as in autism and other PDDs. According to many investigators these criteria formally exclude children with a semantic-pragmatic language disorder from the category of SLI.

6. Deprivation or otherwise inadequate or absent exposure to language, as in the case of emotional deprivation and ill treatment. These factors are difficult to delineate and to quantify, and remain underestimated and understudied.

The inclusion criteria for SLI are as follows:

1. Language test scores falling more than 1 standard deviation (SD) below the mean of age-matched peers. These tests cover different areas of language (*i.e.* phonology, morpho-syntax, and lexicon), and evaluate production as well as comprehension. There are no standardized tests, originally created to evaluate Italian-speaking children, which can be applied from preschool age through adolescence to obtain a detailed characterization of comprehension and production abilities. Most of the testing instruments available in current practice are translations adapted from English; they often have not yet been standardized and do not cover the entire developmental age.

2. Measures and analyses of language abilities that are derived from samples of the child's spontaneous speech, as the measure of the mean length of utterance (MLU) computed in terms of words. A concordance between MLU and nonverbal test scores has been demonstrated in English-speaking children with SLI.

3. The identification of 'clinical markers' of SLI, that is grammatical morphemes that children with SLI have particular difficulty acquiring compared to normal children. Two possible markers regarding the grammatical morphology of verbs have been identified in English (Leonard *et al.*, 1997; Rice *et al.*, 1998). The nonsense words repetition task also appears to be a promising index (Dollaghan & Campbell, 1998). In a recent study, Bortolini, Caselli, Deevy and Leonard (2002) demonstrated that the use of singular definite articles and the inflection of verbs for the third plural person is a sensitive and specific marker to differentiate Italian-speaking children with SLI from their normally developing peers.

Leonard (1998) questions whether a nonverbal IQ score of 85, falling 1 SD below the mean, is the best estimate of nonverbal intelligence to select, and may be provisionally acceptable. Children with SLI achieving this score often perform below their age-mates on other kinds of nonlinguistic activities, such as symbolic play and mental imagery. On the other hand, a cut-off score needs to be established for diagnostic purposes. From the standpoint of diagnostic categories, the 70–84 range constitutes a sort of no-man's-land; it defines the borderline range of intelligence, being too low for normal children, but too high to be considered an index of mental retardation.

Moreover, it should be pointed out that the nonverbal IQ score can decline with age, as the nonverbal tasks become more abstract and conceptual, and that language deficits probably limit the degree to which children can rely on verbal reasoning to assist them in solving problems that are nonverbal in nature. Adhering strictly to the cut-off criterion of a nonverbal IQ score of 85, such children should not be included in the category of SLI. Furthermore, if the decline in nonverbal IQ stems from a language disorder, the rigid application of this criterion becomes even more questionable. In a study on the efficacy of early treatment and on the relationship between the degree of improvement and the baseline nonverbal IQ, Fey et al. (1994) demonstrated that children with SLI scoring in the 70–84 range on performance tests made gains that were comparable to, if not greater than, those made by children with nonverbal IQs above 85, and therefore met the criteria for SLI. It is conceivable that the children whose nonverbal IQ at preschool is high and is maintained throughout childhood, present with a different language disorder than that of the children whose scores fall within average levels at first, but then decline.

From a clinical standpoint, it is not always easy to differentiate SLI from the disorders of social interaction and communication. In this respect, the main issue regards the differential diagnosis between the 'semantic-pragmatic' language disorder and high-functioning autism, and between verbal auditory agnosia and typical autism. With the exception of Asperger syndrome, in which language is normally structured but repetitive in content and deviant in prosody, autistic children are usually characterized by their deficient and idiosyncratic use of language.

Rapin and Allen (1983, 1987) have identified 14 different criteria for the diagnosis of semantic-pragmatic dysphasia, and Bishop and Rosenbloom (1987) added still other criteria. These children show deficits in communicative ability marked by difficulties with comprehension in conversational contexts and especially severe problems in the semantic and pragmatic domains. Some of these children exhibit age-appropriate non-verbal IQ scores along with normal hearing and no signs of frank neurological impairment; their social interactions are, however, odd. According to Lemay (2004), when applying the criteria by Rapin and Allen together with those proposed by Bishop (1989), these children fulfill diagnostic criteria for a mild form of autistic disorder (high-functioning autism). In this respect the two syndromes, SLI and PDD, seem somehow to merge. In terms of DSM-IV criteria, these children would also fall in the category of PDD not otherwise specified (PDD-NOS).

Reaching a correct diagnosis may be even more difficult when considering children with a severe language disorder involving both comprehension and expression, and characterized by verbal auditory agnosia. To these children, the words spoken by others have no meaning; the children tend to withdraw into self-sensory activities, yet manifesting the willingness to communicate through non-verbal modalities (eye contact, mimicry and gesticulation, search for body contact). Lemay (2004) describes how difficult, if not impossible, a correct diagnosis may be in these cases, if one relies only on the questionnaires for autism and/or on neuropsychological tests. A prolonged clinical observation is mandatory in such children, with particular attention paid to selected clinical clues that may correctly direct the diagnosis of an selective language disorder. Some of these clues are as follows:

- The willingness to communicate which is manifested when the child is exposed to verbal stimuli that are appropriate as to quantity, rhythm, and complexity. It may be compensated through mimicry and gesticulation, which are employed for understanding other people and making oneself understood.
- The production of jargon or words that are close to an adult target.
- The possibility of emerging from sensory fixations and repetitive activities, when the examiner gradually attempts to participate in the child's activities.
- The ability to answer the questions of peers, despite of the tendency to isolation; the ability to understand mimicry and emotions.
- The possibility of improving the quality of drawings, symbolic play, and mental imagery through the imitation of others.
- The gradual reduction of autistic features following educational treatment and family support, despite the persisting impairment of expressive language.

The language characteristics of SLI

As mentioned earlier, the generative grammar theories have modified the understanding of language development in normal and impaired children.

As late as the 1960s, the approach to language development was mainly descriptive; based on operant behavioral theories, the development of language was conceived as a process setting up complex 'habits', taking place under the effect of environmental models. Current logopaedic treatments still rely on this concept.

The first studies of the language of English-speaking children with SLI, referring to the so-called standard theory proposed by Chomsky (1957), started to appear in the 1960s.

The further elaboration of generative theories led to the 'principles and parameters' framework of universal grammar, which was first proposed by Chomsky in 1981. This theory considers two different abstract entities: the principles of universal grammar, that is the properties and operations which characterize the grammar of all natural languages; and the parameters, which are binary sets of characteristics that vary systematically from language to language, and represent the limited space in which a variation is possible. The acquisition of language came to be regarded as the result of a process which, on the basis of the linguistic experience, selects grammar from a variety of different possibilities established by the universal grammar. For instance one a principle of universal grammar is that all sentences need a subject, although in Italian the subject of a sentence may in some cases be implicit, contrary to English where the absence of a subject represents a mistake and a lack of information. One of the main sources of variation between the various languages is the grammatical morphology which characterizes each language. It is well known that young normally developing children and children with SLI have difficulties with the use of grammatical morphemes (Leonard, 1992).

Different hypotheses have been proposed to explain this phenomenon which, besides being interesting from a theoretical point of view, may address the choice of rehabilitation treatment. Jakubowicz (2004) has identified two hypothetical mainstream hypotheses, one suggesting an *deficit in implicit grammatical use* and the other a *limitation in language processing capacities*.

According to the theories based on the first hypothesis, the difficulties with the use of grammatical morphemes stem from a deficit in the acquisition of grammatical rules, that is transient in the young normally developing child and putatively permanent in children with SLI.

Various investigators view the defective use of grammatical morphemes as either generalized or selective. Gopnik (1990), Gopnik and Crago (1991), and Guilfoyle *et al.* (1991) are strongly inclined towards a generalized deficit in the use of grammatical morphemes. These authors suggested that grammatical morphemes and elements of functional categories are missing from the underlying grammar of individuals with SLI. As a result, these children's grammar is qualitatively different and frankly deviant from the universal grammar. Although they noted occasional productions having the appearance of grammatical morphemes in the speech of children with SLI, they assumed that these forms were simply memorized lexical items with no grammatical significance. Yet Leonard (1995), reporting on English-speaking preschoolers with SLI having difficulties in the use of grammatical morphemes, brought out evidence for the presence of at least some functional categories, including pronominal determiners, some pronominal possessive forms, some verb inflections, and so forth.

Studies supporting the hypothesis of a selective deficit in the use of grammatical morphemes have focused mainly on English- and German-speaking children. Some investigators proposed that both young normally developing children and children with SLI go through a stage in which a quite normal grammar coexists with a grammar selectively deficient in the use of some morphemes and syntactic rules. This period is transient in normally developing children; whereas children with SLI are assumed to remain in this early stage for an extended period, or perhaps permanently.

Wexler (1994, 1998) has noted that English-speaking children with SLI fail to mark tense as required and show an improper use of infinitive forms. Clahsen (Clahsen, 1989; Clahsen & Hansen, 1993; Clahsen et al., 1997) reported that children with SLI acquiring German show a selective impairment in the grammatical agreement of verbs with the person and number of the subject. Van der Lely & Stollwerck (1996; 1997) found English-speaking children with SLI to have great difficulties with syntactic relations.

The theories viewing SLI as a limitation in general processing capacity include the so-called 'surface hypothesis' proposed by Leonard, and the hypothesis by Tallal and colleagues of a nonlinguistic deficit affecting temporal processing.

The accounts proposed by Leonard and colleagues (Leonard, 1989; Leonard et al., 1992; 1997) assume a general limitation of processing capacity in children with SLI. This limitation affects the perception of phonetically weak grammatical morphemes that are short in duration, at least relative to adjacent material. This holds for grammatical inflections in the form of single consonants and of unstressed syllabic morphemes that rarely, if ever, appear in sentence positions in which significant lengthening occurs. Leonard observed that most of the closed-class morphemes that distinguished English-speaking children with SLI from their MLU controls are morphemes of relatively short duration. These included the third-person singular -s and paste tense -ed inflections, possessive 's, copula and auxiliary be forms, the conjunctions infinitival to and complementizer that.

Italian-speaking children with SLI, by contrast, do not have particular problems with inflections that, in Italian, are syllabic and occur frequently in utterance-final and phonological phrase-final position. Bortolini, Caselli and Leonard (1997) noted that Italian children with SLI acquiring language show lower percentages of use of articles and direct object clitic pronouns than their MLU-matched peers. These monosyllabic forms are unstressed and usually occur in phrase-initial or phrase-medial position, where they are short in duration.

According to the surface hypothesis, children with SLI are capable of perceiving word-final consonants and weak, non-lengthened syllables, but have a limited processing capacity in terms of reduced speed of processing that is severely taxed. When these forms play a morphological role, the child must perform additional operations, such as discovering the grammatical functions of the forms and placing the forms in the proper cell of a morphological paradigm. This, of course, must occur while processing the rest of the sentence that is being heard. It is assumed that such operations require a large number of exposures before these brief grammatical forms are established in the language.

According to Leonard, the organization of grammar in children with SLI is no different from that seen in normally developing children. Furthermore, assuming that the speed of processing limitation affects grammatical morphology, this same processing limitation may lead to a different type of linguistic profile in those languages whose morphology is not as fragile as it is in English.

The surface hypothesis, however, does not answer for some of the data reported by other investigators. As noted by Gopnik and Crago (1991), English-speaking children with SLI show significant differences in their use of grammatical morphemes that have identical phonetic values, such as the plural -s and the third-person singular verb inflection -s. The same difference in degree of use was reported by Bottari and colleagues (Bottari et al., 1998) in Italian-speaking children with SLI regarding the use of the definite article lo/la and the direct object clitic lo/la. On the other hand, Leonard himself has identified several limitations in his account regarding the use of grammatical morphemes.

The hypothesis proposed by Tallal and colleagues (Tallal & Piercy, 1973, 1974; Tallal *et al.*, 1985, 1996) is based the finding that children with SLI, when compared to normal children, perform quite poorly on tasks that require the processing of brief stimuli and the processing of stimuli that are presented in rapid succession. The same difficulties were observed whether children responded to verbal or nonverbal stimuli. Children performed better when the duration of each non-verbal stimulus exceeded 250-ms or when the rate of presentation of succeeding stimuli lasting 75-ms each exceeded 300-ms. According to Tallal, children with SLI exhibit a selective deficit in auditory temporal processing that hampers the formation of the phonetic prototypes typical of each language. This processing deficit, however, is assumed to be malleable by training aimed at speeding the temporal processing of auditory verbal and nonverbal stimuli. Tallal and colleagues (1996) report on impressive gains as a result of concentrated practice over a very short period of time.

The hypothesis proposed by Tallal has not been supported by studies by other investigators, who have criticized it for the poor specification of the language characteristics of the children in their case series (Studdert-Kennedy & Mody, 1995).

In conclusion, recent decades have witnessed a great progress in the understanding of SLI. Nevertheless, definitive data on this disorder and on the interpretation of its linguistic basis are still lacking. These are required in order to reach a correct diagnosis and apply appropriate treatment.

References

American Psychiatric Association (1980): Diagnostic and Statistical Manual of Mental Disorders (3rd edn.) (DSM-III). Washington, DC: APA.

American Psychiatric Association (1994): Diagnostic and Statistical Manual of Mental Disorders (4rd edn.) (DSM-IV). Washington, DC: APA.

Bird, J., Bishop, D.V. & Freeman N.H. (1995): Phonological awareness and literacy development in children with expressive phonological impairments. *J. Speech Hear. Res.* **38**, 446–462.

Bishop, D. (1989): Autism, Asperger's syndrome and semantic-pragmatic disorder: where are the boundaries? *Br. J. Disord. Commun.* **24**, 107–121.

Bishop, D.V. & Adams, C. (1990): A prospective study of the relationship between specific language impairment, phonological disorders and reading retardation. *J. Child Psychol. Psychiatry* **31**, 1027–1050.

Bishop, D. & Rosenbloom, L. (1987): Classification of childhood language disorders. In: *Language, development and disorders*, eds. W. Yule & M. Rutter, pp. 16–41. London: Mc Keith Press.

Bortolini, U., Caselli, M.C. & Leonard, L.B. (1997): Grammatical deficits in Italian-speaking children with specific language impairment. *J. Speech Hear. Res.* **40**, 809–820.

Bortolini, U., Caselli, M.C, Deevy, P. & Leonard, L.B. (2002): Specific language impairment in Italian: first steps in the search of a clinical marker. *Int. J. Lang. Commun. Disord.* **37**, 77–93.

Bottari, P., Cipriani, P., Chilosi, A.M. & Pfanner, L. (1998): The determiner system in a group of Italian children with SLI. *Lang. Acquisition.* **7**, 285–315.

Chévrie-Muller, C. (2000): Troubles spécifiques du développement du langage 'dysphasies de développement'. In: *Le langage de l'enfant: aspects normaux et pathologiques*, eds. C. Chévrie-Muller & J. Narbona, pp. 262–291. Paris: Masson.

Chomsky, N. (1957), *Syntactic structures*. Mouton & Co., The Hague.

Chomsky, N (1981): *Lectures on government and binding*. Dordrecht, The Netherlands: Foris.

Clahsen, H. (1989): The grammatical characterization of developmental dysphasia. *Linguistics* **27**, 897–920.

Clahsen, H., & D. Hansen. (1993): The missing agreement account of specific language impairment: evidence from therapy experiments. *Essex Research Reports in Linguistics* **2**, 1–36.

Clahsen, H., Bartke S. & Göllner S. (1997): Formal features in impaired grammars: a comparison of English and German SLI children. *Journal of Neurolinguistics* **10**, 151–171.

Dollaghan, C. & Campbell, T.F. (1998): Nonword repetition and child language impairment. *J. Speech Lang. Hear. Res.* **41**, 1136–1146.

Fey, M. & Leonard, L. (1983): Pragmatic skills of children with specific language impairment. In: *Pragmatic assessment and intervention issues in language*, eds. T. Gallagher & C. Prutting. San Diego: College-Hill Press.

Fey, M., Long, S.H. & Cleave, P.L. (1994): Reconsideration of IQ criteria in the definition of specific language impairment. In: *Specific language impairments in children*, eds. R.V. Watkins & M.L. Rice, pp. 161–178. Baltimore: Paul H. Brookes.

Gerard, C.L. (2003): Place des syndromes dysphasiques parmi les troubles du développement du langage chez l'enfant. In: *Les dysphasies*, eds. C.L. Gérard & V. Brun, pp. 1–15. Paris: Masson.

Gopnik M. (1990): Feature blindness: a case study. *Language Acquisition* **1**, 139–164.

Gopnik, M. & Crago, M.B. (1991): Familial aggregation of a developmental language disorder. *Cognition* **39**, 1–50

Guilfoyle, E., Allen, S. & Moss. S. (1991): Specific language impairment and the maturation of functional categories. Paper presented at the Boston Conference of Language Development in Boston.

Jakubowicz, C. (2004): Hypothèses psycho-linguistiques sur la nature du déficit dysphasique. In: *Les dysphasies*, eds. C.L. Gérard & V. Brun, pp. 23–70. Paris: Masson.

Lemay, M. (2004): Les problèmes soulevés par le diagnostic différentiel. In: *L'autisme aujourd'hui*, ed. M. Lemay, pp. 229–249. Paris: Odile Jacob.

Leonard, L. (1989): Language learnability and specific language impairment in children. *Appl. Psycholinguistics* **10**, 179–202.

Leonard, L. (1992): The use of morphology by children with specific language impairment: evidence from three languages. In: *Processes in language acquisition and disorders*, ed. R. Chapman, pp. 186–201. St. Louis: Mosby-Yearbook.

Leonard, L. (1995): Functional categories in the grammars of children with specific language impairment. *J. Speech Hear. Res.* **38**, 1270–1283.

Leonard, L. (1998): *Children with specific language impairment*, pp. 1–339. Cambridge, MA: MIT Press.

Leonard, L.B., McGregor, K.K. & Allen, G.D. (1992): Grammatical morphology and speech perception in children with specific language impairment. *J. Speech Hear. Res.* **35**, 1076–1085.

Leonard, L.B., Eyer, J.A., Bedore, L.M. & Grela, B.G. (1997): Three accounts of the grammatical morpheme difficulties of English-speaking children with specific language impairment. *J. Speech Lang. Hear. Res.* **40**, 741–753.

Rapin, I. & Allen. D. (1983): Developmental language disorders: nosological consideration. In: *Neuropsychology of language, reading and spelling*, ed. U. Kirk, pp. 155–184. New York: Academic Press.

Rapin, I. & Allen. D. (1987): Developmental dysphasia and autism in preschool children: characteristics and subtypes. In: *Proceedings of the first international symposium of specific speech and language disorders in children*, pp. 20–35. Brentford, UK: Association for All Speech Impaired Children.

Records, N.L., Tomblin, J.B. & Freese, P.R. (1992): The quality of life of young adults with histories of specific language impairment. *Am. J. Speech Lang. Pathol.* **1**, 44–53.

Rice, M.L., Wexler, K. & Hershberger, S. (1998): Tense over time: the longitudinal course of tense acquisition in children with specific language impairment. *J. Speech Lang. Hear. Res.* **41**, 1412–1431.

Studdert-Kennedy, M. & Mody, M. (1995): Auditory temporal perception deficits in the reading-impaired: a critical review. *Psychol. Bull. Rev.* **2**, 508–514.

Tallal, P. & Piercy, M. (1973): Defects of non-verbal auditory perception in children with developmental aphasia. *Nature* **241**, 468–469.

Tallal, P. & Piercy, M. (1974): Developmental aphasia: rate of auditory processing and selective impairment of consonant perception. *Neuropsychologia* **12**, 83–93.

Tallal, P., Stark, R.E. & Mellits, E.D. (1985): Identification of language-impaired children on the basis of rapid perception and production skills. *Brain Lang.* **25**, 314–322.

Tallal, P., Miller, S.L., Bedi, G., Byma, G., Wang, X., Nagarajan, S.S., Schreiner, C., Jenkins, W.M. & Merzenich, M.M. (1996): Language comprehension in language-learning impaired children improved with acoustically modified speech. *Science* **271**, 81–84.

Tomblin, J.B., Freese, P.R. & Records, N.L. (1992): Diagnosing specific language impairment in adults for the purpose of pedigree analysis. *J. Speech Hear. Res.* **35**, 832–843.

van der Lely, H.K.J. (1997): Narrative discourse in grammatical specific language-impaired children: a modular language deficit? *J. Child Lang.* **24**, 221–256.

van der Lely H.K.J. & Stollwerck L. (1996): A grammatical specific language impairment: an autosomal dominant inheritance? *Brain Lang.* **52**, 484–504.

van der Lely, H. K. J., & Stollwerck, L. (1997). Binding theory and specifically language-impaired children. *Cognition* **62**, 245–290.

Wexler, K. (1994). Optional infinitives, head movement and the economy of derivations. In: *Verb Movement*, eds. D. Lightfoot & N. Hornstein. Cambridge, MA: Cambridge University Press.

Wexler, K. (1998): Very early parameter setting and the unique checking constraint: a new explanation of the optional infinitive stage. *Lingua* **106**, 23–79.

World Health Organization (1992): Tenth Revision of the International Classification of Diseases and Related Health Problems (ICD-10). Geneva: WHO.

Chapter 16

Developmental language delay in early childhood: differential diagnosis between specific language delay and language delay secondary to other communication disorders

Bruna Molteni, Gloria Airaghi, Giulia Mantegazza and Daniela Sarti

Service for the Diagnosis and Rehabilitation of Language and Learning Disorders, Department of Developmental Neurology, National Neurologic Institute 'C. Besta', via Celoria 11, 20133 Milan, Italy
lingapp@istituto-besta.it

Summary

Developmental language delay is one of the main reasons for seeking medical advice in preschool children. Language delay is widely recognized as being a symptom of various childhood developmental disorders, including specific language impairment, mental deficiency, various disorders affecting social interaction, neurological diseases, and sensory deficits.

Thanks to the increasing awareness of physicians, school staff, and parents, the age at which a child is first referred has decreased and referral is no longer delayed in the hope of spontaneous recovery.

Common to all international classifications, a diagnosis of language delay or specific language impairment still rests on exclusion rather than inclusion criteria, the latter implying deficits in the production and/or comprehension of language. When dealing with children who do not speak or who speak very little, the first diagnostic issue to address does not relate to the type of language disorder, but rather to the presence of a specific language problem, in contrast to a problem secondary to hearing deficit or other psycho-developmental disorders. As it is impossible to assess language and communication properly without considering their pragmatic and social aspects, an early and reliable diagnosis relies on the availability of observational instruments which allow one to demonstrate, quantify, and analyze the child's extra-verbal communicative abilities, parent-child interactions and the possible modifications of these aspects over time.

We present data derived from a longitudinal evaluation of four children with language delay, collected using a controlled observational method. The data regarding verbal and non-verbal communicative abilities were analyzed using custom-made software specifically created to allow both quantitative and qualitative analysis. The criteria used to make a diagnosis are discussed and evaluated.

Introduction

Verbal language is a specifically human skill, but it is not the only instrument used for efficient communication. In normal children, gestures and language are tightly interconnected from the first stages of development (Iverson *et al.*, 1994). Vocal and manual babbling are recognized as being linked and related to the unitary capacity for language (Petitto & Marentette, 1991). Normal children develop their first communicative gestures at the same age as their first words. Moreover, the emergence of pointing predicts the acquisition of the first words and the development of the first word-plus-gesture combinations predict the emergence of the first word associations (Bates & Dick, 2002). The experimental withholding of gestures has a negative influence on the production of words, and when blind people speak to other blind people they produce gestures together with words (Iverson & Goldin-Meadow, 1998).

Different functional neuroimaging studies have shown that, both in monkeys and humans, the motor representations of oral and manual movements are adjacent or partially overlapping in several frontal and parietal regions, including the primary motor, ventral premotor (F4 and F5) regions, intraparietal sulcus (AIP and VIP), and inferior parietal gyrus (Rizzolatti *et al.*, 1988; Rizzolatti & Arbib, 1998; Matelli & Luppino, 2001). It is worth remembering that these same F5 and AIP areas contain mirror neurons, a specific class of visuomotor neurons that discharge both when we observe another individual performing a particular action or experiencing certain emotions, and when we ourselves perform a similar action and experience a similar emotion. The discovery of this neurophysiological system has paved the way for a better comprehension of those 'learning' processes underlying the human capacity to learn by imitation, and to understand and share other people's emotions (Gentilucci *et al.*, 1988; Gallese *et al.*, 1996; Rizzolatti *et al.*, 2001; Buccino *et al.*, 2004; Gallese, 2004; Rizzolatti & Craighero, 2004). Perception, imitation, and spontaneous production of language are therefore superimposed on a set of neural systems that are shared with the perception, imitation, and spontaneous production of manual gestures (Bates & Dick, 2002).

In particular situations, such as children who are 'late talkers' or have focal brain injuries, a dissociation between language and gesture development, and between comprehension and expression within language itself may be observed (Bates *et al.*, 1997; Bates & Dick, 2002). Late talkers in whom word comprehension and gesture production are spared but who have a selective delay in word production usually have a favourable prognosis and eventually move into the normal range. By contrast, late talkers who are also delayed in word comprehension and gesture production tend to remain delayed, in some cases manifesting a more serious language disorder.

Children with focal brain injury involving the left temporal lobe display a severe delay in language production, with sparing of both word comprehension and gesture production. By contrast, children with right parietal focal lesions appear to be mildly delayed in both word comprehension and production, while being severely delayed in gesture production (Bates & Dick, 2002).

Taken as a whole, these observations suggest that the right hemisphere (especially the parietal lobe) plays a crucial role in the first phases of development, when language is still not mastered and context-derived information provides robust proprioceptive and visual support for language comprehension and gesture production. By contrast, less context is available to infants for the successful achievement of speech production, a skill that will later be mastered by the left hemisphere. This hypothesis fits with the observation that gesture-related communication emerges very early in life, suggesting its crucial role in sustaining the mediation of extrinsically driven information and, eventually, the emergence of language.

Language delay may be a symptom of a wide range of developmental disorders of infancy, including autistic spectrum disorders, disorders secondary to severe early global deprivation, severe mental impairment, and specific language disorders. The difficulty distinguishing between such a range of different disorders is attributable to the fact that, in very young children, different aetiological factors may result in the same overt symptoms. Furthermore, the behavioral neuropathology differs somewhat among children, both because of the high degree of plasticity of the infant brain and because the same behavior may reflect the involvement of neuronal networks specific to each individual. This means that there is no universal basis for either of the three levels of causality – aetiological, neuropathological, or neuropsychological – because both localization of function and plasticity are strongly influenced by experience and the environment. For this reason, children may 'shift' from one diagnosis to another over time, making the formulation of a diagnosis a dynamic process. Rather than consisting of a mere cataloguing of symptoms and description of surface behaviors, formulating a diagnosis actually involves the analysis of hidden factors, including environmental risk and protection factors, the child's potential, possibly deviant modes employed in establishing relationships, and mechanisms of defense. In this respect, it is worth underlining that the causes of developmental neuropsychological disorders are virtually always multiple and interacting.

The diagnosis of specific language delay in very young children who do not speak, or whose verbal production is too scanty to allow a complete formal language assessment, rests on the need to exclude definitively sensory – especially hearing – deficits, impairment of reciprocal social interaction, and the presence of mental retardation. The psycholinguistic diagnostic model we refer to is a cognitive-interactional one, according to which the communicative 'function' always precedes the linguistic 'structure'. The aim of the clinical evaluation, carried out by different professionals, is to assess the child's verbal and non-verbal potential in the context of a communicative interaction. The observational setting, ideally to be videotaped, must take into account the child's age and level of cognitive and emotional development. The evaluation may be carried out through observations of the child's play in free situations, with or without the parents, or in a semistructured setting in the presence of the parents. The use of prearranged settings makes possible an easier longitudinal analysis of the clinical data and a better evaluation of the therapeutic results. Moreover, it is advisable to use questionnaires exploring the child's communicative development and, when possible, standardized test material.

In our department, data collection encompasses the objectives that we consider most important for reliable clinical observations. These include:

(1) Assessment of verbal and non-verbal comprehension, derived from the analysis of all behavioural and verbal responses. Comprehension must be evaluated with and without contextual support, in order to amplify a possible dissociation between verbal and gestural production and comprehension.

(2) Assessment of verbal and non-verbal communicative expression, achieved by considering different competences:
- Communicative functions, including actions aimed at regulating other people's behaviour, actions exclusively aimed at social interaction, and actions aimed at sharing attention with others
- Communicative roles, assessing whether the child's communication is spontaneous, in reply, or imitative
- Communicative means, including eye gaze and mimicry, vocal and verbal production, and gestures.

(3) The evaluation of three different features of play:
- Decontextualization – that is, the increasing presence of representational skills
- Ability to integrate separate actions in coordinated behavioral sequences
- Decentralization, that is the ability to involve other individuals besides oneself in the play.

In this chapter, we report features of the clinical course of four children who presented with a delay in language development secondary to various disorders. Our goal in describing their clinical verbal and non-verbal communicative behaviours, assessed applying the observational method just described, was to identify the most significant features for making a diagnosis.

Method

We evaluated four boys with severe language delay. Their ages ranged from 29 to 49 months (Table 1). All children underwent a thorough neurological, psychological, and logopaedic evaluation, and other tests: electroencephalography (EEG), brain magnetic resonance imaging (MRI), standard audiometric screening, brain-stem auditory and slow vertex evoked potentials, to exclude other disorders, including sensorineural hearing loss, CNS malformations, and EEG abnormalities.

The parents were asked to complete the Italian version of the MacArthur Communicative Developmental Inventory (Caselli & Casadio, 1995), which documented that all children scored in the 12-15 months range for word expression, and in the 12-30 months range for word comprehension. They all had normal non-verbal intelligence scores on the Griffiths Developmental Scale (Griffiths, 1970).). At the time of the initial observation, the two possibly autistic children were also evaluated with the Child Autism Rating Scale (CARS) (Schopler et al., 1980) for a better assessment of their behavioral features.

Following the initial clinical evaluation, a tentative diagnostic hypothesis was formulated for each child, including autism of severe and mild degree in two of the children (#1 and 2) based on their CARS scores, specific language impairment in one child (#4); and language delay associated with psychomotor delay in one case (#3).

All children were subsequently treated. The two autistic children (Cases 1 and 2) underwent psychomotor treatment in other centres; Case 3, who presented with psychomotor and language delay, was given logopaedic therapy; and Case 4 who had a specific language disorder was treated in our institute, focusing first on the mother-child interaction, then shifting to formal logopaedic therapy.

All the boys were evaluated serially with videotaped recordings lasting 1 hour each, following the criteria outlined above. A 10-minute fragment showing an episode of symbolic play with a toy house was selected from the videotapes of the first and last clinical observation and was used to analyze in detail the communicative-linguistic abilities of each child. According to Bonifacio & Stefani (2004), this context is the most effective one for soliciting the child's speech production.

Table 1. Results of language tests and diagnosis at the first evaluation

Children	Age (months)	Verbal production (MacArthur CDI)	Verbal comprehension (MacArthur CDI)	Diagnostic hypothesis
1	33	14-15 months	12-13 months	Severe autism
2	29	14-15 months	16-17 months	Mild autism
3	49	14-15 months	30 months	Psychomotor and language delay
4	33	12-13 months	30 months	Specific language delay

MacArthur CDI: MacArthur Communicative Developmental Inventory (Caselli & Casadio, 1995)

The last observation took place 16 to 24 months after the first, and included quantitative language tests including *Primo Vocabolario del Bambino* (PVB) (Caselli & Casadio, 1995), the *Peabody Picture Vocabulary Test* (PPVT) (Dunn & Dunn, 2000), the *Syntactic Comprehension Test* (Rustioni Metz Lancaster, D. 1993), and a new diagnosis was formulated (Table 2).

Given the severe delay in language development, which precluded the analysis of more complex features of language, we selected and analyzed only some of the domains included in our observational method (Table 3). The data were then processed using custom-made software which yielded both qualitative analysis and longitudinal comparison of each child's communicative skill.

Table 2. Results of language tests and diagnosis at the final evaluation

Children	Age (months)	Lexical Production (PVB)	Lexical Comprehension (PPVT)	Syntactic Comprehension (Rustioni)	Diagnosis
1	53	26-27 months	–	–	Mild autism
2	53	28-29 months	–	–	Mild autism
3	65	26-27 months	QV 80	4.0-4.6 years level	Psychomotor and language delay
4	56	28-29 months	QV 93	4.6-5.0 years level	Specific language delay

PVB: Primo Vocabolario del Bambino (Caselli & Casadio, 1995); PPVT: Peabody Picture Vocabulary Test (Dunn & Dunn, 2000); QV = verbal quotient; -: not determined.

Table 3. Features of language evaluated in our observational method

A. Communicative intents
- Request for attention, for action and for information
- Declarative utterance regarding an object
- Declarative self-referential utterance

B. Communicative means
- Eye gaze towards the social partner
- Joint attention
- Eye gaze towards the social partner plus pointing: requesting or declarative pointing followed or preceded by eye gaze
- Total verbal-plus-gesture mixed production
- Verbal production: spontaneous, in reply, imitative, echolalic
- Gesture production: spontaneous, in reply, imitative, echopraxic
- Mixed verbal and gesture production: spontaneous, in reply, imitative, echopraxic/echolalic
- Mean length of utterance
- Verbal production/unit of time
- Total number of different words
- Total pointing to request and to declare
- Total different referential gesture

C. Syntactic structure
- Total word-plus-gesture associations with same or different meaning
- Total gesture-plus-gesture associations with different meaning
- Total two-word utterances
- Total complete or incomplete simple nuclear phrases
- Total complete or incomplete expanded nuclear phrases
- Total complete or incomplete complex phrases

Results

Requesting and declarative utterances

Table 4 details the frequency with which the boys used verbal language to request or comment. Case 2, the more severely autistic boy, never uttered a *request for attention* either at baseline or at outcome. Cases 1 and 3 expressed a few but the least severely affected boy, Case 4, made the most. All the boys produced *requests for action* and *requests for information* at observation 2, even the two autistic boys who had made none at baseline. The numbers of utterances tended to increase most in Case 4 who, with a specific language delay, was the least severely affected child of the four; this remained true throughout most of this study.

Declarative utterances regarding an object were absent in all the children at baseline but, except for Case 3, were documented during the last observation, especially in Cases 2 and 4. None of the boys produced *self-referential declarative utterances* at the first observation; at the last, only the two non-autistic boys did so: the boy with overall delay once only, whereas the boy with specific language delay did so frequently.

Means of communication

Table 5 provides details on the ways the boys used language and gestures communicatively. *Eye gaze towards the social partner* was documented at the first observation only in the two non-autistic children in whom it remained sparse at outcome, whereas it had increased most dramatically in the boy with overall delay. *Joint attention* increased dramatically with time in all the boys, including in the less severely autistic one where it had been completely lacking at baseline. Only the boy with specific language d
elay was *pointing to request preceded by eye gaze towards the social partner* at the first observation and he was the only one to show *declarative pointing preceded by eye gaze towards the social partner* at the last observation. Neither of the autistic boys developed pointing as a communicative skill.

It should be noted that at the first observation, *total verbal production* was highest in the more severely autistic boy (Case 1), but the total included echolalic utterances which were not self-generated or fully meaningful. By the last observation, Case 4, predictably, was the most verbal.

Table 4. Number of the 'communicative intents' at the first and last observation (obs.)

Children and Diagnoses		1 More severe autism		2 Milder autism		3 Delayed development and language		4 Specific language delay	
		1st obs.	2nd obs.	1st obs.	2nd obs.	1st obs.	2nd obs.	1st obs.	2nd obs.
Requesting utterances	For attention	2	3	0	0	3	2	9	9
	For action	0	7	0	2	2	6	4	13
	For information	0	3	0	2	0	4	1	4
Declarative utterances	Regarding an object	0	2	0	12	0	0	0	15
	Regarding subject (self-referential)	0	0	0	0	0	1	0	9

Table 5. Number of different means of communication at the first and last observation

Children and Diagnoses			1 More severe autism		2 Milder autism		3 Delayed development and language		4 Specific language delay	
			1st obs.	2nd obs.	1st obs.	2nd obs.	1st obs.	2nd obs.	1st obs.	2nd obs.
Eye gaze towards the social partner			0	3	0	3	8	33	21	28
Joint attention			9	39	0	22	10	20	22	64
Eye gaze towards the social partner plus pointing	Pointing to request followed by eye gaze		0	0	0	0	0	0	0	0
	Pointing to request preceded by eye gaze		0	0	0	0	0	1	3	2
	Declarative pointing followed by eye gaze		0	0	0	0	0	0	0	0
	Declarative pointing preceded by eye gaze		0	0	0	0	0	0	0	3
Total verbal productions			15	29	2	21	6	20	3	55
Total gesture productions			0	1	0	0	5	22	10	3
Total verbal-plus-gesture productions			0	12	0	0	2	4	11	12
Verbal productions	Spontaneous		2	13	2	16	0	10	1	39
	In reply		1	14	0	3	5	9	2	16
	Non-echolalic imitations		5	2	0	2	1	1	0	0
	Echolalic		7	0	0	0	0	0	0	0
Gesture productions	Spontaneous		0	0	0	0	4	0	2	0
	In reply		0	1	0	0	1	22	8	3
	Non-echolalic imitations		0	0	0	0	0	0	0	0
	Echopraxic		0	0	0	0	0	0	0	0
Mixed verbal and gesture productions	Spontaneous		0	3	0	0	2	3	11	11
	In reply		0	9	0	0	0	1	0	1
	Non-echolalic imitations		0	0	0	0	0	0	0	0
	Echopraxic/echolalic		0	0	0	0	0	0	0	0
Mean length of utterances			0,53	1,44	0,50	2,95	1,00	1,67	0,79	1,90
Verbal productions per unit time			3,8	2,9	0,7	3,5	0,6	0,8	0,4	3,9
Total number of different words			8	32	1	38	3	28	9	85
Total pointing	To request		0	0	0	0	1	1	4	2
	To declare		0	0	0	0	0	0	0	3
Total different referential gestures			0	2	0	0	2	3	7	1

As one might expect, *total gesture production* was absent at both evaluations in the two autistic boys. That gestures paradoxically decreased over time in Case 4 probably reflects his better verbal skills that those of the other three boys. *Total verbal-plus-gesture productions* were absent in Cases 1 and 2; they failed to develop in the less severely autistic boy but increased dramatically in the more severely affected.

Spontaneous verbal productions and *verbal replies*, which were absent or scarce at baseline in all the children, increased significantly in all of them, especially Case 4. Case 2 is the only boy who had no *verbal replies* at baseline and still very few at outcome. *Non-echolalic verbal imitations* and *echolalia* were observed mainly in Child 1, the more verbal and more severely affected autistic boy.

By *spontaneous gesture production*, we refer to communicative gestures used to clarify meaning or substitute for speech. Only the two non-autistic boys produced occasional gestures spontaneously at the first observation. The reason for the sharp increase over time of gestures-as-replies in Case 4, the boy with overall delay, is not clear. Communicative gestures of any type remained virtually absent in the autistic boys. None of the boys *imitated* or *echoed gestures* or *mixed words and gestures*. Only the non-autistic boys produced *mixed verbal utterances and gestures* spontaneously, and it was the more communicative boy with specific language delay who produced the largest number. By the time of the last observation, Case 1 was also producing mixed gestural and verbal productions spontaneously but he did so manly to reply. Extremely sparse or absent gesturing is reflected by virtually absent pointing in the boys with autism. Pointing was noted but infrequent in the other boys and was used essentially only for requesting.

Mean length of utterance (MLU) was one word or less in all the children at baseline. By the last observation it had increased in all the children, but surprisingly it was the less autistic of the two boys, with the lowest MLU at baseline, who had the highest MLU at outcome when it approached 3, compared to below 2 in the other boys. Fluency, expressed as *verbal production per unit time*, was highest in the more severely autistic boy, but this child had produced many echolalic utterances at the time of the first evaluation. It improved a great deal in Cases 2 and 4 but remained essentially unimproved in the boy with global delay.

The *total number of different words*, a measure of the richness of the vocabulary, was extremely small in all the children at the first observation, but had increased in all of them by the time of the last observation, especially in Case 4.

Syntax

Table 6 shows the severity of the boy's language impairment, as no child produced two-word utterances at baseline, and only the two children with language delay (Cases 3 and 4) produced word-plus-gesture associations, whether the gesture had a meaning that was the same as or different from the word. By the last observation all the children produced two-word utterances, with Case 4 producing the most. Simple nuclear phrases were documented in all children, but only at the time of the last observation, and even in Case 4 they were exceptional.

Discussion

The main finding in this study is a confirmation that a number of features clearly differentiate children with delayed language who are also autistic from those in whom delayed language is the chief problem. It also shows that there are features that characterize children with specific

Table 6. Progress in syntactic structure between the first and last observation (obs.)

Children and Diagnoses		1 More severe autism		2 Milder autism		3 Delayed development and language		4 Specific language delay	
		1st obs.	2nd obs.	1st obs.	2nd obs.	1st obs.	2nd obs.	1st obs.	2nd obs.
Two word or gesture utterances	Word-plus-gestures with same meaning	0	4	0	0	0	0	3	1
	Word-plus-gestures with different meanings	0	1	0	0	2	0	6	0
	Gesture-plus-gesture	0	0	0	0	0	0	1	0
	Two word	0	4	0	8	0	7	0	12
Nuclear phrases	Incomplete	0	3	0	2	0	3	0	12
	Complete	0	2	0	5	0	3	0	7
Expanded nuclear phrases	Incomplete	0	0	0	0	0	0	0	0
	Complete	0	0	0	0	0	0	0	2
Complex phrases	Incomplete	0	0	0	0	0	0	0	1
	Complete	0	0	0	0	0	0	0	0

language delay from those with more global delay. Thirdly, it emphasizes the importance of gestural communication in the habilitation of preschoolers with impaired language.

Selected communicative behaviours present from early on are reliable diagnostic indices to distinguish between specific language disorder and pervasive developmental disorder. These include lack of requests for action and information, lack of eye contact, failure to use gestures either spontaneously or to reply, total failure to point, lack of referential gestures, complete lack of word-plus-gesture combination. Persistent absence of self-referential declarative behaviour characterized the autistic children at the time of the last observation.

Analysis of the data over time suggest that certain behaviours are reliable indices of the progressive acquisition of social and communicative abilities in preschoolers with autism. These include an increase in requests for attention and the appearance of requests for action and information, the emergence of utterances related to an object, the development of eye contact (even if rare), progressive ability for joint attention, the appearance of mixed word-plus-gesture communications (whether spontaneous or in reply), and, finally, the appearance of referential gestures.

At the time of the first evaluation, all the children had profoundly immature communicative skills and severely delayed language, as none of them produced declarative utterances. What set apart the two children with language delay is that they were none the less able to produce isolated requests for action, and the less severely impaired could produce rare requests for information, which are signs of communicative intent and pragmatic competence. The two boys with language delay made frequent requests for attention and the more severely autistic child also made some. Pointing preceded by looking at a social partner is widely recognized as the best index for documenting a child's awareness of the importance of sharing attention with a partner (Mundy *et al.*, 1986; Baron-Cohen *et al.*, 1996; Bernabei *et al.*, 1997; Muratori *et al.*, 1992; Camaioni *et al.*, 1997). It serves as a surrogate for robust communicative intention, which remained weak in the two autistic children, notwithstanding the increase in their verbal productions.

Gestures – either produced spontaneously or as a response and whether or not differentiated into indicative and referential gestures – clearly separated children with language disorders from those with impairment of social interaction, and this from the time of the very first clinical observation. It is worth recalling that the markedly echolalic autistic child (Case 1), who initially seemed the more severely affected according to his CARS score, progressively increased the number of his gestures and mixed productions, his joint attention towards a focus, and his requests for action, and started to make requests for information, whereas his non-communicative verbal production decreased progressively. Overall, compared to the other autistic child, this increase in gestures was a sign of a better prognosis for communicative and social competence. Thus our longitudinal analysis showed that, at the two year follow-up, the initially more severely affected child with autism (Case 1) had developed better spontaneous communicative abilities than Case 2, possibly because of more effective language intervention focused on verbal and non-verbal pragmatic abilities of the child and his parents.

These observations provide the bases which guided the clinical and rehabilitative approach to communication disorders in our institute: gesture is essential for soliciting the visual attention of the social partner and for fostering social interaction. Clinical studies (Bates *et al.*, 1997; Bates & Dick, 2002) indicate that gesture is also essential for the subsequent emergence of verbal language, and neurophysiological studies indicate its possible role in the neural basis of intersubjectivity (Gallese, 2003, 2004).

In the two children with language delay, there was a dissociation between the development of gestures and of language observable from the very first. The child with a specific language disorder (4) was delayed in verbal production, but his verbal comprehension and gesture production were in the normal range, according to the criteria of Bates and Dick (2002). By the time of the last observation, 23 months later, this boy had significantly reduced his use of gesture for communication while his language had progressed to the syntactic phase. By contrast, the dissociation between verbal comprehension, which was normal for his mental age, and gesture and language production, which were mildly delayed at the first observation, was less striking in the child with psychomotor delay (3). Sixteen months later, this child was still using significantly more gestures and mixed means of communication. Thus, although delayed, his development appeared to follow the normal course.

In conclusion, our data show that the collection of only verbal indices is inadequate to reach a correct diagnosis in the communication disorders of early childhood; studies must also consider the use of non-verbal communication means such as gestures and direction of gaze, and therapeutic interventions must aim at soliciting the use of gesture and at assisting the care-giver to foster the child's pragmatic competence.

References

Baron-Cohen, S., Cox, A., Baird, G., Swettenham, J., Nightingale, N., Morgan, K., Drew, A. & Charman, T. (1996): Psychological markers in the detection of autism in infancy in a large population. *Br. J. Psychiatry* **168**, 158–163.

Bates, E. & Dick, F. (2002): Language, gesture, and the developing brain. *Dev. Psychobiol.* **40**, 293–310.

Bates, E., Thal, D., Trauner, D., Fenson, J., Aram, D., Eisele, J. & Nass, R. (1997): From first words to grammar in children with focal brain injury. *Dev. Neuropsychol.* **13**, 275–343.

Bernabei, P., Campioni, L., Levi, G., Di Falco, M. & Paolesse, C. (1997): Lo sviluppo socio-comunicativo nei primi due anni di vita di bambini con autismo: possibilità di una diagnosi precoce. *Psicologia Clinica dello Sviluppo* **2**, 245-259.

Bonifacio, S. & Hvastja Stefani, L. (2004): *Il modello INTERACT*. Tirrenia (Pisa): Del Cerro.

Buccino, C., Vogt, S., Ritzl, A., Fink, G.R., Zilles, K., Freund, H.J. & Rizzolatti, G. (2004): Neural circuits underlying imitation learning of hand actions: an event-related fMRI study. *Neuron* **42**, 323-334.

Camaioni, L., Perucchini, P., Muratori, F. & Milone, A. (1997): Brief report: a longitudinal examination of the communicative gestures deficit in young children with autism. *J. Autism Dev. Disord.* **27**, 715-725.

Caselli, M.C. & Casadio, P. (1995): Il primo vocabolario del bambino. Guida all'uso del questionario MacArthur per la valutazione della comunicazione e del linguaggio nei primi anni di vita. Milano: FrancoAngeli.

Dunn, L.M. & Dunn, L.M. (2000): Manuale Peabody Test di vocabolario recettivo, PPVT, Peabody Picture Vocabulary Test-Revised, eds. G. Stella, C. Pizzoli & P.E. Tressoldi. Torino: Omega.

Gallese, V. (2004): Il sistema multiplo di condivisione: la ricerca di un meccanismo neurofisiologico alla base dell'intersoggettività. *Infanzia e adolescenza* **3**, 128-144.

Gallese, V., Fadiga, L., Fogassi, L. & Rizzolatti G. (1996): Action recognition in the premotor cortex. *Brain* **119**, 593-609.

Gentilucci, M., Fogassi, L., Luppino, G., Matelli, M., Camarda, R. & Rizzolatti, G. (1988): Functional organization of inferior area 6 in the macaque monkey: I. Somatotopy and the control of proximal movements. *Exp. Brain Res.* **71**, 475-490.

Griffiths, R. (1970): The abilities of young children. High Wycombe, UK: The Test Agency Ltd.

Iverson, J.M., Capirci, O. & Caselli, M.C. (1994): From communication to language in two modalities. *Cognitive Development* **9**, 23-43.

Iverson, J.M. & Goldin-Meadow, S. (1998): Why people gesture when they speak. *Nature* **396**: 228.

Matelli, M. & Luppino, G. (2001): Parietofrontal circuits for action and space perception in the macaque monkey. *Neuroimage* **14**, S27-S32.

Mundy, P., Sigman, M., Ungerer, J. & Sherman, T. (1986): Defining the social deficit of autism: the contribution of non-verbal communication measures. *J. Child Psychol. Psychiatry* **27**, 657-669.

Muratori, F., Bernazzani, I., Cerri, B. & Conti, P. (1992): L'organizzazione preverbale del linguaggio nelle psicosi precoci. *Gior. Neuropsich. Età Evol.* **12**, 91-101.

Petitto, L.A. & Marentette, P.F. (1991): Babbling in the manual mode: evidence for the ontogeny of language. *Science* **251**, 1493-1496.

Rizzolatti, G. & Arbib, M.A. (1998): Language within our grasp. *Trends Neurosci.* **21**, 188-194.

Rizzolatti, G. & Craighero, L. (2004): The mirror-neuron system. *Annu. Rev. Neurosci.* **27**, 169-192.

Rizzolatti, G., Camarda, R., Fogassi, L., Gentilucci, M., Luppino, G. & Matelli, M. (1988): Functional organization of inferior area 6 in the macaque monkey: II. Area F5 and the control of distal movements. *Exp. Brain Res.* **71**, 491-507.

Rizzolatti, G., Fogassi, L. & Gallese, V. (2001): Neurophysiological mechanisms underlying the understanding and imitation of action. *Nat. Rev. Neurosci.* **2**, 661-670.

Rustioni Metz Lancaster, D. (1993): Prova di valutazione della comprensione linguistica. Firenze: O.S. Organizzazioni Speciali.

Schopler, E., Reichler, R.J., De Vellis, R.F. & Daly, K. (1980): Toward objective classification of childhood autism: Childhood Autism Rating Scale (CARS). *J. Autism Dev. Disord.* **10**, 91-103.

Chapter 17

The natural history of early language delay: from late talking to specific language impairment

Anna Maria Chilosi, Paola Cipriani, Lucia Pfanner, Chiara Pecini and Tiziana Fapore

Department of Developmental Neurosciences, Fondazione Stella Maris-University of Pisa, via dei Giacinti 2, 56018 Calambrone (Pisa), Italy
achilosi@inpe.unipi.it

Summary

An important question in the field of language disorders is whether late talkers and preschool children with specific language impairment (SLI) belong to fundamentally different categories. Until recently, however, there have been few consistent longitudinal data on which to base diagnostic and prognostic statements for children under age 3 and for identifying the early manifestations of later language impairment.
The aim of the present study was to provide some diagnostic and prognostic guidelines by analysing language development longitudinally in 52 late-talking children (39 boys and 13 girls) followed from the third to the fourth year of life. Language testing was done through a combination of indirect (parental report) and direct procedures. At the first evaluation (mean age 28 months) all the late-talking children had deficits affecting different aspects of linguistic performance such as phonology, lexicon, and syntactic skills. However at the short-term follow-up (38 months), three different developmental trajectories emerged from the analysis of language outcome, which suggests three different clinical conditions. By 28 months of age it was already possible to detect some significant differences among groups on tests of productive vocabulary and receptive and expressive grammar, but the predictive value of linguistic measures changed with age and stage of language acquisition. The careful monitoring of language-delayed children through the 30 to 44 months age period is therefore warranted to ensure that significant progress in lexical and grammatical development has occurred.

Specific language impairment (SLI) refers to a selective failure to develop language at a normal rate in the absence of frank cognitive, neurological, or sensory deficits and psychiatric disorders, and in spite of adequate social and educational opportunities for learning language (*Diagnostic and Statistical Manual of Mental Disorders*, 4th edition, DSM-IV). The pathophysiology of SLI is still poorly defined but recent research suggests that genetic mechanisms play a major role, although it is still not known how this genetic influence operates (for a review see Bishop, 2000). Although different subgroups of children with SLI have been widely described (Rapin & Allen, 1988; Haynes & Naidoo, 1991; Robinson, 1991; Rapin 1996, Chilosi et al., 2002), most of the research on the clinical characterization of the disorder has been cross-sectional. It is therefore still unclear whether the patterns of difficulty identified at an early age are stable over time or whether children tend to move from one subgroup to another in terms of the types of linguistic profile delineated by the available systems of classification (*International Classification of Diseases*, ICD 10 and DSM-IV).

The incidence of SLI varies with age and is highest in 24- to 36-month-old children; however, the prevalence of persistent disorders is estimated to be 3 per cent (Silva, 1987; Whitehurst & Fischel, 1994; Stella & Marini, 2002). SLI is a complex area of investigation because of the broad interindividual variability that characterizes normal language development, and because linguistic competence includes a set of abilities that can be delayed or deficient depending on different lines of investigation or dimensions of development. Moreover, the pattern of impairment tends to change with age, so that a longitudinal perspective is needed for an understanding of the early origins of the disorder.

Early language delay has been the focus of research by several investigators in the past 15 years (Fischel *et al.*, 1989; Thal *et al.*, 1991; Paul, 1993; Paul & Alforde, 1993; Paul *et al.*, 1997; Rescorla *et al.*, 1997; Rescorla, *et al.*, 2000; Rescorla, 2002; Bishop *et al.*, 2003; Dale *et al.*, 2003; Rescorla, 2005), as late-talking children are known to be at risk for persistent language problems, emotional disorders, and later learning disabilities. Follow-up studies have found that approximately half the toddlers with delayed onset of language catch up with their peers by 3 years and have no further language difficulties (Bishop & Edmundson, 1987; Rescorla & Schwartz, 1990). Until recently, however, there have been few consistent data on which to base diagnostic and prognostic statements for children under 3 with circumscribed language delay, as the issue of what factors best predict later language outcome is still controversial.

The term 'late talker' (as currently used by many investigators) is applied to a child aged between 18 and 30 months with an expressive vocabulary score at or below the 10th centile at 24 months and/or with no multiword combinations at 30 months. Few clinical studies with formal assessment of receptive language skills have been published, on the assumption that before 28 months production tasks which tap into the vocabulary burst (typically occurring between 18 and 24 months) may themselves tap into processes that also involve aspects of comprehension (Bates *et al.*, 1988). This assumption supports the view that reliable and valid measures of expressive language would detect not only children with expressive delay but also the vast majority of those with comprehension problems (Whitehurst & Fischel, 1994). However, in toddlers with delayed language acquisition the evaluation of comprehension may be highly informative, given their limited repertoire of expressive skills, which may confuse different types of possible underlying dysfunction.

Among the early predictors of language outcome in young children, three have received most attention: the severity of initial expressive language delay; the degree of impairment of receptive as well as expressive abilities; and the degree of impairment of gestural communication.

In this chapter we report on the results of an ongoing project involving a large sample of late-talking children who were tested repeatedly from an early age through the preschool years, with the aim of providing some diagnostic and prognostic guidelines based on early linguistic profiles and their modes of development.

Methods

Subjects

Subjects were selected from a large population of children referred for language delay to the Department of Developmental Neuroscience of the Stella Maris Scientific Institute, according to the following criteria:

- expressive vocabulary, evaluated using the Italian version of the MacArthur-Bates Inventories (Questionario 'Il Primo Vocabolario del Bambino' (PVB), Caselli & Casadio, 1995), at or below the 10th centile and/or absence of combinatorial language at 24 to 30 months;
- comprehensive longitudinal linguistic assessment with at least two evaluations between the second and the fourth year of life (T1 and T2), and an interval of at least 6 months between the two consecutive observations;
- normal cognitive development: full-scale developmental quotient (80) at the time of the first evaluation (Griffiths scales; Griffiths, 1954, 1984), and absence of auditory deficits and behavioural and socio-emotional disorders.

On the basis of these criteria, we selected 52 children (39 boys and 13 girls). Their mean age at the first observation (T1) was 28 months (range 18 to 34) and at the second observation (T2) 38 months (range 34 to 49). The mean interval between T1 and T2 was 10 months. Thirty-five children were followed to a mean age of 49 months (range 40 to 65) (T3) as their language was still delayed at T2 (for four persistently delayed children at T2, the T3 follow-up data were not available because evaluation could only be carried out at an older age).

The children were divided into three groups: in group 1, none of the children received direct language intervention. In group 2, only four children underwent language intervention, while in group 3 all the children received direct language treatment. In particular, 22 children were followed during intensive language treatment in our department (mean age at intake, 38.7 months).

Linguistic assessment

Language evaluation was done through a combination of indirect (parental report) and direct procedures.

Expressive vocabulary was tested by means of the MacArthur-Bates Infant and Toddler Communication Development Inventories (Italian version, PVB) which cover the age from 8 to 30 months. For children markedly delayed in language development well past the age range normally covered by the PVB, assignment of scores was based on language level rather than on chronological age. The analyses presented here are based on raw scores for total words and on lexical quotient (LQ), corresponding to the ratio between lexical age (assigned by determining the age at which a particular score corresponds to the median in the normative sample) and chronological age.

Expressive grammar was evaluated by analysing language samples collected in our laboratory during a standardised play situation involving the child and the child's parents. Speech was transcribed independently by one of us (L.P.) and by a trained research assistant (interobserver agreement reached 90 per cent). The level of grammatical development was defined on a six-level rating system [the Grid for the Analysis of Spontaneous Speech (GASS)] developed by Cipriani *et al.* (1993), ranging from level 0 (prelinguistic stage) to level 5 (complex grammar). Level 0 corresponds to a prelinguistic stage, as spontaneous language production is limited to babble, sounds, and sporadic single words, while at level 1 (holophrastic stage), though true words are few in number, single-word utterances begin to be used consistently. Level 2 corresponds to the emergence of combinatorial speech, but single word utterances clearly prevail. At level 3 multiword utterances are far more common, though many grammatical rules are still missing. The following two levels mark the transition from ungrammatical or telegraphic speech to the emergence of grammar, because in the normal 28- to 36-month-old child they lead to a fairly complete control of complex grammar. At level 4 children are able to control the basic rules of the main clause, and at level 5 their competencies extend over many types of complex sentences.

Verbal comprehension was examined with a receptive language test that includes 56 items of increasing complexity, consisting of verbal commands that the child is required to act out with a set of toys and familiar objects. Complexity varies with respect to sentence length (from one to two and three words), semantic complexity (predictable *vs.* unpredictable or anomalous sentences), agency (child *vs.* object agent of the action). Individual z scores were obtained on the basis of Italian norms available for children aged from 16 to 36 months (Chilosi *et al.*, 2003).

Language measures at T3 were as follows:

- *Peabody, Picture vocabulary test (PPVT)* (Dunn & Dunn, 1997; Stella *et al.*, 2000; standardized Italian version) for the assessment of lexical comprehension in children from 3 years 9 months to 11 years 6 months;
- One-word picture vocabulary test (Brizzolara *et al.*, 1994), a picture matching test of lexical production that has been standardized on Italian-speaking children aged between 4 years 6 months and 10 years;
- Test of Comprehension of Grammar for Children (TCGB) (Chilosi & Cipriani, 1995), a multiple choice test that assesses the child's ability to understand orally presented grammatical structures and contrasts (percentile and standard scores are available for children aged from 3 years 6 months to 8 years);
- Test of sentence repetition (De Vescovi & Caselli, 2001) and test of repetition of clitic pronouns (Bottari *et al.*, 1998);
- Spontaneous language analysis according to the five levels of the GASS grading (see above).

Results

First observation (T1)

At group level the children showed a severe expressive delay that involved phonology, vocabulary and grammar (Table 1).

Vocabulary

The mean number of words produced by the whole sample at T1 was 61.3, with high interindividual variability (SD=68). The above value corresponds to a mean age equivalent score of about 18 to 19 months, reflecting an average delay of about 10 months. The mean lexical quotient was 62.8 (range 40.7 to 89); in 75 per cent of the cases the lexical quotient fell below 70; in the remaining children it did not reach a score of 90.

Table 1. Means (standard deviations) of scores obtained by the whole sample at T1

	Mean (SD)
Word production (number)	61.3 (68)
Lexical quotient	62.8 (11.4)
Verbal comprehension (z score)	−1.7 (1.7)
Grammatical level*	Median=1; range 0 to 3

* Grammatical level was measured on an ordinal scale, thus the median instead of the mean was calculated.

Grammatical production

The median expressive grammatical score for the whole sample was 1 (range 0 to 3). None of the children scored at a normal level for their age, showing a variable degree of delay in expressive grammar: 80 per cent of children had very primitive language organization (pre-verbal or holophrastic speech), and only 20 per cent were starting to combine words.

Verbal comprehension

The mean receptive z score of the whole sample was –1.7. Receptive abilities were delayed in 60 per cent of the sample, with 27 per cent showing moderate delay (scores 1 SD below the mean) and 33 per cent scoring more than 2 SD below the mean; 40 per cent of the sample had normal verbal comprehension skills.

Linguistic follow-up

At T2 most of the children (41) had persistent language delay, while 11 showed rapid language growth with a spurt in both vocabulary and grammar. Thirty-five of the 41 children with persistent delay at T2 were followed up to a mean age of 49 months to evaluate their linguistic development further. At the third assessment (T3), 10 children (28.5 per cent) showed normalization of language performance, while 25 (71.5 per cent) had persistent impairment in one or more linguistic domains.

On the basis of these three different developmental patterns, we re-examined the data at T1, subdividing the original sample into three groups to verify whether and which of the linguistic measures at intake were predictive of language outcome. Expressive and receptive scores and statistical analyses are reported for each group in Tables 2 to 4.

Table 2. Group 1 (N=11): Mean (standard deviations) of scores at T1 and T2 and statistical comparisons (Student *t* test and Wilcoxon tests) between times

	T1	T2	*t* Test
	Mean (SD)	Mean (SD)	
Word production (number)	92.8 (84.2)	538.8 (115.2)	$t(9)=-7.5, p<0.001$
Lexical quotient	73.5 (10.4)	91.8 (11.8)	$t(9)=-4.5, p<0.001$
Verbal comprehension (z score)	–0.61 (0.9)	0.06 (0.7)	$t(6)=-2.2, p=0.07$
Grammatical level*	Median=1; range 1 to 2.5	Median=4.5; range 3 to 5	$z=-2.99, p<0.005$

* Median, range, and Wilcoxon test.

Table 3. Group 2 (N=13): Mean (standard deviation) of scores at T1 and T2 and statistical comparisons (Student *t* test and Wilcoxon tests) between times

	T1	T2	*t* Test
	Mean (SD)	Mean (SD)	
Word production (number)	78.46 (66.2)	328.5 (161.6)	$t(9)=-4.7, p<0.001$
Lexical quotient	65.89 (6.6)	70.5 (12.5)	$t(9)=-1.1$, NS
Verbal comprehension (z score)	–0.87 (1.6)	–0.52 (1.3)	$t(7)=-1.2$, NS
Grammatical level*	Median=1.5; range 1 to 3	Median=3; range 2 to 5	$z=-3.2, p<0.001$

* Median, range, and Wilcoxon test.

Table 4. Group 3 (N=28): Mean (standard deviation) of scores at T1 and T2 and statistical comparisons (Student t test and Wilcoxon tests) between times

	T1	T2	t Test
	Mean (SD)	Mean (SD)	
Word production (number)	40.3 (55.9)	265.0 (167.6)	$t(22)=-7.4, p<0.001$
Lexical quotient	57.2 (10.1)	61.8 (12.2)	$t(23)=-2.5, p<0.05$
Verbal comprehension (z score)	−2.35 (1.6)	−1.5 (2.2)	$t(22)=-2.3, p<0.05$
Grammatical level*	Median=1; range 0 to 2.5	Median=3; range 0.5 to 4	$z=-4.5, p<0.001$

* Median, range, and Wilcoxon test.

Analyses of variance conducted on chronological age at T1 and T2 showed no significant differences among the three groups at either time.

Comparisons across groups at different times of development

To test whether linguistic measures at T1 could differentiate the three groups, we used one-way analysis of variance on the numerical variables and the Kruskal-Wallis test for non-parametric measures (grammatical level). When the main effect of the group was significant, paired comparisons were undertaken with *post-hoc* correction for multiple comparisons. Statistical results obtained at T1 and at T2 are reported in Table 5 and Table 6.

A significant group effect was found at T1 on all the linguistic measures: paired comparisons showed that these differences resulted from a better performance by group 1 and group 2 in comparison with group 3; the differences between group 1 and group 2 were not statistically significant (Table 5).

At T2 the lexical quotient and the level of spontaneous language organization differentiated the three groups significantly. On both measures, paired comparisons showed a better

Table 5. Statistical differences across groups at T1

	Group effect	Post-hoc comparisons
Word production (number)	$F(2,48) = 3.1, p=0.05$	NS
Lexical quotient	$F(2,49) = 12.7, p<0.001$	G1 and G2 > G3
Verbal comprehension (z score)	$F(2,44) = 6.1, p<0.005$	G1 and G2 > G3
Grammatical level*	$\chi^2 (2)=10.5, p<0.05$	G1 and G2 > G3

* Median, range, and Wilcoxon test.

Table 6. Statistical differences across groups at T2

	Group effect	Post-hoc comparisons
Word production (number)	$F(2,41)=10.9, p<0.001$	G1 > G2 and G1 > G3
Lexical quotient	$F(2,41)=21.4, p<0.001$	G1 > G2 and G1 > G3
Verbal comprehension (z score)	$F(2,37)=2.5$, NS	NS
Grammatical level*	$\chi^2 (2)=25.7, p<0.001$	G1 > G2 > G3

* Median, range, and Wilcoxon test.

performance by group 1 in comparison with both group 2 and group 3, while group 2 scored better than group 3 only on the grammatical level (Table 6).

As children from group 1 showed rapid recovery, comparisons at T3 were conducted only between group 2 and group 3 (Table 7). Although some results may have been affected by the small number of children in group 2, statistical comparisons at T3 showed significantly worse performance by group 3 than group 2 in terms of grammatical level and phonology.

Table 7. Mean (standard deviation) of the scores obtained by group 2 and group 3 at T3

	Group 2	Group 3	t Test
	Mean (SD)	Mean (SD)	
Word production high frequency (z score)	0.62 (1.1)	−0.58 (1.6)	t(21)=1.9, p=0.08, NS
Word production low frequency (z score)	0.09 (2.3)	−1.43 (0.7)	t(11)=1.8, p=0.09, NS
Verbal comprehension (z score)	−0.4 (0.9)	−0.65 (0.9)	t(25)=0.7, NS
Repetition (z score)	−1.8 (2.8)	−3.68 (2.9)	t(14)=0.86, NS
Grammatical level*	Median=4.2; range 3.5 to 5	Median=3.5; range 1.5 to 4.5	z=−2.7, p<0.01
Phonological level*	Median=3; range 2 to 3	Median=3; range 2 to 3	z=−2.4, p<0.05

* Median, range, and Mann-Whitney U test.

The linguistic trajectory of group 1 children appears to be characterized by a mild delay in lexical and grammatical development, with normal comprehension, followed – after a slow start – by acceleration of the development rate around 33 months with catch-up in language acquisition within the third year of life. These children seem to correspond to the so-called 'late bloomers' or transiently delayed children.

The group 2 children similarly presented a language delay restricted to the expressive domain with substantially good comprehension skills. However, delay of vocabulary and grammar was still present at 3 years, in spite of a significant increase in expressive vocabulary. Nonetheless the prognosis for these children appeared to be quite favourable. In fact, between the third and the fourth year of life a rapid improvement in lexical and grammatical attainments with complete recovery of language skills occurred. These children could be defined 'slow learners', because of the pace of development.

Group 3 included children who continued to show a generalized deficit of both lexical and grammatical language abilities that did not resolve by age 4 and persisted well into the preschool years (SLI children). The initial linguistic profile was characterized by impaired verbal comprehension and by a more severe lexical and grammatical delay than in the other two groups.

Discussion

An important question in the field of language disorders is whether late talkers and preschool children with SLI belong to fundamentally different categories. Because late talkers generally have a relatively good outcome (Paul, 1996; Rescorla et al., 2000; Rescorla, 2002), they do not appear to be as 'disordered' as preschool children with SLI (Whitehurst & Fischel, 1994). Thus, from a categorical point of view late talkers are assumed to have difficulties that are different from those of SLI children whose language problems do not resolve. Viewed as belonging to a continuum of language ability (Rescorla et al., 2000; Rescorla, 2002), late talkers occupy a position that is closer to average than the position of children with SLI. In Rescorla's view, young children who are significantly delayed in expressive language after 2 years have a diathesis for weak language abilities. The most mildly impaired outgrow their delay by age 4, those with an intermediate level of SLI recover by age 5, and those most severely impaired continue to have language problems for many years.

A question of considerable clinical importance is how to distinguish early transient from persistent language difficulties in young children – that is, how to identify the early manifestations of later language impairment.

Most studies of late talkers refer to children with specific expressive language delay (SELD) and exclude children with a receptive delay. Because a primary aim of our study was early diagnosis and a better understanding of the origins of specific language impairment, children with verbal comprehension deficits were included in the experimental sample.

Our subjects also differed from those enrolled in community-based projects (in which late-talking children were recruited through questionnaires distributed in paediatric offices or through newspapers and radio advertisements) because they were referred to our clinic for language delay. The lower incidence of good short-term language outcome in our sample in comparison with published reports probably reflected this methodological bias.

At an early age all the late talking children had deficits affecting different aspects of linguistic performance such as phonology, lexical and syntactic skills. The short-term follow-up (38 months) showed three different developmental trajectories that suggest three different clinical conditions. The predictive value of linguistic measures changed with age and stage of language acquisition. By 28 months of age it was already possible to detect differences among groups. In particular, vocabulary and receptive and expressive grammar differentiated groups 1 and 2 from group 3. However at this age we did not find any significant difference between children who outgrew their language delay by age 3 (group 1) and children with a low language performance continuing past age 3 (group 2). By age 3, lexical quotient and expressive grammar were still significant indices, while verbal comprehension missed statistical significance, although group 3 children scored more than one standard deviation below the mean. At this age the level of expressive grammar was the best predictor that differentiated children with an unfavourable outcome (group 3) from both late-blooming (G1) and slow-learning children (G2).

From a clinical point of view, one implication of our study is that children who present with severe receptive-expressive language delay and more severe vocabulary lag around 24–30 months are at major risk of SLI, especially when lexical and grammatical difficulties persist past four years of age.

These data are in agreement with published reports (Paul, 1996) suggesting that careful monitoring through the 30- to 44-months period is warranted to ensure that significant progress in lexical and grammatical development has occurred. Careful monitoring may also provide decision-making criteria for selecting children who may benefit from early intervention.

This assumption relates to the issue of defining reliable guidelines for clinical management and for deciding whether and when to start treatment. From previous experience on the effects of early treatment in 20 preschool children with severe language delay (Cipriani et al., 2002), we concluded that direct intervention before 36 months is advised in the following situations: severe specific language delay of the receptive-expressive subtype; specific expressive language delay complicated by verbal dyspraxia; and severe expressive language delay in a child at a high genetic risk for SLI.

Even if the role of intervention in our group of late talking children did not appear to be a primary determinant of outcome, the results suggested that early language intervention may modify the pattern of language disorder within a relatively short time by providing external support that could act as a protective factor, with possible long-term effects (Stothard *et al.*, 1998).

References

Bates, E., Bretherton, I. & Snyder, L. (1988): *From first words to grammar*. Cambridge: Cambridge University Press.

Bishop, D.V.M. (2000): How does the brain learn language? Insights from the study of children with and without language impairment. *Dev. Med. Child Neurol.* **42**, 133–142.

Bishop, D.V.M. & Edmundson, A (1987): Language-impaired 4-year-olds: distinguishing transient from persistent impairment. *J. Speech Hear. Disord.* **52**, 156–173.

Bishop, D.V.M., Price, T.S., Dale, P.S. & Robert, P. (2003): Outcomes of early language delay: II. Etiology of transient and persistent language difficulties. *J. Speech Lang. Hear. Res.* **46**, 561–575.

Bottari, P., Cipriani, P. & Chilosi, A.M. (1998): Dissociations in the acquisition of clitic pronouns by dysphasic children: a case study from Italian. In: *The acquisition of scrambling and cliticization*, eds. C. Hamman & S. Powers. Amsterdam: Kluwer.

Brizzolara, D., Chilosi, A.M., Cipriani, P. & De Pasquale, L. (1994): L'apprendimento del linguaggio scritto nei bambini con difficoltà di acquisizione del linguaggio: continuità o discontinuità? In: *Apprendimento e patologia neuropsichica nei primi anni di scuola*, eds. G. Masi & A. Martini. Rome: Borla.

Caselli, M.C. & Casadio, P. (1995): *Il primo vocabolario del bambino*. Milan: FrancoAngeli.

Chilosi, A.M. & Cipriani, P. (1995): *TCGB: Test di Comprensione Grammaticale per Bambini*. Tirrenia: Del Cerro.

Chilosi, A.M., Cipriani, P. & Fapore, T. (2002): I disturbi specifici del linguaggio. In: *I disturbi dello sviluppo*, eds. S.Vicari & M.C. Caselli, pp. 59–76. Bologna: Il Mulino.

Chilosi, A.M., Cipriani, P., Villani, S. & Pfanner, L. (2003): Capire giocando: uno strumento per la valutazione verbale precoce (TCVP). Technical Report, Italian National Research Council, CNR002D39–004.

Cipriani, P., Chilosi, A.M., Bottari, P. & Pfanner, L. (1993): *L'acquisizione della morfosintassi in italiano: fasi e processi*. Padova: Unipress.

Cipriani, P., Fapore, T., Massei, M., Pfanner, L., Salvadorini, R.& Chilosi, A.M. (2002): Early treatment of late-talking children. *Dev. Med. Child Neurol.* suppl. 92, 44.

Dale, P.S., Price, T.S., Bishop, D.V.M. & Plomin, R. (2003): Outcomes of early language delay: I. Predicting persistent and transient language difficulties at 3 and 4 years. *J. Speech Lang. Hear. Res.* **46**, 544–560.

De Vescovi, A. & Caselli, M.C (2001): Una prova di ripetizione di frasi per la valutazione del primo sviluppo grammaticale. *Psicologia Clinica dello Sviluppo* **3**, 2001.

Dunn, L.M & Dunn, L.M (1997): *Peabody Picture Vocabulary Test-PPVT, Third Edition*. American Guidance Service Inc., Circle Pines, Minnesota, USA.

Fischel, J.E., Whitehurst, G.J., Caulfield, M.B. & DeBaryshe, B. (1989): Language growth in children with expressive language delay. *Pediatrics* **82**, 218–227.

Griffiths, R. (1954): *The ability of babies*. London: London University Press.

Griffiths, R. (1984): *The abilities of young children*. Buckingham: The Test Agency.

Haynes, C. & Naidoo, S. (1991): Children with specific speech and language impairment. *Clin. Dev. Med.* **119**, 1–289.

Paul, R. (1993): Outcomes of early expressive language delay. *J. Child. Commun. Disord.* **15**, 7–14.

Paul, R. (1996): Clinical implications of the natural history of slow expressive language delay. *Am. J. Speech Lang. Pathol.* **5**, 5–21.

Paul, R. & Alforde, S. (1993): Grammatical morpheme acquisition in 4-year-olds with normal, impaired, and late-developing language. *J. Speech Hear. Res.* **36**, 1271–1275.

Paul, R., Murray, C., Clancy, K. & Andrews, D. (1997): Reading and metaphonological outcomes in late talkers. *J. Speech Lang. Hear. Res.* **40**, 1037–1047.

Rapin, I. (1996): Practitioner review: developmental language disorders – a clinical update. *J. Child Psychol. Psychiatry* **37**, 643–655.

Rapin, I. & Allen, D.A. (1988): Syndromes in developmental dysphasia and adult aphasia. In: *Language, communication and the brain*, ed. F. Plum, pp. 57–75. New York: Raven Press.

Rescorla, L. (2002): Language and reading outcomes to age 9 in late-talking toddlers. *J. Speech Lang. Hear. Res.* **45**, 360–371.

Rescorla, L. (2005): Age 13 language and reading outcomes in late-talking toddlers. *J. Speech Lang. Hear. Res.* **48**, 459–472.

Rescorla, L. & Schwartz, E. (1990): Outcome of toddlers with expressive language delay. *Appl. Psycholinguistics* **11**, 397–407.

Rescorla, L., Roberts, J. & Dahlsgaard, K. (1997): Late-talkers at 2: outcome at age 3. *J. Speech Lang. Hear. Res.* **40**, 556–566.

Rescorla, L., Dahlsgaard, K. & Roberts, J. (2000): Late-talking toddlers: MLU and IPSyn outcomes at 3;0 and 4;0. *J. Child Lang.* **27**, 643–664.

Robinson, R. (1991): Causes and association of severe and persistent specific speech and language disorders in children. *Dev. Med. Child Neurol.* **33**, 943–962.

Silva, P.A. (1987): Epidemiology, longitudinal course and some associated factors: an update. In: *Language development and disorders*, eds. W. Yule & M. Rutter, pp. 1–15. London: MacKeith Press.

Stella, G. & Marini, A. (2002): Studio epidemiologico sulla prevalenza dei disturbi del linguaggio nei bambini in età prescolare. In: *Indici di rischio nel primo sviluppo del linguaggio*, eds. M.C. Caselli & O. Capirci, pp. 124–135. Milan: FrancoAngeli.

Stella, G., Pizzoli, C. & Tressoldi, P. (2000): *Peabody Test di Vocabolario Recettivo*. Torino: Omega.

Stothard, S.E., Snowling, M.J., Bishop, D.V., Chipchase, B.B. & Kaplan, C.A. (1998): Language-impaired preschoolers: a follow-up into adolescence. *J. Speech Lang. Hear. Res.* **41**, 407–418.

Thal, D., Tobias, S. & Morrison, D. (1991): Language and gesture in late talkers: a 1-year follow-up. *J. Speech Hear. Res.* **34**, 604–612.

Whitehurst, G.J. & Fischel, J. (1994): Practitioner review: early developmental language delay – what, if anything, should the clinician do about it? *J. Child Psychol. Psychiatry* **35**, 613–648.

Chapter 18

A follow-up study of reading and writing in Italian children with specific language impairment

Daniela Brizzolara*°, Claudia Casalini°, Filippo Gasperini*, Silvia Roncoli°, Sara Mazzotti*, Paola Cipriani*° and Anna Maria Chilosi°

* Division of Child Neurology and Psychiatry, University of Pisa, via dei Giacinti 2, 56018 Calambrone, Pisa, Italy;
° Department of Developmental Neuroscience, 'Stella Maris' Scientific Institute, Pisa, Italy
daniela.brizzolara@inpe.unipi.it

Summary

Children with specific language impairment (SLI) are at high risk for developing literacy problems – about half of them have problems in acquiring written language, thus demonstrating a continuity between oral and written language development. However, it has not been clarified which oral language deficits cause literacy problems and which aspects of the complex acquisition of literacy skills are more compromised by the linguistic deficits of SLI children. Moreover, few studies have focused so far on the literacy outcome of children with different types of SLI.
In this chapter we complement some of the problems in the development of reading and writing a group of children with SLI (n = 33) encountered in the first stages of literacy (first and second grades) with longitudinal data. We also address the problem of differential literacy outcomes in children with different types of SLI (according to DSM-IV criteria); the linguistic impairment affected morphosyntactic and phonologic domains at the input and output level (mixed receptive-expressive language disorder) or at the output level only (expressive language disorder) and the phonological domain only (phonological disorder).
Children with SLI appear to have a slow start in learning to read and write; however, not all children with SLI in the preschool years have problems with reading and writing. Our data confirm the evidence that children with morphosyntactic and phonologic deficits have a higher risk of difficulties in literacy acquisition than those with isolated phonological problems who have a better outcome.

Introduction

The relation between specific language impairment and dyslexia

Children with specific language impairment (SLI) are at high risk for developing reading disabilities; it is estimated that about 50 per cent of children with SLI have problems acquiring written language (Catts, 1993). Longitudinal data on English-speaking children show that, when the language problems persist into school age, literacy difficulties are very common, whereas literacy outcome is far better and often normal when the children have resolved their language problems by the start of elementary school (Bishop & Adams, 1990;

Catts et al., 2002). These data seem to support a continuity between oral and written language development; however, it is not yet clear which oral language deficits cause literacy problems and which aspects of the complex acquisition of literacy skills are more likely to be compromised by the linguistic deficits of SLI. Both SLI and specific reading and writing difficulties (dyslexia and dysgraphia) are heterogeneous disorders. SLI includes a wide range of difficulties – phonological, morphosyntactic, lexical, and semantic at the expressive or receptive level, or both. On the other hand, there are different subtypes of dyslexia depending on whether the difficulties affect sublexical procedures of reading (phonological dyslexia) or spare them, affecting semantic/lexical procedures (surface dyslexia).

The relation between SLI and dyslexia is a complex one; for some investigators, SLI and dyslexia are manifestations of the same pathology, a 'language learning impairment' that manifests itself in different ways at different developmental stages (Catts, 1991; Tallal et al., 1997). For others they are distinct disorders which share many similarities (Bishop & Snowling, 2004).

The research on the linguistic deficits shared by children with SLI and children with dyslexia has focused mainly on the phonological aspects of language, stimulated by the 'phonological core deficit' hypothesis of dyslexia (Stanovich & Siegel, 1994). There are substantial experimental data documenting the presence of oral language deficits in dyslexic children (reviewed in Snowling, 2000). McArthur & Bishop (2001), in a study examining 110 children with a specific reading disability, used a battery of oral language tasks widely used to identify children with SLI (CELF-R, Semel et al., 1987), and found that the scores of over half the sample of dyslexic children was 1 SD or more below the mean on the CELF-R. In many children deficits may be subtle and not clinically evident, and may be restricted to areas of language development that are particularly relevant for learning an alphabetical written code. It is well documented that phonological analysis and phonological memory are areas of weakness among dyslexic individuals, as well as among children with SLI (reviewed in Snowling, 2000). There is concern in the case of phonological analysis that poor metaphonological skills may depend on poor reading rather than being its cause, although they remain subnormal even in compensated dyslexic adults (Frith, 1997). The ability to segment words at the phoneme level seems particularly crucial for the first stages of learning to read and write in alphabetical systems, in which it is necessary to categorise the phonemes and match them to the orthographic signs; the activated sublexical units need to be maintained in memory for the time necessary to synthesise the phonemic sequences and access the lexical entries. Phonological deficits are common among children with SLI and have been extensively demonstrated in Italian children with specific disorders of language acquisition (Brizzolara et al., 1999; Chilosi et al., 2002; Casalini et al., 2006). Moreover, severe difficulties in the representations of complex syllabic structures (CCV) have been demonstrated in Italian children with SLI who tend to simplify and transform the complex structures into simple CV syllables (Orsolini et al., 2003).

The nature of the phonological deficits in dyslexic children is still debated (reviewed in Ramus, 2003); while the locus of the difficulties is, for some investigators, at the level of an underspecified phonological representation (Snowling, 2000), there are data supporting the hypothesis that the deficit is at the level of acoustic processing (Tallal et al., 1985). A representational deficit may cause problems of explicit phoneme segmentation (metaphonological) and of memorising new phonemic sequences (for example, non-word repetition); on the other hand, low level acoustic processing deficits in the temporal resolution of sounds could be the basis of difficulties in forming segmental phonological representations both in SLI and in dyslexic children (Tallal, 2000). Beside the phonological component, however, other linguistic abilities are involved in reading and writing (lexical, morphosyntactic, and semantic).

These non-phonological linguistic abilities may interfere with both decoding and comprehending written sentences and texts. As children with SLI have problems affecting different linguistic domains, we can expect that their problems in literacy may extend beyond the level of decoding and may affect reading comprehension and written narratives. The SLI children's behavioural profiles in reading and writing may thus differ from those of dyslexic children. The process of reading and writing acquisition may then follow a different developmental trajectory.

Learning to read and write with SLI

How do children with SLI read and write? Are their reading and writing profiles different from those of children with dyslexia without oral language impairment? Does reading disability occur more often in children with specific types of SLI? Few studies have focused on how children with SLI read different types of material, which require the activation of different reading procedures. We know from studies in adult and young readers (Castles & Coltheart, 1993) that reading and writing non-words requires sublexical processes and the establishment and activation of connections between orthography and phonology. When reading words – and especially irregularly spelt words (as in English) or, in a language with quasi-transparent orthography (as in Italian) – assigning a correct accent to the words requires a procedure of direct access to the orthographic lexicon, based on the connections between orthography and lexical-semantic components of the reading process. We have no data in Italian children with SLI that examine their reading and writing processes in terms of sublexical or lexical reading and writing procedures. There are few data on English-speaking children with SLI who seem to have difficulty reading both words and non-words (Bishop & Adams, 1990; Catts, 1993; Briscoe *et al.*, 2001). If we compare the behavioural reading profile of SLI children with that of dyslexic children, we note one important difference: the behavioural marker of English dyslexic children is a severe difficulty in reading non-words compared to words (Snowling, 2000).

Regarding the question of the developmental trajectory of literacy in children with SLI, we need follow-up data, given the large variability found in samples of SLI children in terms of type, severity, and developmental trajectory of the language impairment. In a follow-up study of a small number of children with SLI, we found that delay in reading and writing acquisition was present in the first year of elementary school and was correlated with the persistence and severity of the language impairment at school entrance (Brizzolara *et al.*, 1999).

Another interesting aspect of the relation between literacy and oral language problems is whether the nature of the language impairment (expressive/receptive, phonological, lexical/semantic, morphosyntactic) is related to reading outcome, namely which SLI subtypes are more likely to be associated with reading problems.

Some studies have suggested that children with morphosyntactic and semantic/lexical difficulties are at greatest risk of reading and writing problems (Bishop & Snowling, 2004). This is an important area of research that may provide insights into the differences between literacy problems that derive from language problems and literacy problems that are independent of language. For instance, dyslexic children often have comprehension abilities far superior to their decoding abilities (Zoccolotti *et al.*, 1999). If one takes into account the multicomponent nature of reading and writing, in terms not only of decoding and encoding processes but also of grammatical and lexical/semantic processes, it is reasonable to expect that children with deficits extending beyond the phonological component may encounter major difficulties in written comprehension and written narrative abilities.

What is really unexpected in terms of 'phonological' theories of reading is the fact that children with phonological deficits (as defined in the *Diagnostic and Statistical Manual of Mental Disorders*, DSM-IV) are not specifically impaired in the acquisition of reading and writing unless the phonological deficits are severe, persistent, and associated with other non-phonological language deficits (Bishop & Adams, 1990; Catts, 1993). Moreover, it is not clear whether impairments affecting phonological output or input/output processes differentially affect literacy acquisition, and whether atypical *versus* delayed phonological processes are differentially related to the literacy outcome in SLI children (Dodd, 1995).

Recent long-term studies in adults who had isolated phonological problems in childhood have shown that the literacy abilities of these populations are inferior to those of normal adult readers, even though superior to those of adults who had presented phonological problems associated with other language impairments (Lewis & Freebairn, 1992).

We have very little information on how children with SLI write. Writing requires fine-grained phonological representations activated in working memory, especially in the first stages of learning the alphabetic principles when an orthographic lexicon is not yet built up. In the first stages, writing is based on phonological segmental analysis, for which there is evidence that children with SLI have difficulties (Tallal *et al.*, 1997). We would expect, therefore, that children with SLI would be likely to have even greater difficulty learning to write (spell) than to read. The few data available support the idea that writing both English and Italian is difficult for children with SLI (Bishop & Clarkson, 2003; Brizzolara *et al.*, 1999). In this chapter we attempt to clarify some of the problems regarding the development of reading and writing in children with SLI at the first stages of literacy. We used a longitudinal design with a larger group than in our previous research. We also address the question of differential literacy outcome in children with different types of SLI, and present data on both reading and written language.

Methods

Subjects

From a larger population of children referred for language problems to the Division of Child Neurology and Psychiatry of the University of Pisa-Scientific Institute Stella Maris, we selected a group of 33 children (11 girls and 22 boys, mean non-verbal IQ = 108) who had a diagnosis of SLI during the preschool period according to DSM-IV diagnostic criteria (American Psychiatric Association, 1994), as follows:

- absence of sensory deficits, neurological disorders, or psychiatric abnormalities;
- normal hearing sensitivity threshold, as determined by pure tone audiometry, and absence of structural or motor impairment of the speech apparatus affecting the speech or non-speech movements of the articulators;
- non-verbal intelligence, as measured by IQ performance [Leiter International Performance Scale (Leiter, 1979) or Wechsler Intelligence Scale for Children-Revised (Wechsler, 1974)], in the normal range (IQ $\geq$ 85);
- clinical history of significantly delayed language development that interfered with academic achievement and social communication;
- deficient performance (two or more standard deviations below the mean value expected for chronological age) on at least one (or more) standardised test of expressive or receptive language, or both.

Language assessment included tests standardised for Italian children which measure phonetic discrimination (Pinton, 1998), receptive grammar [Test di Comprensione Grammaticale per

Bambini (TCGB); Chilosi & Cipriani, 1995], receptive vocabulary [Peabody Picture Vocabulary Test (PPVT); Dunn & Dunn, 1997; Italian adaptation, Stella *et al.*, 2000], sentence repetition [Test di Ripetizione Grammaticale per Bambini (TRGB); Benassi *et al.*, 1997], expressive lexicon (Brizzolara *et al.*, 1994), phonology [Prove per la Valutazione Fonologica del Linguaggio Infantile (PFLI); Bortolini, 1995], and the level of morpho-syntactic organisation of spontaneous language production (Cipriani *et al.*, 1993).

On the basis of the results of the language assessment, performed at school entrance, three different subtypes of SLI were diagnosed according to DSM-IV criteria: Mixed Receptive-Expressive language disorder (n = 11, mean non-verbal IQ = 104); Expressive language disorder (n = 11, mean non-verbal IQ = 105); Phonological disorder (n = 11, mean non-verbal IQ = 114).

We are aware that this classification system is an oversimplification and does not describe the linguistic core deficits of the different subtypes; moreover in each group there are children who vary in degree of severity of the impairment and typical *versus* atypical linguistic profiles. In order to characterise the language status of the children at school entrance, we provide a brief description of their linguistic profiles based on the results of both standardised tests and spontaneous language analysis (see Table 1). SLI children classified as receptive-expressive and expressive subtypes (according to DSM IV) share a phonologic – syntactic deficit (as described by Rapin and Allen, 1988 and Rapin, 1996) but differ in their language comprehension; SLI children with phonological disorder do not show any syntactic deficit when evaluated at school entrance, and probably might be assigned to the Rapin (1996) 'speech programming deficit' subtype. As can be observed in Table 1, the three groups also differ in phonological working memory, a cognitive marker of SLI, confirming previous data from our group (Pecini *et al.*, 2005; Casalini *et al.*, 2006) which demonstrated that different typologies of SLI may be subsumed by different cognitive and neurobiological organizations.

Material and procedure

The children's spelling and reading abilities were tested in first grade (age between 5.9 and 8 years; mean age = 6.9); 17 of them (three girls and 14 boys, age between 7.2 and 9.3 years; mean age = 7.9) were also tested in second grade (Receptive-Expressive disorder, n = 7; Expressive disorder, n = 6; Phonological disorder, n = 4).

Table 1: Linguistic characterisation of the three subtypes of SLI of our sample

Mixed Receptive/ Expressive disorder (RE)	Children with RE-SLI were characterised by deficient performance in the test of receptive grammar and in at least one of the other measures of receptive abilities (phonetic discrimination, receptive vocabulary) and in two or more expressive language tests (morpho-syntactic organisation in a narrative task, sentence repetition and expressive lexicon). Grammatical acquisition during the preschool years was characterized by a slow pace and an atypical profile. All the children showed a deficit of phonological working memory.
Expressive disorder (Ex)	Children with Ex-SLI were impaired in at least two expressive domains (morpho-syntactic organization in a narrative task, sentence repetition and expressive lexicon) and had normal (or only mildly delayed) comprehension skills. The children in this group were heterogeneous in terms of degree of severity and typical *versus* atypical grammatical profiles associated with delayed or impaired phonological working memory skills.
Phonological disorder (Ph)	Children with Ph-SLI were impaired only in the phonetic-phonological domain. Generally all the children were severely delayed in the acquisition of speech and most of them showed immature and deviant phonological processes; lexical and syntactic abilities developed normally after a slow start in the earliest years. Most children had delayed or normal phonological working memory.

Spelling and reading abilities were tested with a word dictation task and with a test of reading word lists aloud. Four lists of words, each including 10 words, were selected from a standardised Italian battery (Martini, 1995). The first two lists were composed of bisyllabic (B) words (for example, *luna*) and bisyllabic words with a consonant cluster (Bc) (for example, *prato*); the second two lists were formed of trisyllabic (T) words (such as *balena*) and trisyllabic words with a consonant cluster (Tc) (for example, *spirale*). The number of spelling errors and the speed of reading were scored. Raw scores were converted to z scores. A z score lower than -2 (either in accuracy or speed, or both) was taken as the cut-off for pathological performance.

A qualitative analysis of spelling errors was also carried out. Spelling errors were classified as follows:

- minimal distance substitutions (Mdsub) (substitutions of consonant or vowels that differ only in a single distinctive feature, for example sonority, as in *vilo* instead of *filo*);
- non-minimal distance substitutions (Nmdsub) (all the substitutions of phonemes which differ in more than one distinctive feature, for example *cilo* instead of *filo*);
- omission of phonemes (Omis) (such as *pato* instead of *prato*);
- addition of phonemes (Add) (such as *camapo* instead of *campo*).

Results

Figures 1 to 3 show mean z scores and percentage of subjects showing deficits (z score <-2) on the spelling and reading tests for first-grade children.

In first grade, the groups with receptive-expressive disorder and expressive disorder showed deficient performance in both spelling and reading, the children with receptive-expressive disorder usually being the more impaired. For both these groups, spelling and reading accuracy were deficient approximately to the same extent, whereas reading speed was relatively spared. The group with phonological disorder performed within the normal limits for each of the written language measures (Figs. 1a, 2a, 3a).

Approximately half the children with receptive-expressive disorder had impaired performance in spelling or reading accuracy. About half of the expressive disorder group was also deficient in spelling compared to reading accuracy, which was less often impaired. Reading speed was less likely to be deficient than reading accuracy in both receptive-expressive disorder and expressive disorder groups. In most children from the phonological disorder group, written language abilities were within the normal range (Figs. 1b, 2b, 3b).

Figures 4 to 6 show mean z scores on spelling and reading tests for second grade children. Because most children's written language skills were adequate, percentages of deficient performances are not shown for this group. The figures show that by the second grade children with receptive-expressive disorder had overcome their spelling and reading deficits, whereas in the expressive disorder group only reading skills normalised; these children improved their spelling abilities significantly, but a deficit was still evident in writing words with consonant clusters. The phonological disorder group continued to show normal ability in both reading and spelling.

Mean z scores for the different types of errors in the spelling test are shown in Fig. 7.

In the first grade, children with phonological disorder made an abnormal number of Mdsub errors, while other types of error were virtually absent in this group. Children with receptive-expressive disorder and expressive disorder made abnormal numbers of errors of all kinds (Mdsub, Nmdsub, Omis, and Add errors).

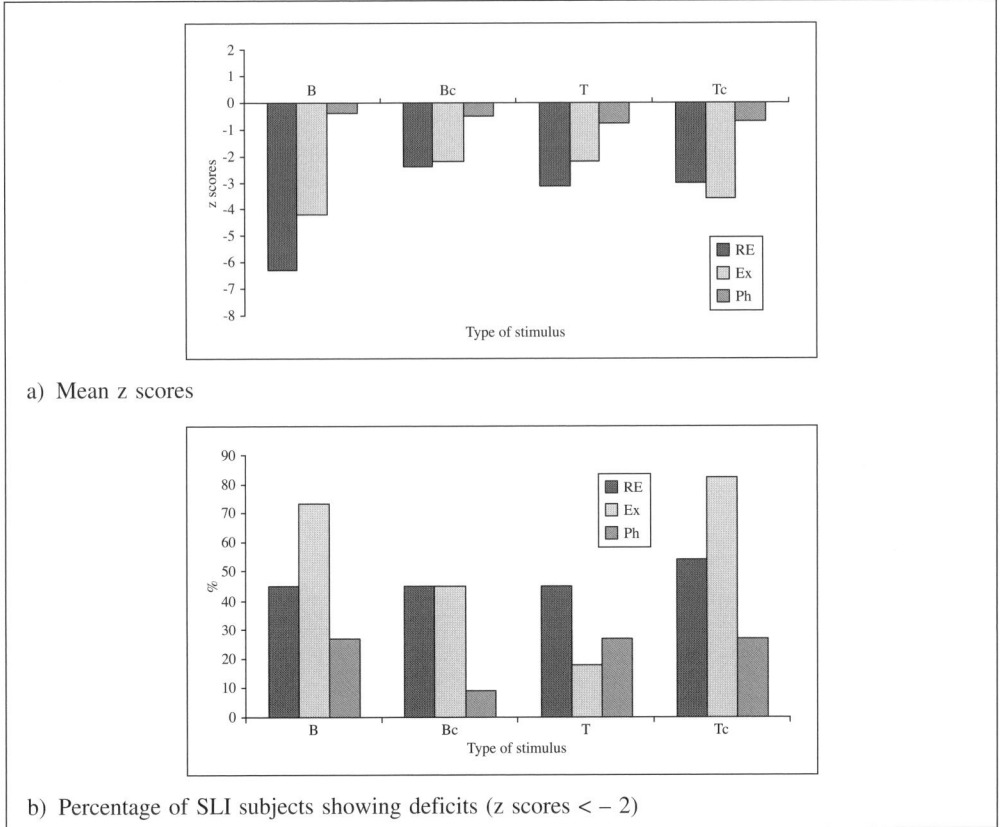

a) Mean z scores

b) Percentage of SLI subjects showing deficits (z scores < − 2)

Fig. 1. Performance of SLI groups on the spelling test (1st grade).
RE: children with Mixed Receptive-Expressive language disorder
B: bisyllabic words
Ex: children with Expressive language language disorder
Bc: bisyllabic words with a consonant cluster
Ph: children with Phonological disorder
T: trisyllabic words
Tc: trisyllabic words woth a consonant cluster

In the second grade, all types of errors were markedly reduced in all three groups. Only the children with expressive disorder continued to have a high rate of Mdsub and Nmdsub errors.

Data analysis was carried out using analysis of variance (ANOVA). It should be noted that given the small size of the SLI subgroups (11 subjects in each) the statistical power of the analysis was reduced, resulting in a high probability of not detecting effects that were in fact significant.

ANOVAs with group (receptive-expressive disorder, expressive disorder, phonological disorder) as the unrepeated factor and the type of stimulus (B, Bc, T, and Tc words) as the repeated factor were carried out separately on z scores for spelling, reading accuracy, and reading speed. These analyses were performed for children in both first and second grade.

In first grade, ANOVAs indicated a tendency for the group effect to be significant as to both spelling ($F_{(2,30)} = 3,01$, $p = 0.06$) and reading accuracy ($F_{(2,28)} = 2,94$, $p = 0.07$). Bonferroni *a posteriori* comparisons showed that children with receptive-expressive disorder tended to

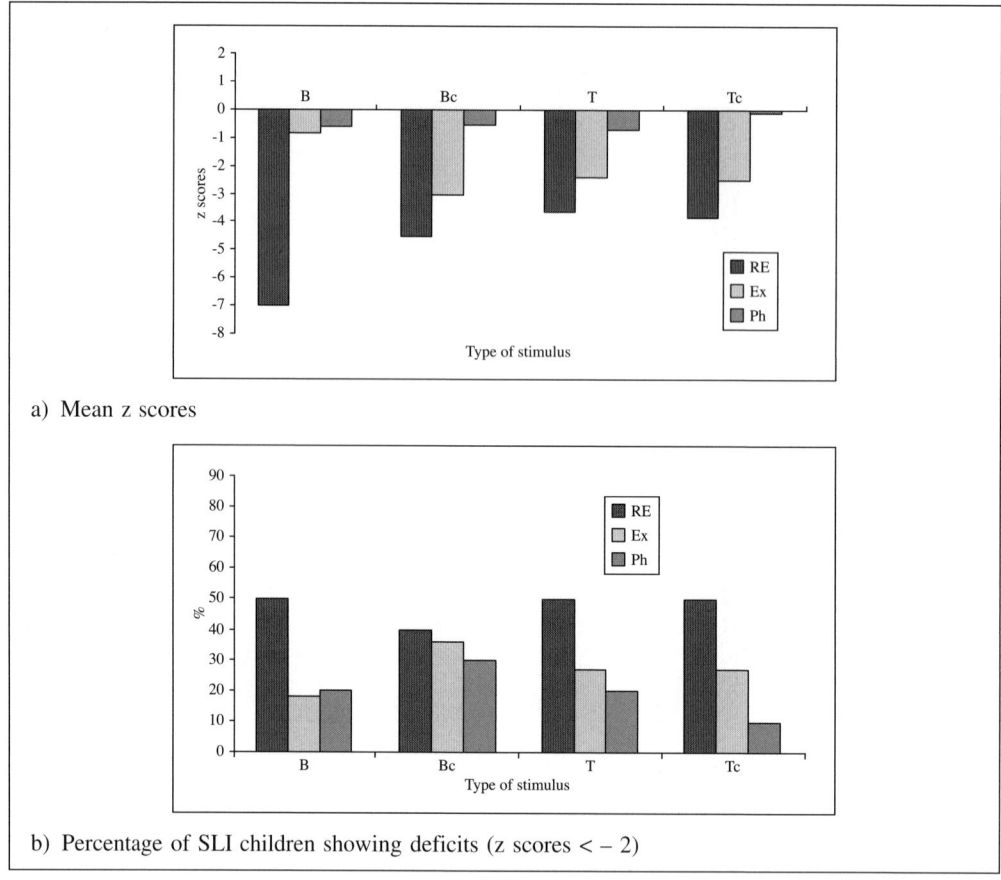

a) Mean z scores

b) Percentage of SLI children showing deficits (z scores < – 2)

Fig. 2. Performance of SLI groups in reading accuracy (1st grade).

perform worse than children with phonological disorder ($p < 0.10$); in the case of reading accuracy, a group by type of stimulus was also evident ($F_{(6,84)} = 2,26, p < 0.05$): the difference in reading accuracy between the receptive-expressive disorder and phonological disorder groups was more evident for B words. The group main effect for reading speed was not significant.

In second grade, the group main effect was significant only for spelling ($F_{(2,12)} = 4,86, p < 0.05$): Bonferroni *a posteriori* comparison showed that children with expressive disorder performed worse than children with phonological disorder ($p < 0.05$); group by type of stimulus interaction proved significant ($F_{(6,36)} = 3,09, p < 0.05$): the difference between the expressive disorder and phonological disorder groups was greater for Bc and Tc words than for B and T words.

Discussion

Children with SLI appear to have a slow start in learning to read and write. However, not all children with SLI in the preschool years develop problems with reading and writing. Our data confirm that expressive and receptive-expressive disorders are associated with a higher risk of difficulty in learning to read than SLI children with isolated phonological problems who have a better outcome. Yet not all children with expressive and receptive-expressive SLI at preschool have difficulty grasping the alphabetical principles. These are the main results of our study.

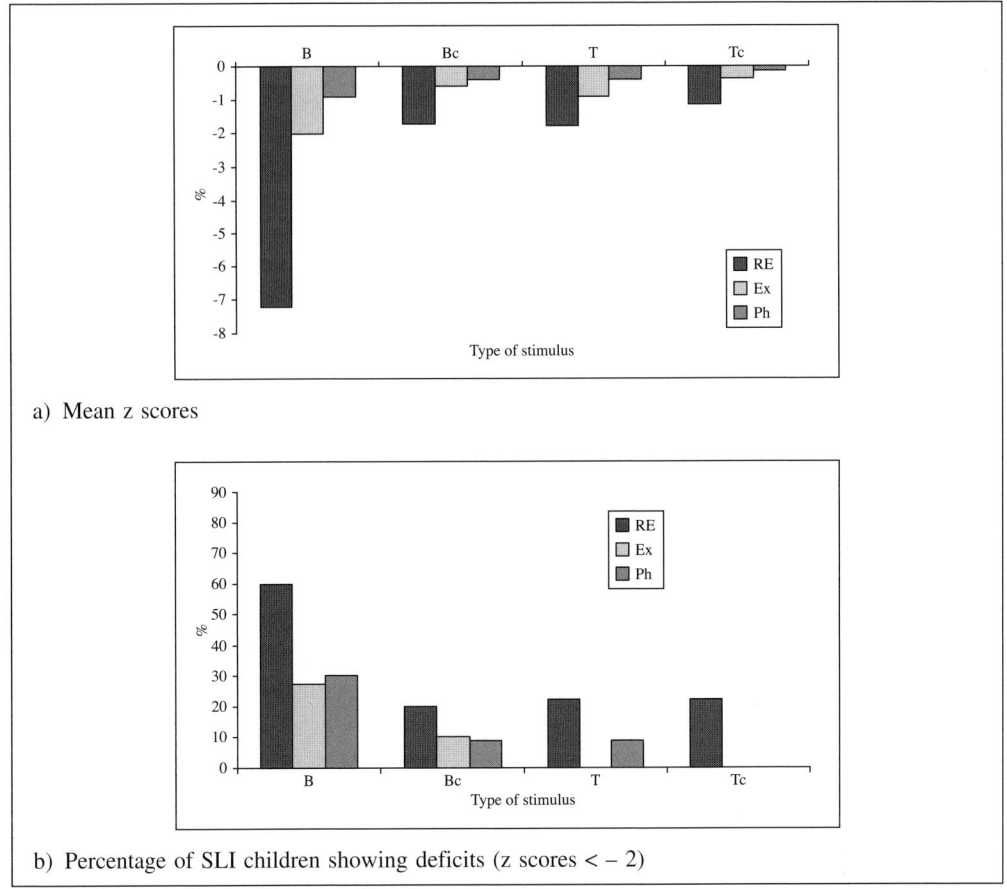

Fig. 3. Performance of SLI groups in reading speed (1st grade).

We now examine each of them in greater detail. The main finding of our study is that children with SLI are 'late readers and writers', which echoes their slow start in language acquisition. We know that there are children, defined as 'late talkers,' who may become children with SLI, although not necessarily so. Difficulties may emerge at various points in development when complex new abilities must be acquired on the solid base of already mastered language competencies.

The slow start of children with SLI in reading acquisition supports the continuity between oral and written language, yet poses many problems on the relation between the two domains. If continuity exists and the relation is a causal one, it should be apparent in all children with SLI, at least in those subgroups sharing common deficiencies. If this is not so – and it was not the case in our data, as about half our sample of children with receptive/expressive and expressive SLI had a normal start in reading acquisition – the problem is to identify the differences between children with SLI who are normal readers from the start and children with SLI who are 'late' readers and writers. Is there a general cognitive difference? In our sample, all the children had normal non-verbal cognitive abilities, although individual variability was high, as is usual in clinical material.

Another possibility is that children with SLI who have problems acquiring the written code have a more severe language impairment than those who are normal readers from the start.

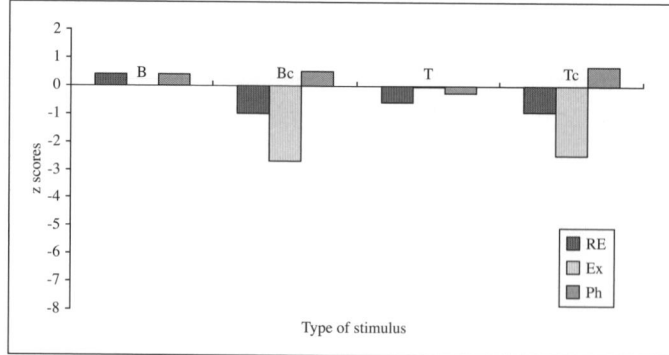

Fig. 4. Performance (mean z scores) of SLI groups on the spelling test (2nd grade).

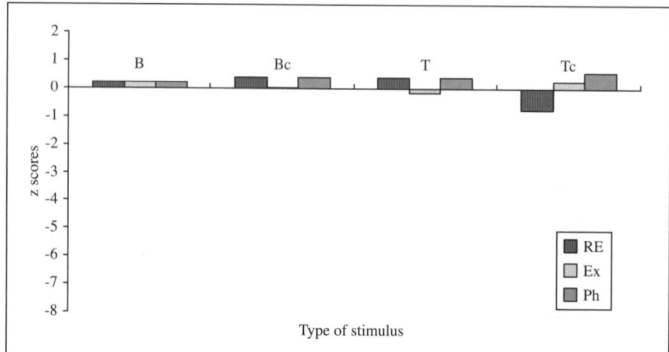

Fig. 5. Performance (mean z scores) of SLI groups in reading accuracy (2nd grade).

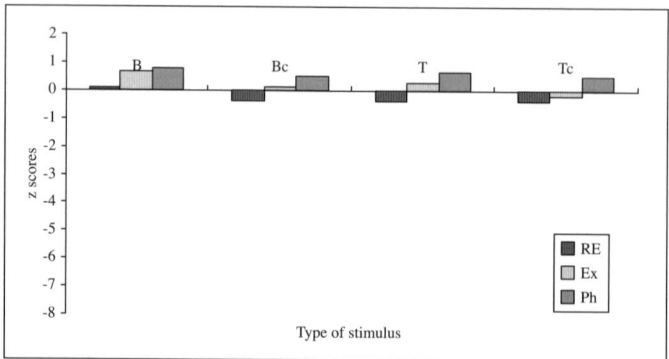

Fig. 6. Performance (mean z scores) of SLI groups in reading speed (2nd grade).

Those children who have decoding and spelling problems in first grade may be children in whom a genetic risk for reading disability is associated with oral language impairment. The two disorders may be correlated but not causally related. This might explain why not all the SLI children become poor readers and writers. If this were the case, the behavioural profile of this subsample of SLI children should be similar to that of dyslexic children – namely, children with specific reading difficulties not diagnosed as SLI in the preschool years. The behavioural profile of the SLI children who have difficulties in reading and writing is characterised by inaccuracy in decoding single words, but not specifically by slowness in decoding the text by

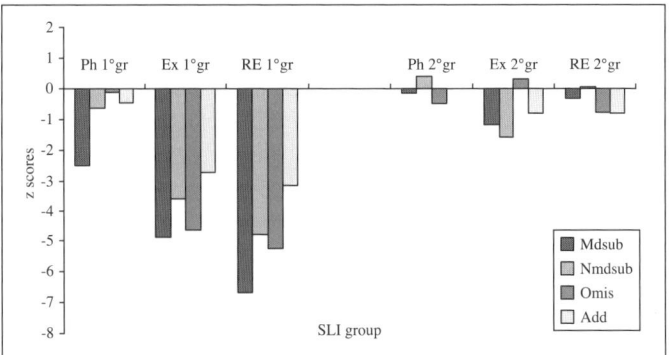

Fig. 7 Different typologies of spelling errors for SLI groups in 1st and 2nd grade.
Mdsub: minimal distance substitutions
Nmdsub: non-minimal distance substitutions
Omis: omissions of phonemes
Add: additions of phonemes

the end of second grade. We know from other studies (Zoccolotti *et al.*, 1999) that the behavioural marker of Italian dyslexic children is slow speed, with speed being much more compromised than accuracy. Slow speed does not seem to be the persistent marker in our sample of SLI children who mostly had poor accuracy. A warning is necessary concerning the age of the children in this study: dyslexia is not usually diagnosed before the end of second grade, and we lack sufficient data on the behavioural reading profiles of dyslexic children in first grade. Inaccuracy in decoding might, however, be a marker for dyslexic children who have had language problems in the preschool years. Although this hypothesis needs to be supported by larger samples of children, recent data from our group suggest that dyslexic children with retrospectively documented language delay in the preschool years are worse decoders in terms of accuracy than dyslexic children without a history of slow language development (Chilosi *et al.*, 2003). However, both groups (dyslexic children with and without a history of language delay) are slow decoders.

The fact that children in our clinic with a diagnosis of SLI in the preschool years and who were followed up in the first two grades of elementary school were slow readers but not dyslexic may be interpreted tentatively as supporting the view that their reading problems differ from those of dyslexic children and are related to their language problems. The type of SLI seems relevant for literacy acquisition: in our sample, children with expressive and receptive/expressive disorders made significantly more errors in reading and writing and were slower developers in first grade than children with an isolated phonological impairment whose performance was within normal limits.

Our data are thus in agreement with studies of English SLI children (Bishop *et al.*, 2003) and support the idea that impairment in multiple components of language is a risk factor for literacy, compared with an isolated phonological impairment. Thus, language impairment in the preschool years affects not only comprehension of written narratives, but also the basic procedures of phoneme-grapheme and grapheme-phoneme mapping. Children with expressive/receptive impairment also have phonological deficits which may contribute to their difficulty in 'cracking the code', but phonological deficits *per se* are not sufficient to cause a barrier to literacy. The question left unanswered is whether the phonological deficits of children with phonological impairment either alone or associated with expressive/receptive impairment are of the same nature. The latter may be more severe and may involve input as well as output processes.

Another result of our study that is worth discussing and raises new questions is the fact that writing is also affected in children with SLI. Writing to dictation requires good phonological analysis of the input, good segmentation abilities, and maintenance of a string of phonemes in working memory. All these cognitive abilities are impaired in children with SLI, as has been shown in a recent study by Casalini *et al.* (in press) on a sample that included most of the children of the present study: children with expressive/receptive deficits were more severely impaired than children with isolated phonological impairment in non-word repetition. SLI children with expressive/receptive disorders also had difficulty with spelling, in agreement with a recent study by Kemp & Bryant (2003) who showed that knowledge of grammatical morphology influences spelling abilities.

Finally it is important to consider the favourable reading outcome in second grade of many children who were 'late readers and writers' at the end of first grade. In second grade many of these children seem to have caught up and resumed a normal rate of development; thus the disorder in the first phase of written language acquisition seems to be transitory. We already know that this result does not apply to the entire population of SLI children. Children in our sample in fact received language therapy during the first 2 years of school, which included training in alphabetisation. This may have been a protective factor. A study with a control group of children who have not received this specific training would need to be performed to test this hypothesis. We know that specific reading deficits in dyslexic individuals can be very resistant to treatment, although compensation is possible in a percentage of cases. The presence of reading and writing problems can be interpreted as a transient difficulty at the developmental phase requires the learning of new 'language-based' complex skills. The presence of a previous language impairment in the preschool years makes these children particularly vulnerable at this developmental stage. Other developmental challenges in the acquisition of complex literacy skills may well await these children – for example, comprehension of texts and written narratives may be other obstacles to face. Data on complex written language abilities besides decoding and encoding in SLI children support the view that these children may go through an 'illusory recovery' (Scarborough, 1990) in acquiring the basic literacy skills and that new difficulties may emerge at a later stage of their academic careers.

References

American Psychiatric Association (1994): *Diagnostic and statistical manual of mental disorders*, 4th edn. Washington: American Psychiatric Association.

Benassi, C., Chilosi, A., Cipriani, P., Pfanner, L. & Bottari, P. (1997): Lo sviluppo delle abilità di ripetizione in età prescolare: prospettive applicative per lo studio dei disturbi specifici del linguaggio. *Psichiatria dell'Infanzia e dell'Adolescenza* **64**, 323–338.

Bishop, D.V.M. & Adams, C. (1990): A prospective study of the relationship between specific language impairment, phonological disorders, and reading retardation. *J. Child. Psychol. Psychiatry* **21**, 1027–1050.

Bishop, D.V.M. & Clarkson, B. (2003): Written language as a window into residual language deficits: a study of children with persistent and residual speech and language impairments. *Cortex* **39**, 215–237.

Bishop, D.V.M. & Snowling, M.J. (2004): Developmental dyslexia and specific language impairment: same or different? *Psychol. Bull.* **130**, 858–886.

Bortolini, U. (1995): *PFLI. Prove per la valutazione fonologica del linguaggio infantile*. Padova: Edit Master.

Briscoe, J., Bishop, D.V.M. & Norbury, C. (2001): Phonological processing, language, and literacy: a comparison of children with mild-to-moderate sensorineural hearing loss and those with specific language impairment. *J. Child Psychol. Psychiatry* **42**, 329–340.

Brizzolara, D., Cipriani, P., Chilosi, A. & De Pasquale, L. (1994): L'apprendimento del linguaggio scritto nei bambini con difficoltà di acquisizione del linguaggio orale: continuità o discontinuità? In: *Apprendimento e patologia neuropsichica nei primi anni di scuola. Modelli interpretativi della clinica*, eds. G. Masi & A. Martini. Rome: Borla.

Brizzolara, D., Casalini, C., Sbrana, B., Chilosi, A. & Cipriani, P. (1999): Memoria di lavoro fonologica e difficoltà di apprendimento della lingua scritta nei bambini con disturbo specifico di linguaggio. *Psicologia Clinica dello Sviluppo* **3**, 465–488.

Casalini, C., Brizzolara, D., Chilosi, A., Cipriani, P., Marcolini, S., Pecini, C., Roncoli, S. & Burani, C. (in press): Non-word repetition in children with specific language impairment: a deficit in phonological working memory or in long-term verbal knowledge? *Cortex*.

Castles, A. & Coltheart, M. (1993): Varieties of developmental dyslexia. *Cognition* **47**, 149–180.

Catts, H. (1991): Early identification of dyslexia: evidence from a follow-up study of speech-language impaired children. *Ann. Dyslexia* **41**, 163–177.

Catts, H. (1993): The relationship between speech-language impairments and reading disabilities. *J. Speech Hearing Disord.* **36**, 948–958.

Catts, H., Fey, M., Tomblin, J. & Zhang, X. (2002): A longitudinal investigation of reading outcomes in children with language impairment. *J. Speech Lang. Hearing Res.* **45**, 1142–1157.

Chilosi, A. & Cipriani, P. (1995): *TCGB, Test di comprensione grammaticale per bambini*. Pisa: Del Cerro.

Chilosi, A., Cipriani, P. & Fapore, T. (2002): Disturbi specifici del linguaggio. In: *I Disturbi dello sviluppo. Neuropsicologia clinica e ipotesi riabilitative*, eds. S. Vicari & M.C. Caselli, pp. 59–71. Bologna: Il Mulino.

Chilosi, A., Lami, L., Pizzoli, C., Pignatti, B., D'Alessandro, D., Gruppioni, B., Cipriani, P. & Brizzolara, D. (2003): Profili neuropsicologici nella dislessia evolutiva. *Psicologia Clinica dello Sviluppo* **2**, 269–285.

Cipriani, P., Chilosi, A., Bottari, P. & Pfanner, L. (1993): *L'acquisizione della morfosintassi in italiano: fasi e processi*. Padova: Unipress.

Dodd. B. (1995): *Differential diagnosis and treatment of children with speech disorder*. London: Whurr.

Dunn, L.M. & Dunn, L.M. (1997): *Peabody Picture Vocabulary Test- PPVT-Third Edition*. Circle Pines, MN: American Guidance Service.

Frith, U. (1997): Brain, mind and behavior in dyslexia. In: *Dyslexia: biology, cognition and intervention*, eds. C. Hulme & M. Snowling, pp. 1–19. London: Whurr.

Kemp, N. & Bryant, P. (2003): Do bees buzz? Rule-based and frequency-based knowledge in learning to spell plurals. *Child Dev.* **74**, 63–74.

Leiter, R. (1979): *Leiter international performance scale*. Chicago: Stoelting Co.

Lewis, B. & Freebairn, L. (1992): Residual effects of pre-school phonology disorders in grade school, adolescence and adulthood. *J. Speech Hearing Res.* **35**, 819–831.

Martini, A. (1995): *Le difficoltà di apprendimento della lingua scritta. Criteri di diagnosi e indirizzi di trattamento*. Tirrenia: Del Cerro.

McArthur, G. & Bishop, D.V.M. (2001): Auditory perceptual processing in people with reading and oral language impairments: current issues and recommendations. *Dyslexia* **7**, 150–170.

Orsolini, M., Fanari, R., Serra, G., Cioce, R., Rotondi, A., Dassisti, A. & Maronato, C. (2003): Primi progressi nell'apprendimento della lettura: una riconsiderazione del ruolo della consapevolezza fonologica. *Psicologia Clinica dello Sviluppo* **3**, 403–436.

Pecini, C., Casalini, C., Brizzolara, D., Cipriani, P., Pfanner, L. & Chilosi, A. (2005): Hemispheric specialization for language in children with different types of specific language impairment. *Cortex* **41**, 157–167.

Pinton, A. (1998): La valutazione. In: *La valutazione della comunicazione linguistica. Teorie, metodi, prove*, eds. A. Pinton & L. Lena, pp. 15–29. Padova: Imprimenda.

Ramus, F. (2003): Developmental dyslexia: specific phonological deficit or general sensorimotor dysfunction? *Curr. Opin. Neurobiol.* **13**, 212–218.

Rapin, I. (1996): Practitioner review: developmental language disorders: a clinical update. *J. Child Psychol. Psychiat.* **37**, 643–655.

Rapin, I. & Allen, D.A. (1988): Syndromes of developmental dysphsia and adult aphasia. In: *Language, communication, and the brain*, ed. F. Plum, pp. 57–75. New York: Raven Press.

Scarborough, H. (1990): Very early language deficits in dyslexic children. *Child Dev.* **61**, 1728–1743.

Semel, E., Wiig, E. & Secord, W. (1987): *Clinical Evaluation of Language Fundamentals – Revised*. San Antonio: Psychological Corporation.

Snowling, M.J. (2000): *Dyslexia*, 2nd edn. Oxford: Blackwell Science.

Stanovich, K. & Siegel, L. (1994): Phenotypic performance profile of reading-disabled children: a regression-based test of the phonological-core variable-difference model. *J. Educ. Psychol.* **86**, 24–53.

Stella, G., Pizzoli, C. & Tressoldi, P. (2000): *Peabody. Test di vocabolario recettivo.* Torino: Omega.

Tallal, P. (2000): Experimental studies of language learning impairments: from research to remediation. In: *Speech and language impairments in children: causes, characteristics, intervention and outcome*, eds. D.V.M. Bishop & L.B. Leonard, pp. 131–155. Hove: Psychology Press.

Tallal, P., Allard, L., Miller, S. & Curtiss, S. (1997): Academic outcomes of language impaired children. In: *Dyslexia: biology, cognition and intervention*, eds. C. Hulme & M. Snowling, pp. 167–181. London: Whurr.

Tallal, P., Stark, R. & Mellits, E. (1985): Identification of language-impaired children on the basis of rapid perception and production skills. *Brain Lang.* **25**, 314–322.

Wechsler, D. (1974): *Wechsler Intelligence Scale for Children – revised.* New York: Psychological Corporation.

Zoccolotti, P., De Luca, M., Di Pace, E., Judica, A., Orlandi, M. & Spinelli, D. (1999): Markers of developmental surface dyslexia in a language (Italian) with high grapheme-phoneme correspondence. *Appl. Psycholinguistics* **20**, 191–216.

Chapter 19

Developmental language disorders and behavioural disorders

Charles Njiokiktjien

*Stichting Dysphatische Ontwikkeling (Developmental Dysphasia Foundation),
WG-Plein 316, NL-1054 SG Amsterdam, The Netherlands*
cn@suyi.nl

Summary

Since behaviour, including skill (praxis) starting in the first year, is shaped by the language of the mother and later the inner language of the child, it is only logical that behavioural disorders should accompany language disorders. Researchers in this field usually describe what is observed, sometimes venturing to provide an explanation, and only in rare cases do they address brain function. From published reports and own observation it seems that developmental language disorders (DLD) are very frequent in children under treatment for a psychiatric diagnosis. Conversely very few children with DLD have no behavioural problems. The inability to express adequately and the lack of inner language are thought to be the key deficiencies that lead to these problems.

Introduction

In a volume on children with language disorders, attention should also be devoted to comorbidity. In this chapter I will deal with behavioural disorders that often occur in children with comorbidities. The relation between behaviour and language and between language disorders and behavioural disorders is a complex one. If we are to understand behavioural and language disorders, we have to go back to the source of the behaviour, and in this case to its relation to early language development. For this reason I will address the following topics: behaviour under the influence of spoken language during normal development, language disorders accompanying psychopathology, behavioural disorders accompanying language disorders, and the relation between language disorders and behavioural disorders.

Behaviour under the influence of spoken language in normal development

The speaking mother, the acquisition of object knowledge and spoken language, and the early ontogenetic change in thinking*

Soon after birth, the baby sees and recognizes the mother's voice, face and body scent. The baby also recognizes the mother's footstep, her way of picking him up and holding him when she changes his nappy, and the speed of her reactions. These sensory impressions enable the baby to know the mother and predict her physical functioning. Simultaneously with the gratification of vital needs (for example warmth, nourishment, hunger reduction), the continuous flow of maternal stimuli reaching the baby, particularly their emotional features, and the signs the baby himself conveys, lead in turn to what is called *attachment*. From a developmental neurology perspective, one can imagine that attachment is the first multi-modal (multi-sensory) synaptic connection with an object that is, the living *mother* object. Simple verbal assignments or exclamations, gestures, touchings, eye and body contact and voice intonations are often the means of contact in this connection. The mother or care-giver is the starting engine for the emotional connection with the world, with people and through her, with inanimate objects and animals. The process of attachment occurs predominantly in the right hemisphere (Schore 2003), as does early speech development (Bates *et al.* 1992; Dehaene-Lambertz *et al.* 2004; Locke 1997; Tan 1990, 2005).

The mother labels various events, objects and feelings (for example bottle, thirst, hunger, pain, sleep, sweet, naughty, nappy, dirty, delicious, water, bath, cold, warm). In the first stage of spoken language development, the child hears a prosodic flow of sounds, passively learns these words and links them associatively to the appropriate multimodally perceived object, situation, emotion or feeling. The words themselves – phonetic associations – are not symbols yet. For a more extensive description of early development, particularly of language and the neural networks that play a role in its development, the reader is referred to Dutch literature (Tan, 1990, 2005).

Up until his death in 1934, the Byelorussian literary psychologist Vygotsky (translations 1962, 1977, 1978) worked on conceptualizing spoken language development, behaviour and the development of the use of instruments and objects (or actions, with a neurological term praxis). His work was continued by his school, especially his student Luria (1977). Vygotsky held that praxis and speech are typically higher human brain functions that determine the relation between man and his environment and, consequently, his behaviour. He and Luria rejected the concept of maturation as a passive process, an unfolding of mental qualities and of language acquisition as an effect of Pavlovian training. They felt there was no foundation for a mental life that exists *a priori* from birth. Praxis and language acquisition are strongly affected by upbringing and thus develop the child's concepts and thinking. Recent work tends to confirm these ideas (Dominey & Dodane, 2004).

Before Vygotsky, psychologists viewed the development of the symbol as an example of pure intellect and not a product of developmental history. No careful study was conducted on speech development. Speech and praxis were viewed as totally independent – that is *mental* and *physical* functions. In part this was due to the influence of Descartes, who viewed the physical as solely appropriate for scientific study, and the mental as solely appropriate for philosophical reflection. Piaget never attributed great value to speech as an organizer of childhood behaviour.

---

* The mother can be replaced in this sense by the father or some other permanent care-giver.

The beginning of practical intelligence (technical thinking) in children is comparable to the simple actions adult chimpanzees can also perform and is not dependent on speech. Often these early actions even precede speech. In fact, according to Vygotsky, symbolic activity (spoken language) serves an organizing function with regard to praxis and unchains fundamentally new and different behaviours.

There are also other ways in which spoken language influences behaviour that Vygotsky and Luria barely considered. The major criticism expressed by Tan (2005) is that Vygotsky and Luria devote so little attention to the effect of poor inner language on the emotional development of the child. Language development can reduce separation anxiety, provide consolation, decrease impulsiveness, channel aggression and make a differentiated expression of other feelings possible. Early childhood feelings in language, referred to by Tan as the affect-linguistic paradigm and probably still steered by the right hemisphere, can be expressed in a differentiated fashion (and less primitively and physically) in language once the child has entered the left hemisphere stage of language development. The waving bye bye of the eighth month is expressed more subtly in language – for example by saying 'bye bye' at a year and a half, and 'I'll be back, see you tomorrow' a few years later.

If, through her attachment with her baby, the mother is the 'starter' of the baby's relationship with the world in the first 6 months, the early speech and language relationship with the mother is 'driving in first gear'. As a result of the attachment, there is now a basis for the determinants of spoken language development (see below). Language is essential if one is to internalize social codes, self-regulate behaviour, express emotions and feelings, and exert influence on other people's behaviour.

The use of objects (praxis, speech and language)

In the course of a child's development, according to Vygotsky, spoken language is integrated into practical thinking. Language plays a role in organizing *higher* psychological functions and penetrates in a sense the actions – praxis – themselves. The use of scissors, for example, can be modified by words like 'hold the scissors tight', 'cut carefully', 'cut a little more to the right' or 'stop now'. The words can emanate from outside or from the child whose words can accompany his action (egocentric speech). Later the words are internalized as inner language.

Vygotsky viewed egocentric speech as the transition between communicative or social speech from outside and inner language. Inner language does not occur before the age of 4 and only exists with regards to the words a child can say (T. Akhutina, student of Luria, personal communication).

Speech and praxis converge and in part the child becomes master of his environment, including objects and instruments, by way of language. The example of the scissors is no different from the influence of language on social behaviour; speech and social behaviour also converge. Nowadays Barkley (2001) speaks of rule-governed behaviour. Language becomes a grammatical sentence and story structure, and formally a left hemisphere function. Praxis becomes automatic and also turns into a left hemisphere function. As soon as situations or actions become complicated, Vygotsky held that either accompanying language or inner language occurs that can organize the behaviour, or the child falls back on social speech and asks for help. Speech not only accompanies, it also regulates and controls.

Vygotsky held that speech and action are part of one and the same problem-solving psychological process. Speech, hands and eyes solve practical problems and this also leads to an internalization of the visual field. The influence of inner language leads to a greater freedom of action and independence from the concrete visual field. Together with inner language, visual imagination can lead to the preparation of future actions. In a stationary store, the child says to himself, 'I need small scissors for the little things and big scissors for very large pieces of paper because we are going to have an assignment at school next week'. The time element (time axis) also plays a role in the acting; formal time is always expressed in language. In the absence of an object or instrument, the child can also create one under the influence of controlling inner language.

The influence of inner language makes one act less impulsively and directly and makes mental planning possible so that motivation, intentions and alternatives can be considered. Action can also be postponed or cancelled altogether. It facilitates smooth switches from one activity to another ('I am going to stop cutting now because Mother says it is dinner time'). Social speech turn inwards, Vygotsky noted, and becomes inner language so that the child is no longer dependent on social speech. Social speech is internalized and acquires an interpersonal function. In complicated situations though, speech enables the child to call upon another person, thus influencing the other person's behaviour.

Vygotsky noted the following sequence in the influence of speech: first, there is a primitive act without speech (young children label their drawings or what they have cut later), this is followed by a more differentiated but poorly structured act accompanied by speech; and then the act is preceded by organizing inner language (older children say what they are going to cut). The older child first performs an act in his imagination, directed by inner language (she says to herself, 'which scissors and which paper should I use?').

The transition from feelings only to affective and social speech and then egocentric speech and subsequently inner language is a long and complex process. In young children there often remains a fusion between speech and action, which are still closely connected to each other, for example in the holophrase of word with gesture.

Other functions are also involved in the relation between speech and action. Vygotsky emphasizes the role of attention in upbringing. The adult who is bringing up a child constantly directs attention to important things in the child's surroundings. Things and events are endowed with a significance and emotional value and structure the child's mental life through inner language.

In a recent article, Dominey and Dodane (2004) criticize the nativistic idea that language is *automatically* acquired in a *linguistic bath* and is essentially pre-programmed. They demonstrate that speech that is truly directed to the child directs the child's attention to important aspects of the speech signal. Joint attention then focuses the child's eye on relevant aspects of the world. There is thus a double event: language is learned better in a real contact with the mother, and at the same time the child learns the things about the world that the adult feels are relevant.

The mother's speech starts by labeling an object to distinguish it from other objects ('ball', not 'moon'). The word isolates the object from something else, categorizes, generalizes, abstracts and gives the object a function: using language, links are drawn and relations are created. Conversely, perception is not only visual – inner language also becomes perception of the world. Visual perception is often integral and pertains to shapes and forms, whereas speech perception of the world is sequential and analytic. The visual perception of a baby in the prelinguistic stage is factual (that is the toothbrush as object), but in the older child perception becomes a semantic event because seeing the toothbrush opens up a functional world in language ('Is it a toothbrush for a child or a big person?' 'Is it mine or my sister's?' 'How am I supposed to hold it?' 'What is it for and how do you do that?' 'It is dirty, how do I clean it?' 'It is old, I need a new one'). Language not only structures the act of brushing teeth, the act and the object can also be replaced by a *pretend* act. The physical temporal and spatial field of attention can be replaced by an imaginary event. Outside the direct structuring of actions, inner language serves other functions as well: the child can remember spatial and non-spatial events and actions and make imaginary comparisons with reality ('I know I put the toothbrush on top of the cabinet.' 'The dentist said I don't brush my teeth long enough.' 'I lost my last toothbrush'. 'This toothbrush is better than the last one').

Although speech and language influence actions, there are essential differences between language and the instrument. The child uses the instrument to influence and change the physical world. Language is often inwardly directed and influences mental processes. In the first year, Leroi-Gourban (1964) noted that a differentiation is coming into being between the hand and oral functions that enable praxis and speech to ensue. The hand can manipulate and make gestures, and the mouth can manipulate food and speak. Both these functions, speech and praxis, are not merely products of pure maturation of a pre-determined system such as learning to roll over and sit up. These higher psychological functions require upbringing and reinforce each other; they bring each other up.

Looking at something becomes grabbing for it and if it is too far away, pointing at it so the other person gets it. In this case, the external action is internalized. Pointing or speaking as a symbol now influence the other person's behaviour. Through a social system, influence is indirectly exerted on the object. At a later time, the interpersonal process is internalized into an intrapersonal process so that signs (inner language) now solve the problem via tools ('I am going to get that chair and stand on it to get the toothbrush').

Classic French child psychiatrists have long noted that the development of speech has certain consequences for the inner language aspect of children's mental, emotional and social development (De Ajuriaguerra *et al.* 1976). This has consequences with regard to the differentiated verbal expression of feelings and thought contents.

One might rightly wonder what happens to these processes if a child has a language disorder such as developmental dysphasia, or a child lacks social relatedness, as in autism, and also has a language disorder. What happens to the child's social behaviour and what happens to the child's actions even if the child is not overtly dyspraxic?

Developmental language disorders in psychopathology

Terminology

When I refer to developmental language disorders (DLD), or in short language disorders, I mean clinical developmental disorders defined within a classical aphasiological context (Rapin & Allan, 1982). DLD does not include the category semantic-pragmatic language syndrome (SPLS). DLD have also been referred to as developmental dysphasias and entail expressive and mixed receptive and expressive disorders. We use the term 'developmental dysphasia' in a more restricted sense than used by other investigators...*. Tan (2005) defined it as an expressive problem in children who cannot say adequately what they know and understand. So, in developmental dysphasia there is by definition a discrepancy in tests between expression and comprehension – there are word-finding problems, problems in answering on verbal command, and often dysgrammatism and problems in discourse cohesion. Developmental dysphasia is

---

* When the terms "we" or "our" are used, the author is speaking on behalf of his fellow team members at the Developmental Dysphasia Foundation.

similar to (pure) expressive dysphasia, and is very frequent in the category of mixed receptive and expressive language disorders when there is a discrepancy between expression and higher comprehension. SPLS does not meet this definition.

Whereas in young children DLD are nearly always accompanied by deviant speech, we often use the term speech-language disorders; nevertheless, in this chapter we will use DLD. The term 'speech' in DLD usually means a problem in phonological production, either because of a phoneme perception problem or because of verbal/speech dyspraxia, which is a deviant implementation of speech sounds in the articulatory muscles. Apart from these speech problems there are articulation disorders such as the dysarthrias or speech problems accompanying oral dyspraxia for non-speech movements. In the SPLS speech as well as grammar are usually normal.

The diagnostic terms are usually given after linguistic analysis of spontaneous speech-language and examinations using logopaedic language tests.

As regards autism, this disorder in social relatedness is considered today to occur on a spectrum, from subtle to severe autistic behaviour. Autistic behaviour may occur in highly functioning people; the majority of autistic subjects (60 per cent), however, are low functioning, that is mentally retarded. All autists have DLD, but not pure expressive dysphasia. Most autists, especially the lower functioning ones, have mixed expressive and receptive language disorders. The higher-functioning autistic subjects, especially those with Asperger syndrome, have fewer formal expressive language disorders; they do have signs of SPLS.

How often do language disorders occur in psychiatric disorders?

In retrospect, children with psychiatric diagnoses have often had language problems or still have them at the time of treatment. The more subtle the language disorder in a child with a psychiatric disorder, the less likely it is that the language disorder will be diagnosed, so that the behaviour will be interpreted erroneously. Intelligence tests are inadequate to detect language disorders; for this purpose there are specially designed language tests.

In a retrospective study, I examined the prevalence of premorbid and present DLD among inpatients at two child psychiatric hospitals (Njiokiktjien, 2004). In the more than 1000 patients whom I examined (Pedology Institute of the Free University, Amsterdam, 190 children from 1978 to 1982, and Child Psychiatric Center Triversum, Alkmaar, 850 children from 1974 to 2000), 45 per cent had a language disorder, mostly a mixed receptive and expressive disorder, with a higher percentage in the kindergarten age group than among older children. It should be noted that the figures pertain to patients seen by a paediatric neurologist. The reason for referral was often not specifically a language-related problem, and the referred patients were only a fraction of the patients at these hospitals. These percentages coincide with other investigators' findings: 50 per cent in a study by Gualteri *et al.* (1983), 53 per cent in one by Cantwell and Baker (1977), and 50–80 per cent in one by Vallance *et al.* (1999). Cohen *et al.* (1998a) noted that 40 per cent of the children undergoing psychiatric treatment have a language disorder that had never been diagnosed.

The frequent occurrence of language disorders does not, however, mean there is always a causal relation between deviant language development and later psychiatric disorders, nor do the figures indicate which language disorder occurs with which psychiatric disorder. Vallance *et al.* (1999) describe children with psychiatric and language disorders. They frequently have problems with dialogue, impairments with pronouns and causal cohesion. This can be indicative of either developmental dysphasia or a SPLS (personal observation).

Beitchman *et al.* (1986) held that language disorders are a risk factor for psychiatric problems, and that this risk factor is even greater than environmental factors. Cohen *et al.* (1998b) studied 380 children with psychiatric disorders in the 7- to 14-year age group. The children who had language disorders in addition to their psychiatric disorders had more difficulty with social cognition and social problem-solving. Based on a literature survey, Blankenstijn and Scheper (2003) concluded that language disorders are more severe in children with psychiatric disorders than in children without them, and the same is true the other way around – that is, comorbid disorders reinforce each other. This is the subject of the following section.

Very little comprehensive research has been conducted using categories from the field of linguistics (non-conventional language tests) among groups of psychiatric patients. In the Netherlands, Blankenstijn and Scheper (2003) conducted research of this type among 120 children in the 4- to 19-year age group diagnosed with a psychiatric disorder, but not autism or schizophrenia. At least 82 per cent of the children made morphological and syntactic (MS) errors. Many of these children, including children without MS, showed a SPLS. In a third of the 120 children, the language disorder was a combination of MS and SPLS and was severe; this was particularly the case in children with externalizing disorders such as attention deficit hyperactivity disorder (ADHD). Children with pervasive developmental disorder-not otherwise specified (PDD-NOS) had the most severely affected language. These linguists described the children's language systematically without classifying the cases into clinical diagnoses. It is clear from the descriptions that the disorders were variable and mixed and coincided with the clinical categories cited in the section on terminology.

The consequences of coinciding psychiatric and language disorders

Strongly language-related behavioural psychology tests are not suitable for the field of psychiatry, as they assess language more than behaviour. Gualtieri *et al.* (1983) cautioned that children with language disorders can be erroneously diagnosed as having symbiotic psychoses. It can be difficult to differentiate between psychotic and severely dysphasic speech (Diatkine, 1984). This is why a logopaedic examination is always called for. If language comprehension decreases and the child's behaviour in non-structured situations is disorganized and agitated, an erroneous impression of psychotic behaviour may result.

In conclusion, before children are diagnosed as having a psychiatric disorder, their speech and language abilities should be tested. A comorbid language disorder is so common in child psychiatry that a comprehensive logopaedic language examination is indispensable and treatment of the language disorder must be part of the psychiatric treatment.

Behavioural disorders concomitant with language disorders

Behavioural disorders are quite common among children whose primary referral is for language disorders (Table 1). Blankenstijn and Scheper (2003) held that children with a language disorder have a 4.5-fold increased chance of behavioural disorders compared with children without a language disorder. Richman and Stevenson (1977) noted behavioural disorders in 57 per cent of a total group of 705 children of preschool age, compared with 14 per cent in the control group. In a group of 142 children, Beitchman *et al.* (1986) noted that behavioural disorders occur in 48.7 per cent of the children with speech and language disorders and in only 12 per cent of the children without them, but that the prevalence of psychiatric disorders was far higher in the case of predominantly language disorders (95 per cent) than with speech-only disorders

(29 per cent) or speech and language disorders (45 per cent). These children had attention deficit disorders (30.4 per cent), unspecified emotional disorders (12.8 per cent) and antisocial behavioural disorders (5.5 per cent). The attention disorders were not further differentiated. Predominantly language disorders without phonologic (speech) disorders suggest the existence of a SPLS, as affected children usually have no phonology problems.

In a classic study on disorders of speech, Ingram (1959) noted that among 80 children with this diagnosis, 40 also had expressive language problems. Of the 80, 25 (34 per cent) had a psychiatric disorder, and their IQ was not especially low. They often exhibited withdrawn, explosive, and slight autistic behaviour.

Tan (1990; 2005) noted various determinants of language acquisition: the relation with the parent, body language by the parent, body contact, imitation and play. The absence of these determinants can contribute towards psychopathology; while, it is never the cause of the language disorder, it does aggravate it. Important psychiatric syndromes such as childhood depression or autism are never the cause of developmental language disorders (Cantwell & Baker 1977, Tan 1990). The reverse is more likely to be the case.

If Vygotsky's and Tan's ideas on the influence of language on behaviour hold true, a child who cannot express himself well and consequently has poor inner language runs a considerable risk of developing abnormally in his interpersonal relations and actions. Various investigators (Cantwell & Baker, 1977, 1987, 1991; Cantwell *et al.*, 1980; Paul & Cohen, 1984) feel that emotional development is retarded. This is all the more so if there are also body schema and dyspraxic disorders. Afferent information from the body and limbs plays an important role in the body awareness and, in turn, the sense of ego and self-consciousness (Samuels, 1986). Spoken language development affects inner language, the semantic aspects of cognitive, emotional and social development, play, praxis and the differentiated expression of feelings and thoughts (De Ajuriaguerra *et al.*, 1976; Menyuk, 1986).

Our own research

In a retrospective study on 100 children referred to us from 2002 to 2005 with developmental dysphasia in whom this diagnosis was confirmed by tests, I examined the frequency of behavioural comorbidity in the history and assessment. Children who were mentally retarded or handicapped (non-verbal IQ lower than 70) or exhibited autism were excluded. The age distribution was 48 per cent older than 6 years and 52 per cent 6 years or younger.

If AD(H)D is not viewed as a behaviour disorder, 20 per cent of the children had no behavioural disorder, and if it is, only 8 per cent of the children had no behavioural problems at all. Table 1 presents an overview. The Table does not show in what combinations the symptoms occurred. The right column does, however, show how often a symptom occurred in isolation. Categories 7 and 8 probably overlap, but also occurred separately. Category 13 is included because chronagnosia – virtually no conception of time above age of 6 – in itself can cause problems in communication.

Nature of behavioural disorders accompanying developmental language disorders

It has been my experience that various types of behavioural disorders can accompany DLD, depending on whether the disorder is the result of deficient expression or a lack of comprehension. The behavioural disorders can occur together or in isolation (see Table 1).

Table 1. Behavioural disorders in 100 children with predominant developmental dysphasia

	percentage	isolated
1. No behavioural problems at all including AD(H)D or chronagnosia	8	
2. Behavioural disorders not including AD(H)D or chronagnosia	80	
3. Mental inflexibility, 15 clear (6 above age of 6), 28 slight (9 above age of 6)	43	4 clear 5 slight
4. Play inadequate, poor symbolic playing or none at all	21	1
5. ADD, usually in the verbal domain	16	4
6. ADHD, half of which so severe that medication was required	12	4
7. Anxieties often including separation anxiety	15	4
8. Silent, shy, withdrawn, socially fearful	11	2
9. Autistic-like	10	0
10. Impulsive, usually with other symptoms	9	2
11. Aggressive, explosive, very angry, temper tantrums	9	5
12. Proxemics (physical social distance) abnormal	4	0
13. Chronagnosia, virtually no conception of time (above the age of 6)	5	4

Legends: ADD, attention deficit disorder; ADHD, attention deficit-hyperactivity disorder.

- First, there is sometimes acting out, frustration with what has failed to be understood and the inability to express oneself, sometimes accompanied by aggressive behaviour. Temper tantrums are not unusual in these children. Clinical studies of children with developmental dysphasia indicate behaviour that is oppositional and unmanageable.

This behaviour is not uncommon among children who are impulsive and temperamental or children with ADHD, and also occurs in children with separation anxiety. Conversely, ADHD can be reinforced by receptive language problems (Beitchman, 1986). In the light of Vygotsky's ideas, attention is likely to be poor if it is not steered by the language of the other or by inner language; attention deficit within the verbal domain is frequent, but this does not amount to ADHD. ADHD is sometimes observed in children with developmental dysphasia (table 1), but less frequently than in children with non-verbal developmental disorders (Njiokiktjien & Verschoor, 1998). The prevalence of ADHD in a population with DLD is higher in a child psychiatric clinic than in private logopaedic practice; there is often a selection bias.

- Second, flight or withdrawal is sometimes observed, and can be so extreme that – particularly in children of preschool age – the child can be prematurely and erroneously diagnosed as having autism. Especially in children with developmental dysphasia, Caulfield et al. (1989) note shy, fearful and withdrawn behaviour that can already begin at the age of 2. These children are generally very quiet, avoid eye contact, and only say what is absolutely necessary. They are inhibited, lack assertiveness, and their peers are apt to dominate them. It is our experience that after early treatment of these children, the 'autistic' symptoms disappear. The differential diagnosis between reactive withdrawal in a dysphasic child and autism in a dysphasic child is, though often not easy, essential for subsequent treatment.

Richman et al. (1983) noted that language disorders led later to increasing introversion and withdrawal. Due to longstanding habit formation on this basis, depression is in my view not uncommon in such children in adolescence and keeps them from realizing their potential. This behaviour in older children is often predictable at pre-school age and exhibits a strong correlation with the language structure at this age (Stevenson et al. 1985). Cohen et al. (1993) stated that 99 of 399 children who were psychiatric day patients exhibit this premorbid language disorder. They were mainly children with high scores on anxiety and social withdrawal scales.

- Third, Mahler's separation and individuation stage (Mahler, 1969) – that is, separation from the mother as the child becomes independent, can deviate if there is deviant language development. Concomitant dyspraxia or learning to walk late – the latter does not occur often in children with developmental dysphasia – make it impossible for the child to perform symbolic communicative gestures or to approach the mother, and aggravates the situation (Tan, 1990). The result is inadequate separation ability and individuation for the child's age, which is often erroneously interpreted as excessive concern and anxiety about separation on the part of the mother. Separation problems cause difficulties in day-to-day interaction with others, including teachers and therapists. Rubin (1982) gave a striking example of a child with developmental dysphasia and separation anxiety, but wrongly suggests that the separation anxiety is a cause of the language disorder.

- Fourth, children with language comprehension disorders run a greater risk of expressing themselves in an autistic fashion (Cantwell & Baker, 1977). I would add here that these authors had probably cases of autism with SPLS in mind.

Children who do speak, albeit late, yet without any content and who have no communicative language are also referred to as echolalic autistic or diagnosed later as having a SPLS (Rapin & Allen, 1982) or an atypical pervasive childhood developmental disorder. It is true that the SPLS is not a behavioural problem, but this kind of language use does disturb interaction.

- Fifth, another aspect pertains to symbolic and representative play, which is sometimes disturbed in children with language disorders (see table) and, probably due to deficient egocentric and inner language, can be a separate aspect of deviant symbolization (Inhelder, 1976; Largo and Howard, 1979). This is unfavourable for the child's emotional development and ability to play with other children. Deviant play in dysphasic children is different from deviant play in autistic children, whose play is in addition disordered due to a lack of imagination and mentalising.

- Sixth, attention disorders as disorders of executive function also include mental rigidity and an inability to switch language from one topic to another. In developmental dysphasia and certainly in severe SPLS, this is not rare. It is striking that 43 per cent of the children with developmental dysphasia appear in the history to be mentally rigid, most of them to a minor degree (Table 1). In an absolute as well as a relative sense, the majority only have this problem until the age of 6, so the problem appears to be age-related. Only two of the children required treatment with medication. An inability to make a smooth switch from one activity to another can be the result of deficient inner language with inadequate rule-governed behaviour (Barkley, 2001). Although mental rigidity is not uncommon among children with developmental dysphasia, most of them are not autistic.

- Finally, the emotional prosodic and linguistic prosodic aspects of language use deserve mention as well. Each can each be individually disturbed and contribute towards disorders of social contact without any other symptoms of autism.

What is the probable causal relation between language and behavioural disorders?

Baker and Cantwell (1985) noted three possibilities for the probable causal relation between language and behavioural disorders. I have added another two. They are as follows.

(1) Psychiatric disorders can lead to DLD. This is very rare, but it does occur partly in the pragmatic aspect of SPLS in autism. It occurs in cases of selective mutism as well, although recent literature points to the reverse; certain children with DLD are at risk of selective mutism.

(2) Neuropsychiatric and language disorders can have a common cause. The psychiatric disorders autism, PDD-NOS, Asperger syndrome and sometimes ADHD are accompanied by deviant semantic-pragmatic language use, attention deficits, cognitive rigidity and deviant emotion/cognition. These are predominantly right hemisphere disorders. It should not be surprising that these psychiatric disorders are concomitant with SPLS, as the same neural networks are involved in part.

(3) DLD can lead to behavioural disorders – for example, if they are not treated (Baker & Cantwell, 1985). This connection is the most frequent. There are several ways in which deviant language can lead to behavioural disorders.

- Deviant language comprehension leads to misunderstandings on the part of the child and in social contact with other people.

- There are problems of bringing up a child whose inner language is deficient; behavioural control of such a child is detrimentally affected, including actions; this can have a negative effect on parent-child relationships.

- Interaction with a child with a language disorder often has a decisive effect of the further course of the problem; for example by using a punishing approach or by blaming the child, parents who are not well informed can reinforce the psychopathology.

- The ability to make a smooth switch from one action is facilitated by inner language; this is often slightly deficient in dysphasic children and has to be differentiated from mental rigidity in autists.

(4) A fourth possibility is separation anxiety. Language disorders in preschool and kindergarten-age children lead to separation anxiety (see previous section), which can lead to atypical development of the sense of self (deviant separation and individuation). This in turn causes a lack of motivation. In essence there is often evidence of reinforced and prolonged stage problems as defined by Mahler. This pertains to the stages of separation and individuation, the stubborn stage, and the growing identity.

(5) Another factor that can be important is the language the parents speak. In a child with DLD, learning two languages at the same time can have an inhibiting effect in the language acquisition stage. The language of parents who are deaf, dysphasic or aphasic themselves and adhere to a certain behavioural and conversation pattern can play a negative role (Mattejat, 1980). There are known to be relational problems in families with more than one dysphasic member on a genetic basis. For a more extensive review on the links between deviant language development and other aspects of development, the reader is referred to Howlin and Rutter (1987).

Conclusions

One should always consider the possibility of DLD in a child with psychopathology, as DLD can contribute to the psychopathology. Conversely, given the relationship between language and emotional development, and between DLD and psychiatric disorders, the child psychiatrist has a role in the diagnostic work-up and treatment of DLD. Analysis of behavioural problems in children with DLD may inspire suggestions for an optimal treatment.

References

Baker, D.P. & Cantwell, L. (1985): Psychiatric and learning disorders in children with speech and language disorders: A critical review. In: *Advances in learning and behavior disabilities*. Vol. 1, ed. K.D. Gadow. Greenwich, CT: JAI Press.

Barkley, R.A. (2001): The executive functions and self-regulation: an evolutionary neuropsychological perspective. *Neuropsychol. Rev.* **11**, 1–29.

Bates, E., Thal, D. & Janowsky, J.S. (1992): Early language development and its neural correlates. In: *Handbook of Neuropsychology*, Vol. 7: *Child Neuropsychology*. Part 2, eds. S.J. Segalowitz & I. Rapin, pp. 69–110. Amsterdam: Elsevier.

Beitchman, J.H., Nair, R., Clegg, M. *et al.* (1986): Prevalence of psychiatric disorders in children with speech and language disorders. *J. Am. Ac. Child. Psychiat.* **25**, 528–35.

Blankenstijn, C. & Scheper, A. (2003): *Language development in children with psychiatric impairment*. Thesis, University of Amsterdam.

Cantwell, D.P. & Baker, L. (1977): Psychiatric disorders in children with speech and language retardation. A critical review. *Arch. Gen. Psychiat.* **34**, 583–591.

Cantwell, D.P. & Baker, L. (1987): Psychiatric symptomatology in language-impaired children: a comparison. *J. Child Neurol.* **2**, 128–33.

Cantwell, D.P. & Baker, L. (1991): Association between attention deficit-hyperactivity disorders and learning disorders. *J. Learning Disab.* **24**, 88–95.

Cantwell, D.P. & Baker, L. & Mattison, R.E. (1980): Psychiatric disorders in children with speech and language retardation. Factors associated with development. *Arch. Gen. Psychiat.* **37**, 423–426.

Caulfield, M.B., Fischel, J.E., DeBaryshe, B.D. & Whitehurst, G.J. (1989): Behavioral correlates of developmental expressive language disorder. *J. Abn. Child. Psychol.* **17**, 187–201.

Cohen, N.J., Hincks, C.M., Davine, M. *et al.* (1993): Unsuspected language impairment in psychiatrically disturbed children: prevalence and language and behavioral characteristics. *J. Am. Acad. Child Adolesc. Psychiatry* **32**, 595–603.

Cohen, N.J., Barwick, M.A., Horodezky, N.B. *et al.* (1998a): Language, achievement, and cognitive processing in psychiatrically disturbed children with previously identified and unsuspected language impairments. *J. Child Psychol. Psychiatry* **39**, 865–77.

Cohen, N.J., Menna, R., Vallance, D.D. *et al.* (1998b): Language, social cognitive processing, and behavioral characteristics of psychiatrically disturbed children with previously identified and unsuspected language impairments. *J. Child Psychol. Psychiatry* **39**, 853–64.

De Ajuriaguerra, J., Jaeggi, A., Guignard, F. *et al.* (1976): The development and prognosis of dysphasia in children. In: *Normal and deficient language*, eds. D.M. Morehead & A.E. Morehead, pp. 345–385. Baltimore: University Park Press.

Dehaene-Lambertz, G., Pena, M. & Christophe, A. (2004): Phoneme perception in a neonate with a left Sylvian infarct. *Brain and Language* **88**, 26–38.

Diatkine, R. (1984): Problèmes cliniques et thérapeutiques des dysphasies graves de l'enfance. *Neuropsychiatrie de l'Enfance* **32**, 553–556.

Dominey, P.F. & Dodane, C. (2004): Indeterminacy in language acquisition: the role of child-directed speech and joint attention. *J. Neuroling.* **17**, 121–145.

Gualtieri, C.T., Koriath, U., van Bourgondien, M. & Saleeby, N. (1983): Language disorders in children referred for psychiatric services. *J. Am. Ac. Child Psychiat.* **22**, 165–171.

Howlin, P. & Rutter, M. (1987): The consequences of language delay for other aspects of development. In: *Language development and disorders*, eds. W. Yule & M. Rutter, pp. 271–294. Oxford: Blackwell Scientific Publications and Philadelphia: J.B., Lippincott Co.

Ingram, T.T.S. (1959): Specific developmental disorders of speech in childhood. *Brain* **82**, 450–67.

Inhelder, B. (1976): Oberservations on the operational and figurative aspects of thought in dysphasic children. In *Normal and deficient child language*. eds. D.M. Morehead & A.E. Morehead, pp. 335–343. Baltimore: University Park Press.

Largo, R.H. & Howard, J.A. (1979): Developmental progression in play behavior of children between nine and thirty months: II: Spontaneous play and language development. *Dev. Med. Child. Neurol.* **21**, 492–503.

Leroi-Gourhan, A. (1964): *Le geste et la parole. Technique et langage*. Paris: Albin Michel.

Locke, J.L. (1997): A theory of neurolinguistic development. *Brain Lang.* **58**, 265–326.

Luria, A.R. & Yudovich, F.I. (1977): *De rol van de taal in de geestelijke ontwikkeling van het kind*. Dutch translation, Rotterdam: Kooyker Reeks.

Mahler, M. (1969): *On human symbiosis and the vicissitudes of individuation*, Vol. 1. Infantile psychoses. London: The Hogarth Press and the Institute of Psycho-Analysis.

Mattejat, F. (1980): Sprachauffalligkeiten von Kindern bei aphasicher Störung des Vaters – Eine entwicklungspsycholinguistische Fallstudie. *Praxis Kinderpsychol. Kinderpsychiat.* **29**, 83–89.

Menyuk, P. (1986): Language development in a social context. *J. Pediatrics* **109**, 217–224.

Njiokiktjien, C. (2004): *Gedragsneurologie van het kind*. Amsterdam: Suyi Publicaties.

Njiokiktjien, C. & Verschoor, C.A. (1998): Attention and the right hemisphere. *J. Human Physiol.* **24**, 145–51.

Paul, R. & Cohen, D.J. (1984): Outcome of severe disorders of language acquisition. *J. Autism Dev. Dis.* **14**, 405–422.

Rapin, I. & Allen, D. (1982): Developmental language disorders, nosologic considerations. In: *Neuropsychology of language, reading and spelling*, eds. I. Rapin & A. Allen, pp. 157–186. New York: Academic Press Inc.

Richman, N. & Stevenson, J. (1977): Language delay in 3-year olds. *Acta Ped. Belg.* **30**, 213–19.

Richman, N., Stevenson, J. & Graham, P. (1983): The relationship between language, development and behaviour. In: *Epidemiological approaches in child psychiatry*. II, eds. M.W. Schmidt & H. Remschmidt. New York: Thieme-Stratton.

Rubin, S.S. (1982): Expressive language deficits in preschool children and faulty development of the self. Description and case study. *Am. J. Orthopsychiat.* **52**, 58–64.

Samuels, C.A. (1986): Bases for infants' developing self-awareness. *Hum. Dev.* **29**, 36–48.

Schore, A.N. (2003): The human unconscious: the development of the right brain and its role in early emotional life. In: *Emotional development in psychoanalysis, attachment theory and neuroscience*, ed. V. Green. Hove and New York: Brunner-Routledge.

Stevenson, J., Richman, N. & Graham, P. (1985): Behaviour problems and language abilities at three years and behavioural deviance at eight years. *J. Child Psychol. Psychiat.* **26**, 215–230.

Tan, X.S.T. (2005): *Dysfatische ontwikkeling. Theorie – Diagnostiek – Behandeling*. Amsterdam: Suyi Publicaties.

Tan, X.S.T. (1990): Developmental dysphasia (Dutch). In: *Omtrent Logopedie 6, Proceedings XI Congress V.V.L.* (Belgian Society of Logepedics), eds. P. De Meyere & L. Heylen, pp. 145–166. Antwerp.

Vallance, D.D., Im, N. & Cohen, N.J. (1999): Discourse deficits associated with psychiatric disorders and with language impairments in children. *J. Child Psychol. Psychiat. Allied Discipl.* **40**, 693–704.

Vygotsky, L.S. (1962): *Thought and language*. Cambridge, MA: MIT Press.

Vygotsky, L.S. (1978): Tool and symbol in child development. In: *Mind in society*, eds. M. Cole, V. John-Steiner, S. Scribner & E. Souberman. Cambridge, MA: Harvard University Press.

Vygotsky, L.S. (1978): Mind in society. In: *The development of higher psychological processes*, eds. M. Cole, V. John-Steiner, S. Scribner & E. Souberman. Cambridge, MA: Harvard University Press.

Achevé d'imprimer par Corlet, Imprimeur, S.A.
14110 Condé-sur-Noireau
N° d'Imprimeur : 92754 - Dépôt légal : septembre 2006
Imprimé en France